Active Learning Workbook for
Wilkins'
Clinical Practice of the
Dental Hygienist

JANE F. HALARIS, ASDH, BS, MA
Retired
Department of Periodontics and Oral Medicine
University of Michigan School of Dentistry
Ann Arbor, Michigan

CHARLOTTE J. WYCHE, BSDH, MS
Retired
Department of Periodontics and Oral Medicine
University of Michigan School of Dentistry
Ann Arbor, Michigan

JONES & BARTLETT
LEARNING

World Headquarters
Jones & Bartlett Learning
5 Wall Street
Burlington, MA 01803
978-443-5000
info@jblearning.com
www.jblearning.com

Jones & Bartlett Learning books and products are available through most bookstores and online booksellers. To contact Jones & Bartlett Learning directly, call 800-832-0034, fax 978-443-8000, or visit our website, www.jblearning.com.

Substantial discounts on bulk quantities of Jones & Bartlett Learning publications are available to corporations, professional associations, and other qualified organizations. For details and specific discount information, contact the special sales department at Jones & Bartlett Learning via the above contact information or send an email to specialsales@jblearning.com.

Production Credits
VP, Product Management: Amanda Martin
Director of Product Management: Cathy L. Esperti
Product Manager: Sean Fabery
Product Coordinator: Elena Sorrentino
Senior Project Specialist: Vanessa Richards
Digital Project Specialist: Angela Dooley
Director of Marketing: Andrea DeFronzo
VP, Manufacturing and Inventory Control: Therese Connell

Composition & Project Management: S4Carlisle Publishing Services
Cover Design: Kristin E. Parker
Senior Media Development Editor: Troy Liston
Rights Specialist: Rebecca Damon
Cover Image (Title Page, Part Opener, Chapter Opener): © phyZick/Shutterstock
Printing and Binding: LSC Communications
Cover Printing: LSC Communications

ISBN: 978-1-975106-90-4

6048

Printed in the United States of America
24 23 22 21 20   10 9 8 7 6 5 4 3 2

DEDICATION

To Esther, of course

And, as always
To instructors who ask open-ended questions and encourage the kind of reflection that helps students discover what they do not yet know. They understand that clinical dental hygiene practice is not a multiple-choice test.

and

To students who struggle to find answers for the open-ended questions their instructors ask them. They will soon discover that reflecting on what they don't know and working to find answers to real questions is what leads to real learning.

Contents

Preface

There is no doubt each student learns differently. Therefore, the aim of this workbook is to provide a variety of exercises so you will be able to find something here to help you learn important concepts that are the foundation of the dental hygiene practice. You are always encouraged, of course, to create additional learning experiences and activities that fit with your own learning style.

HOW TO USE THIS WORKBOOK

Some general guidelines for the exercises in the workbook are described here. Exercises in the **Knowledge** sections of the workbook provide lines for you to write your answers. Some chapters include crossword or word search puzzles to help learn terminology. For **Competency**- and **Discovery**-type exercises, a separate computer or handwritten document or a copy of the *Patient-Specific Dental Hygiene Care Plan* template from **workbook** Appendix B may be required to provide a complete answer.

 ### Knowledge Exercises

KNOWLEDGE exercises in each chapter will help you target important information and help you master the introductory material provided in the **textbook**. You will define terms, concepts, and principles in your own words; list the components of larger ideas; and reorganize information from the **textbook** in a variety of ways. Knowledge exercises comprise the largest, but by no means the most important, portion of this workbook.

 ### Competency Exercises

COMPETENCY questions are found in each chapter and also in section summary areas of this workbook. Building competence in translating knowledge to practice is an essential component of becoming a professional dental hygienist. These exercises will ask you to use critical thinking skills to apply basic knowledge to clinical situations, analyze patient assessment data, create components of patient care plans, or document patient care activities. Some of the patient scenarios are written in paragraph form so you can learn to isolate important information, and some are formatted using the Assessment Findings section from the Care Plan template.

 ### Discovery Exercises

DISCOVERY activities are found in some of the chapters and also in each section summary. These exercises will help you learn to think beyond the basic knowledge. The discovery activities will direct you to find and analyze current information about a topic introduced in the **textbook** by, for example, doing a scientific literature search, a Web-based Internet search, or a dental product analysis.

 ### Questions Patients Ask

Questions Patients Ask are also intended to encourage you to practice evidence-based decision-making skills. Reflecting on what additional or new knowledge is needed to address patient concerns is a key skill for lifelong learning and ultimately for providing evidence-based, comprehensive, and effective dental hygiene care.

 ### Everyday Ethics

Everyday Ethics activities will challenge you to reflect on and apply ethical principles. An Everyday Ethics scenario with "Questions for Consideration" is included in each **textbook** chapter. Many of these scenarios were created using real-life ethical situations faced by practicing dental hygienists. Each workbook chapter includes an Everyday Ethics box with **individual learning**, **cooperative learning**, or **discovery** activity prompts that direct you to write about, discuss, or role-play the ethics-related scenario and questions presented in the **textbook**.

 ### Factors to Teach the Patient

Factors to Teach the Patient cases ask you to outline or develop a patient/provider conversation using motivational interviewing (MI) techniques, patient-appropriate language, and knowledge gained from the **textbook**. Those brief conversations can then be compared with conversations written by your student colleagues, used for "role-play" exercises, or placed in your portfolio to illustrate your expertise in patient education.

 ### For Your Portfolio

For Your Portfolio suggestions are located in each section summary and in a few of the chapters. A learning portfolio is a collection of student work and reflection organized in such a way that it demonstrates an increase in student knowledge and professional competence over time. A student portfolio can be compiled simply and creatively using a three-ring binder with tabbed separators to organize the material into appropriate sections. An Internet search will help you locate online portfolio templates that can be used to develop a Web-based portfolio.

Development of a portfolio provides an opportunity for you to reflect on your growth as a dental hygiene professional. A portfolio that highlights your unique talents and provides evidence of special skills, competencies, or learning that goes beyond the requirements of your educational program can be useful during employment interviews or application to graduate education programs.

Answers for the workbook Knowledge questions and rubrics with criteria to help evaluate student responses to competency exercises are available to qualified instructors.

 ## MeSH TERMS

Medical Subject Heading (MeSH) boxes in each chapter contain some headings related to chapter topics under which journal articles are organized within the PubMed database. Combining the terms you find in the MeSH term box in each chapter with other key words related to your topic of interest will help you initiate efficient and effective literature searches.

Competencies for the Dental Hygienist

The American Dental Education Association (ADEA) competencies outline the areas in which a new graduate dental hygienist is expected to be able to apply knowledge to ensure safe and effective patient care is provided. The title page for each section of this workbook lists specific ADEA competencies supported by learning the information from chapters included in that particular section of the **textbook**. The complete list of competency statements found in **workbook** Appendix A will provide a reference point to help you understand why learning specific concepts from each chapter is important for becoming a professional dental hygienist.

As you read the ADEA competency statements, you should note that your school might have adapted them somewhat for use in your dental hygiene program. Your school's competencies may be organized in a slightly different manner but will probably be very similar. You should make a point of receiving a copy of your school's competency statements for reference.

We encourage you to enjoy the process of learning and hope this workbook offers activities that will help you.

Sincerely,
Jane F. Halaris, ASDH, BS, MA
and
Charlotte J. Wyche, BSDH, MS
Dental Hygiene Educators

Acknowledgments

It takes a team to complete a project as big as this workbook. The publishing team is listed at the front of the book, and of course the "main authors" have their names on the cover. However, it doesn't even begin there. The following people gave their knowledge, expertise, experience, and most of all their time to help us make this edition of the workbook what it is. Thank you all for making this workbook possible. We could not have done it without your dedication and help.

Linda D. Boyd, RDH, RD, EdD, and **Lisa Mallonee, RDH, RD, LD, MPH**, leaders of the 13th edition textbook team, and the authors of the textbook chapters, who provided the workbook team with two invaluable tools for revision, the Summary of Changes document and the Key Words documents for each chapter. The 13th edition represents not only the most current knowledge, but also a major reorganization of content. These tools enabled us to develop the workbook revisions in an orderly and efficient manner.

Charlotte Wyche, BSDH, MS, creator of this excellent learning tool, for your mentorship during our years together on the workbook.

Orientation to Clinical Dental Hygiene Practice

Chapters 1–4

SECTION I LEARNING OBJECTIVES

Completing the exercises in this section of the workbook will prepare you to:

1. Identify the characteristics of a dental hygiene professional.
2. Apply ethical, legal, cultural, and personal professional standards to the practice of dental hygiene.
3. Use an evidence-based decision-making process to locate and evaluate current scientific evidence related to dental hygiene interventions.
4. Apply the principles of effective health communication.
5. Describe dental hygiene practice in alternative settings.

COMPETENCIES FOR THE DENTAL HYGIENIST (APPENDIX A)

Competencies supported by the learning in Section I

Core Competencies: C1, C2, C3, C4, C5, C6, C7, C8, C9, C10, C11, C12

Health Promotion and Disease Prevention: HP1, HP2, HP4, HP5, HP6

Community Involvement: CM1, CM2, CM3, CM4, CM6, CM7

Professional Growth and Development: PGD1, PGD3

1

The Professional Dental Hygienist

LEARNING OBJECTIVES

Upon successful completion of these exercises, you will be able to:

1. Identify and define the key terms and concepts related to the professional dental hygienist.
2. Define the scope of dental hygiene practice.
3. Identify and define the components of the dental hygiene process of care.
4. Identify and apply components of the dental hygiene code of ethics.
5. Apply concepts in ethical decision making.

 KNOWLEDGE EXERCISES

Write your answers for each question in the space provided.

1. Briefly describe a dental hygienist using the terminology associated with roles and practice settings, health-care focus, and services provided by dental hygienists.

_____

_____

_____

_____

_____

_____

_____

2. Define *dental hygiene care.*

_____

_____

3. List and (in your own words) briefly define the health-care-related roles your dental hygiene education will prepare you to fulfill.

_____

_____

_____

_____

_____

_____

_____

_____

_____

_____

_____

_____

_____

_____

4. What is the primary goal of each dental hygienist with respect to patient care?

_____

_____

5. What dental hygienist role was originally emphasized by Dr. A. C. Fones, who is considered the father of dental hygiene?

_____

_____

6. Briefly describe at least three factors that affect the way in which the professionalism of an individual dental hygienist is perceived.

_____

_____

_____

7. List three components of self-care important for serving as a healthy model for patients.

_____

_____

8. Define "direct-access" _dental hygiene care._

_____

_____

_____

_____

_____

9. What is the role of the dental hygienist in collaborative interprofessional practice?

_____

_____

10. Briefly define four competency domains necessary for participation in collaborative interprofessional practice.

_____

_____

_____

_____

_____

11. What is a dental therapist?

_____

_____

12. What is advocacy for oral health?

_____

_____

_____

_____

13. List three ways in which a dental hygienist interested in specialty areas of practice can enhance knowledge and skills.

_____

_____

_____

14. List and briefly define each of the six components of the dental hygiene process of care, which together comprise the Standards for Clinical Dental Hygiene Practice.

_____

_____

_____

_____

_____

_____

_____

_____

_____

_____

15. Match each type of supervision with the appropriate requirement for the dentist to be physically present on-site during patient care.

Type of Supervision	Required Dentist Participation
_____ Direct	A. Dentist must be present on-site
_____ Personal	
_____ General	B. Dentist need not be present on-site
_____ Direct access	
_____ Collaborative practice	
_____ Indirect	
_____ Remote	
_____ Independent practice	

16. Which types of supervision allow the dental hygienist to provide for patient needs **without** authorization or supervision by a dentist?

_____

_____

_____

17. What special factors apply to members of a group defined as having a profession?

_____

_____

_____

_____

_____

18. What is a code of ethics?

_____

_____

_____

_____

19. Name at least two professional organizations that have developed codes of ethics for the practice of dental hygiene.

_____

_____

20. In your own words, briefly define each of the seven core values in dental hygiene.

- *Autonomy and respect:*

_____

- *Confidentiality:*

_____

- *Societal trust:*

_____

- *Nonmaleficence:*

_____

- *Beneficence:*

_____

- *Justice and fairness:*

_____

- *Veracity:*

_____

21. What is the difference between an ethical issue and an ethical dilemma?

_____

_____

_____

22. Briefly describe the steps that can help direct your decision making for resolution of an ethical situation.

_____

_____

_____

_____

_____

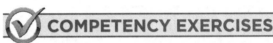 **COMPETENCY EXERCISES**

Use paper and pen or create an electronic document to answer these questions.

1. Write a brief summary of the ways that dental hygiene practice has changed in the more than 100 years since its inception.

2. Use concepts presented related to dental hygiene practice and definitions of key words presented throughout this chapter to describe why a dental hygienist can be considered a primary healthcare professional.

3. Use concepts discussed throughout this chapter to write a reflection on the meaning of dental hygienists' scope of practice.

4. Dental hygienists' interventions play a major role in all levels of prevention of oral disease. Give examples (different from those included in the **textbook**) of a dental hygienist's role in each level of prevention.

DISCOVERY EXERCISES

1. Initiate a review of literature and an Internet search to further investigate the concept of the dental therapist. Describe the relationship between advanced practice dental hygienists and dental therapists.

2. Review a copy of your state's Dental Hygiene Practice Act. List the services dental hygienists may provide and determine the level of supervision required for each service. Explain how the rules in your state enhance or provide a barrier to access to oral health services.

EVERYDAY ETHICS

Before completing the learning exercises below, reread and reflect on the Everyday Ethics Scenario and Questions for Consideration in this chapter of the **textbook**. It may also be useful to review the Dental Hygiene Ethics discussion in Chapter 1, the Ethical Applications in the introduction pages for each section in the **textbook**, as well as the Codes of Ethics in **textbook** Appendices I–IV.

Individual Learning Activity

Imagine that you are the dental hygienist in this scenario. Answer each of the questions for consideration at the end of the scenario.

Collaborative Learning Activity

Work as a group to develop a 2- to 5-minute role-play that introduces the everyday ethics scenario described in the chapter (a great idea is to video record your role-play activity). Then develop separate 2-minute role-play scenarios that provide at least two alternative approaches/solutions to resolving the situation. Ask classmates to view the solutions, ask questions, and discuss the ethical approach used in each. Ask for a vote on which solution classmates determine to be the "best."

QUESTIONS PATIENTS ASK

What sources of information can you identify that will help you answer your patient's questions in this scenario?

Your patient, Jessica Miles, who is a junior in high school, comments, "My mom and I were talking about where I will be going to college after next year. She said to ask you where you went. She thinks what you do would be real cool. What is it that you do, really? Why did you have to take a lot of sciences? Do they have dental chairs and all the equipment right in the school and do people come in for you to learn from? I know you clean our teeth—why do you like working in people's mouths?"

Factors to Teach the Patient

This scenario is related to the following factors listed in this chapter of the **textbook**:

▷ The role of the dental hygienist as cotherapist with each patient and with members of the dental profession.

▷ The moral and ethical nature of becoming a dental hygiene professional person.

▷ The patient's potential state of oral health and how it can be improved and maintained.

Sarah, your really good friend, has agreed to be a patient for your first clinical experience as a dental hygiene student. When you call her to remind her of her appointment tomorrow, she asks you a bit about what you will do during the appointment. You excitedly begin to explain the procedures.

Sarah interrupts saying that it all sounds pretty boring to her. She asks you to tell her why you are studying so hard to become a dental hygienist. Write a statement explaining your knowledge and interest in dental hygiene practice to Sarah.

MeSH TERMS

Use a combination of MeSH terms and other key words to develop an effective and efficient PubMed literature search strategy.

Dental hygienists	Primary health care
Oral health	Standard of care
Health promotion	Codes of ethics
Oral hygiene	Practice guideline

2

Evidence-Based Dental Hygiene Practice

 KNOWLEDGE EXERCISES

Write your answers for each question in the space provided.

1. List four factors that interact to direct selection of patient care interventions in an evidence-based dental hygiene practice.

_____

_____

_____

2. Place the steps for a systematic approach to evidence-based dental hygiene practice in the correct order by placing the numbers 1 through 6 in the space beside each step.

Order	Description of Step
_____	Develop a researchable question
_____	Evaluate outcomes
_____	Search for the evidence
_____	Critically evaluate the evidence
_____	Determine the clinical issue
_____	Integrate and apply the evidence

3. What is a refereed publication?

_____

_____

_____

_____

4. List five types of research studies.

_____

_____

_____

_____

5. What is the difference between qualitative and quantitative research approaches?

_____

_____

_____

_____

_____

6. What type of research looks at the strength and types of relationships between variables?

_____

7. What is the difference between experimental and quasi-experimental research?

_____

_____

_____

_____

8. What is in vitro research?

_____

_____

_____

9. What is the difference between a case report and a case study?

_____

_____

_____

10. What does _retrospective_ mean?

_____

_____

_____

11. Randomized controlled double-blind studies help eliminate _____ by placing study participants randomly in either the experimental or the control group and by "blinding" the researchers to which participant is in which group.

12. Place the levels of evidence in order from the most valuable to support evidence-based practice (1) to less valuable (6) for making decisions related to clinical dental hygiene care.

Order	Type of Evidence
_____	Analysis of all studies that investigate a specific question
_____	Opinions of journal editors or other "expert" practitioners
_____	Cohort and case–control studies
_____	Research that does not involve human subjects
_____	RCT studies
_____	Studies that describe or analyze one or more cases of an unusual condition

13. What six skills can help the dental hygiene practitioner implement EBDH into everyday practice?

_____

_____

_____

_____

_____

_____

14. Informed consent forms and Institutional Review Board approval help protect the rights of _____ in research studies.

15. What is a PICO question?

_____

_____

_____

_____

16. List the components of a PICO question.

_____

_____

_____

_____

17. What is the purpose of the FINER criteria?

_____

_____

_____

18. List the components of the FINER criteria?

_____

_____

_____

✅ COMPETENCY EXERCISES

Use paper and pen or create an electronic document to answer these questions.

1. Your patient is a 1-year-old child who already has evidence of early childhood caries. You know that in order to help decrease risk for further caries activity and help remineralize the white spot lesions, this child needs to be provided with topical fluoride application even at this young age. However, you are unsure whether the topical gel application or the fluoride varnish would be the best choice.

Part 1: Write a PICO question that will help direct your search for information to support the intervention you select for this very young child.

Part 2: Identify the MeSH terms and/or any additional terms you would use to initiate this literature search.

2. Explain why a peer-reviewed journal is more likely than a commercial-based health magazine to contain the type of evidence that is appropriate to support clinical recommendations that a dental hygienist includes in a patient's care plan.

QUESTIONS PATIENTS ASK

What sources of information can you identify that will help you answer your patient's questions?

"I just heard about this cool new dental product from my friend! Do you think it is any good?" "Will it clean my teeth as well as what I am doing now?" "I know my situation is different than some other people, so will it work for me?"

EVERYDAY ETHICS

Before completing the learning exercises that follow, reread and reflect on the Everyday Ethics Scenario and Questions for Consideration in this chapter of the **textbook**. It may also be useful to review the Dental Hygiene Ethics discussion in Chapter 1, the Ethical Applications in the introduction pages for each section in the **textbook**, as well as the Codes of Ethics in **textbook** Appendices I–IV.

Individual Learning Activity

Identify a situation you have experienced that presents a similar ethical dilemma. What did you learn from how the situation was (or was not) resolved at the time it happened?

Discovery Activity

Ask a friend or relative who is not involved in health care to read the scenario and discuss it with you from the perspective of a "patient" who receives services within the healthcare system. Discuss what you learned from the concerns, insights, or difference in perspective that person expressed.

Factors to Teach the Patient

This scenario is related to the following factors listed in this chapter of the **textbook**:

▷ A result from one study doesn't necessarily provide the best answer.

Your patient, Marcus, tells you that he just read a newspaper article citing new research study that contradicts a recommendation you have made for his self-care. How will you respond to his assertion that the research proves that this new technique is probably better than the one that you have recommended?

MeSH TERMS

Use a combination of MeSH terms and other key words to develop an effective and efficient PubMed literature search strategy.

Evidence-based practice
Evidence-based dentistry
Practice guidelines as topic
Clinical trials as topic
Periodicals as topic
Ethics committees, research

Meta-analysis
Randomized controlled trial
Case-control studies
Cohort studies
Case reports
Qualitative research
Reproducibility of results

CHAPTER 2 WORD SEARCH PUZZLE

```
O I N F O R M E D C O N S E N T S Q E F D C Z W
G U I D E L I N E S E N M Q Y N I N N Q O S Z Y
U S Z L E V E L S O F E V I D E N C E J Y U J Q
T E Z N X Q E F Z I G J Z V Q K I Y Y L S R P F
F G U B K C O N F I D E N C E I N T E R V A L H
Q C U D A T A B A S E O X E E J A Z W P U U U A
I X V Z R R C V K O I D Z G R L U T E Y I K D L
S T A T I S T I C A L S I G N I F I C A N C E I
A M R C J D B V I A H P U O H G J G Y E E Y S T
Y O I L C L I N I C A L S I G N I F I C A N C E
R E A S B I O S T A T I S T I C S R S Q U O R R
E V B W N W P A J J W T P S T Y Q H K B O V I A
L B L L Q D W I M F A Q E Q C Z U R E Y H O P T
I R E U O B J R W N L P E E R R E V I E W Q T U
A Z H E F I V Q T P J U Y E V I D E N C E D I R
B I W X Y X V T V A L I D I T Y K F P F F Q V E
I W B E S T P R A C T I C E S Z N E E I E L E R
L J P O S T H O C F A L L A C Y S Y W S B G G E
I D W A L M U A N P F P I P C B U Y F K D H L V
T S L F F F A L C M M F M B O F K S P E H I H I
Y U Z H P F E K S I M P F F O N A F I D D M K E
B S I Y I N F E R E N T I A L S U V J T I X G W
M D K P V A L U E G P J O J U E S C J Y I O R D
K R O U K U E R W U J P T P V A P H U V O Y Z B
```

Puzzle Clues

1. Benchmark practices based on repeatable research over time on large diverse groups of people.

2. Organized collection journal articles, systematic reviews, research reports, theses, and/or dissertations typically in digital form.

3. A branch of statistics directed toward application in the discipline of health sciences.

4. Clinical practice statements that include recommendations intended to optimize patient care.

5. A clinically observable difference rather than statistical difference (two words).

6. A range of values defining a specific probability that the value of a factor lies within it (two words).

7. A type of statistics that describe the main features or characteristics of a particular person, event, or group; determine the frequency with which something occurs; or categorize information.

8. Source of information used to support, determine, or demonstrate the truth of a statement.

9. A scientific, research-supported approach to decide dental hygiene interventions for each patient (acronym).

10. A type of statistical data designed to allow generalization from a sample to a population.

11. Type of consent that requires adequately explaining associated risks and benefits to prospective patients and ensuring that they understand what will happen to them.

12. Hierarchy of evidence based on the strength and types of research studies (three words).

13. Summary and critical analysis of published sources on a particular topic (two words).

14. Review of a journal article by a panel of experts prior to publication.

15. Understanding that correlation does not mean causation between multiple variables.

16. Represents the calculated probability of finding the observed results when the null hypothesis is true.

17. The ability of a measurement instrument or test to get the same results repeatedly.

18. Identifies the extent to which the results are not due to chance; indicated in research by the "p-value" notation (two words).

19. Ability to measure what was intended.

20. Factors in a research study that can be manipulated and measured.

Effective Health Communication

LEARNING OBJECTIVES

Upon successful completion of these exercises, you will be able to:

1. Discuss the skills and attributes of effective health communication.

2. Identify the barriers to effective communication.

3. Explain how the patient's age, culture, and health literacy level affect health communication strategies.

KNOWLEDGE EXERCISES

Write your answers for each question in the space provided.

1. Define *health communication* in your own words.

_____

_____

_____

_____

2. To establish the kind of rapport that enhances communication with a patient of any age, gender, or culture, the dental hygienist will _____ more than _____, especially at the beginning of the appointment.

3. List as many as you can of the abilities/attributes of a dental professional who is able to establish rapport with each patient in order to provide effective health communication.

_____

_____

_____

_____

_____

_____

_____

_____

_____

_____

_____

_____

4. What factors contribute to effective health messages?

_____

_____

_____

_____

_____

_____

5. List and briefly define in your own words the three types of communication.

   _____

   _____

   _____

   _____

   _____

   _____

   _____

   _____

6. What barriers can affect the way health messages are understood during patient's education sessions?

   _____

   _____

   _____

   _____

   _____

   _____

   _____

   _____

   _____

7. The level of a patient's health literacy does not only depend on the individual's reading level, but rather also on the interaction of a complex set of _____ and _____ skills, as well as personal health-related knowledge.

8. List some ways the dental hygienist can address health literacy issues in the dental hygiene practice.

   _____

   _____

   _____

   _____

   _____

   _____

   _____

   _____

   _____

9. Match the age group in column 1 with the correct description of a key point related to communicating with that age group in column 2.

Age Group	Communication-Related Description
___ Infants	A. Marked desire to have their viewpoint and needs considered with respect.
___ Toddlers and preschoolers	B. Like to assert independence and maintain control over situations.
___ School-age children	C. Physical and cognitive changes may impact ability to communicate.
___ Adolescents	D. Communicate primarily through senses.
___ Older adults	E. Developing ability to relate the impact of external events to themselves.

10. True or False (circle one). Using "*terms of endearment*" to address a frail elderly patient is a communication approach that will put the patient at ease as well as demonstrate the care provider's empathy.

11. True or False (circle one). When communicating with a caregiver who is in the treatment room while you are providing oral hygiene instructions for the patient, maintain eye contact with the caregiver as the primary focus of the conversation so that they don't feel left out.

12. In your own words, describe the effect ethnic or cultural background can have on your patients' health status or the way they respond to your dental hygiene interventions.

   _____

   _____

   _____

   _____

   _____

   _____

   _____

   _____

   _____

   _____

13. _____ (two words) delivery of dental hygiene care, including respect for and responsiveness to the unique culturally related characteristics, values, and needs of each patient can make a positive difference in oral health outcomes.

14. _____ (two words) is a skill that can be developed by exploring and learning to appreciate the wide variety of differences among the individuals who are your patients.

15. _____ (two words) is about building relationships that foster understanding.

16. List attributes of a dental hygienist who strives to deliver effective health care for patients of all cultures.

_____

_____

_____

_____

_____

_____

_____

17. List ways to enhance awareness of culture-related needs during patient care.

_____

_____

_____

_____

_____

_____

_____

18. List ways to enhance language-related communication with all patients.

_____

_____

_____

_____

_____

_____

19. List skills that enhance interprofessional communication between healthcare providers.

_____

_____

_____

_____

_____

_____

_____

20. When communicating with a patient while using an interpreter, which one do you speak directly to when asking questions?

_____

_____

21. What factors related to communication and culture are appropriate to document in a patient's permanent record?

_____

_____

_____

_____

_____

_____

_____

_____

_____

COMPETENCY EXERCISES

Apply information from the chapter and use critical thinking skills to complete the competency exercises. Write responses on a paper or create electronic documents to submit your answers.

1. Table 3-1 in the **textbook** lists several factors that can interfere with effective communication and describes or defines what each factor means. Provide a brief example from your own life experience (not necessarily related to dental hygiene) that illustrates each of the types of barriers. For example, an interpersonal barrier to effective communication could be illustrated by describing a time when you could only seem to argue, rather than discuss, with a friend who had taken a political stand opposite yours. After you describe the situation, jot down any thoughts you have about how you might have overcome that barrier and been more effective in communicating.

2. Explain the dental hygienist's role in helping patients understand health-related messages and health information available from popular media and Internet-based sources.

Factors to Teach the Patient

This scenario is related to the following factors listed in this chapter of the **textbook**:

▷ The dental hygienist's ability to provide quality dental hygiene care is affected by the willingness and ability of the patient to communicate accurate and complete information about health status, needs, and concerns.

Mr. Romine has been a patient in the practice for many, many years. You are a new dental hygienist in the practice who is scheduled to provide his regular dental hygiene care today. You discover that his health history form, which notes some significant health history issues including history of an infectious disease, arthritis, hypertension, and an undefined "heart problem," has not been updated in several years. When you politely ask him to fill out a new one, he angrily states, "Information about my health is my private business."

What are some ways that you might approach Mr. Romaine to help build rapport and establish enough trust to help him share the information you need to provide safe and effective dental hygiene care for him? Share your ideas with student colleagues. Was their approach similar to yours or very different? What did you learn from the discussion?

EVERYDAY ETHICS

Before completing the learning exercises below, reread and reflect on the Everyday Ethics Scenario and Questions for Consideration in this chapter of the **textbook**. It may also be useful to review the Dental Hygiene Ethics discussion in Chapter 1, the Ethical Applications in the introduction pages for each section in the **textbook**, as well as the Codes of Ethics in **textbook** Appendices I–IV.

Individual Learning Activity

Imagine the scenario from the patient's perspective. How might the patient's response to the questions following the scenario be different from those of the dental hygienist involved?

Collaborative Learning Activity

Work with a small group to develop a 2–5-minute role-play that introduces the everyday ethics scenario described in the chapter (a great idea is to video record your role-play activity). Then develop separate 2-minute role-play scenarios that provide at least two alternative approaches/solutions to resolving the situation. Ask classmates to view the solutions, ask questions, and discuss the ethical approach used in each. Ask for a vote on which solution classmates determine to be the "best."

MeSH TERMS

Use a combination of MeSH terms and other key words to develop an effective and efficient PubMed literature search strategy.

Health communication
Communication barriers
Health literacy

Cultural competency
Nonverbal
  communication

CHAPTER 3 CROSSWORD PUZZLE

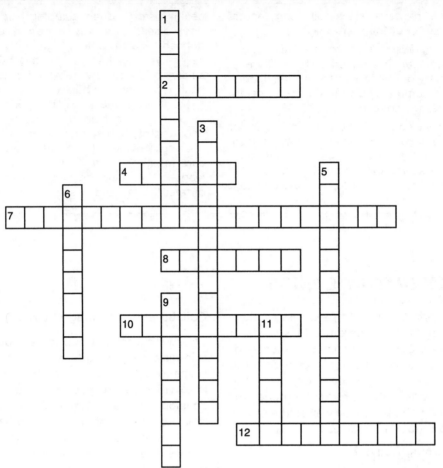

Puzzle Clues

Across

2. Communication disorder; difficult for an individual to read, write, express, or understand language.

4. Communication through sending and receiving messages using words.

7. Social, environmental, and physical circumstances that have an effect on health status (three words).

8. Set of beliefs, values, attitudes, convictions, and behaviors common to a group.

10. Communication through body language, gestures, facial expressions, eye contact, and verbal elements such as rhythm and intonation.

12. Attitude or judgment (either positive or negative), which describes individuals from a population group as though all have the same characteristics.

Down

1. Motor/speech disorder that weakens or paralyzes the muscles of the face, mouth, larynx, and vocal cords, causing slurred, slow, and difficult to understand speech.

3. Ability of a patient to obtain, process, understand, and respond to health messages, and be motivated to make health decisions that promote and maintain good health (two words).

5. Verbal or written health information provided using simplified terminology, clear and to-the-point sentence structure, pictures, or any other method that can enhance understanding for patients with limited language proficiency or health literacy (two words).

6. Receiver's direct response to a communicated message.

9. Translating a thought into words, gestures, or other linguistic; can be verbal or nonverbal, oral, visual, or tactile.

11. Refers to an observed lack of expression or emotional response.

Dental Hygiene Care in Alternative Settings

 KNOWLEDGE EXERCISES

Write your answers for each question in the space provided.

1. What characteristics help identify a person who may not be able to access dental hygiene care in a traditional private practice office setting?

2. What barriers can prevent an individual from receiving oral health they need?

3. How might dental hygienists with direct access be better able to address the needs of individuals who experience barriers to accessing traditional private practice–based oral care?

4. In your own words, describe the advanced dental hygiene practitioner.

5. List objectives of providing dental hygiene care in alternative practice settings for individuals who cannot access the traditional dental practice setting.

_____

_____

_____

_____

6. Identify three unique objects or implements, not usually associated with providing care in a dental office, to include when planning to provide care in alternative practice settings.

_____

_____

_____

7. List three factors that can influence scheduling an appointment time to provide dental hygiene care for a residence-bound patient.

_____

_____

_____

8. Identify unhealthy personal factors that may be associated with inactivity or a monotonous existence of a residence-bound patient.

_____

_____

_____

_____

9. Identify communication and personal approaches that help build a successful relationship with an individual who is relatively helpless, disabled, or ill.

_____

_____

_____

_____

_____

10. When is a firm pillow useful for patient positioning during dental hygiene care?

_____

_____

_____

11. Describe a patient who is comatose.

_____

_____

12. In your own words, define the concept of _interprofessional collaborative practice_.

_____

_____

_____

13. Describe the role of the dental hygienist in providing care for a patient who is critically or terminally ill.

_____

_____

_____

14. Define _palliative care_.

_____

_____

15. What common oral infection is often found in a patient with a terminal illness?

_____

_____

16. What one item is documented in the patient record when the care is provided an alternative practice setting that is not usually documented for care provided in a traditional dental practice setting?

_____

_____

✓ COMPETENCY EXERCISES

Apply information from the chapter and use critical thinking skills to complete the competency exercises. Write responses on paper or create electronic documents to submit your answers.

1. You are one of the dental hygienists on a dental care team that visits the Nightingale Long Term Care Center each month to provide oral care for residents. Your first patient of the day is Ralph Wilkerson, a handsome 29-year-old who has been in a coma since a diving accident 8 years ago. After looking at the information in Ralph's medical record, you enter his room and greet him. As you prepare your armamentarium, position him for oral care, and place towels under his chin, you keep up a cheerful one-sided conversation. Explain why it is important to talk with this patient even though he will definitely not respond to your remarks.

2. Mrs. Malcolm has been a patient in your clinic for about 15 years. She has always had fairly good oral hygiene and a healthy mouth has been important to her. You haven't seen her in quite a while, though, because Mrs. Malcolm has spent a lot of time in the hospital over the last year. You recently heard that she has been receiving hospice care in her home.

   Dr. Gable, the dentist in your clinic, has agreed to provide some basic comfort care at home for Mrs. Malcolm, and she suggests that you accompany her. When you arrive, you find that Mrs. Malcolm, although very weak, is awake and able to speak with you. She complains of having a very dry mouth and you notice that her lips are coated with a dry looking, crusty material. She mentions that her lower partial denture does not fit very well anymore and often slips around whenever she tries to eat. It is rubbing on her left cheek. She says her mouth feels and tastes bad and that her gums were bleeding when her daughter tried to help her brush her teeth a couple of days ago.

   Write at least three dental hygiene diagnosis statements for Mrs. Malcolm's care plan.

3. Write a goal and evaluation method for one of the diagnosis statements you identified in the question above. Include a time frame for meeting that goal.

4. Describe ways that you can arrange your working situation for providing dental hygiene care to Mrs. Malcolm in her the bedroom of her home.

 ## DISCOVERY EXERCISES

1. Use the information in Boxes 4-3 and 4-4 in the **textbook** as well as additional information from dental supply catalogs and websites to put together a plan and a budget for everything you would need to implement a portable dental hygiene practice.

2. Contact a nearby nursing home or senior residence center and ask to talk to someone on the staff about interprofessional collaborative practice. Explain the value of adding a dental hygienist to their patient care team.

 ### Factors to Teach the Patient/Caregiver

This scenario is related to the following factors listed in this chapter of the **textbook**:

▷ Good oral health contributes to good general health and quality of life.

▷ Care for the patient's natural teeth and gums.

▷ Evaluate and address unique patient needs, adapt care as needed.

▷ How to use a suction toothbrush, power brush, or other device to provide oral care for the patient.

Today you are giving hands-on training in providing daily oral care for a group of nurse's aides at the Nightingale Long Term Care Center. You have set up a suction toothbrush at the bedside of Ralph Wilkerson (introduced in Competency Exercises question 1). Besides showing and telling the nurse's aides how to brush someone else's teeth and care for the suction toothbrush afterward, you also want to explain the reasons for providing daily oral cleansing for all of the residents/patients in the center.

Use a motivational interviewing approach (see **workbook** Appendix D) as a guide to write an outline of information you need to present to the group of nurse's aides.

Use the conversation you create to role-play this situation with several fellow students. If you are a nurse's aide in the role-play, be sure to ask questions. If you are the dental hygienist, try to anticipate questions and answer them in your explanation.

QUESTIONS PATIENTS ASK

What sources of information can you identify that will help you answer your patient's questions in this scenario?

"There are so many agencies now that offer health and personal-care services to homebound individuals—why don't they have someone who can come to my house/nursing home so that I could get my teeth cleaned?" "Is there a dentist around here who will make house calls?" "Why doesn't the staff in my mother's nursing home help her brush her teeth every day?" "Can you come to my mother's house to clean her teeth?"

EVERYDAY ETHICS

Before completing the learning exercises below, reread and reflect on the Everyday Ethics Scenario and Questions for Consideration in this chapter of the **textbook**. It may also be useful to review the Dental Hygiene Ethics discussion in Chapter 1, the Ethical Applications in the introduction pages for each section in the **textbook**, as well as the Codes of Ethics in **textbook** Appendices I–IV.

Individual Learning Activities

Imagine that you are the dental hygienist in this scenario. Answer each of the questions for consideration at the end of the scenario.

Imagine that you have observed what happened in the scenario, but are not one of the main characters involved in the situation. Write a reflective journal entry that:

- Describes how you might have reacted (as an observer—not as a participant),
- Expresses your personal feelings about what happened, or
- Identifies personal values that affect your reaction to the situation.

 MeSH TERMS

Use a combination of MeSH terms and other key words to develop an effective and efficient PubMed literature search strategy.

Homebound persons
Terminally ill
Hospice care
Dental care for aged
Dental care for chronically ill
Interdisciplinary communication
Dental care for disabled

Summary Exercises

Orientation to Clinical Dental Hygiene Practice

Chapters 1–4

 COMPETENCY EXERCISES

Apply information from Chapters 1–4 and use critical thinking skills to complete the competency exercises. Write responses on paper or create electronic documents to submit your answers.

SECTION I—PATIENT ASSESSMENT SUMMARY			
Patient Name: *Christopher Michaels*	Age: *10*	Gender: M	☑ Initial Therapy ☐ Maintenance
Provider Name: *D.H. Student*	Date: *Today*		☐ Re-evaluation

Chief Complaint:

Toothache and swollen area in lower left jaw. Ulcerated lesion on left upper lip.

Assessment Findings	
Health History	**At Risk For:** N/A
• No current findings	
• ASA-II and ADL level-0	
Social and Dental History	**At Risk For:**
• No dental exam in 5 years	• Low health literacy (of parents)
• Ulcerated, crusted lesion on left upper lip, spreading to noseHigh sucrose intake (juice, candy)	• Pain and secondary infection due to active herpetic lesion
• Poor dental biofilm control	• Increased incidence of dental caries
	• Increased risk of periodontal infection
Social and Dental History	**At Risk For:**
• Enlarged left submandibular lymph node	• Secondary infection
• Large lesion on mandibular left primary second molar	• Possible endodontic infection and pain from dental caries
• Numerous small carious lesions	• Further incidence of dental caries
• Generalized gingivitis	• Gingival infection/periodontal disease
Social and Dental History	**Caries Management Risk Assessment (CAMBRA) level:**
Gingivitis	☐ Low ☐ Moderate ☐ High ☑ Extreme

Read Section I Patient Assessment Summary to help you answer questions #1 and #2.

1. The clinical issue: The dentist who examines Christopher tells you that the ulcerated lesion you observe on Christopher's upper lip is caused by the herpes virus and is an infectious condition. You are worried that providing treatment for him while the lesion is active can cause the infection to spread or that you could be infected. Write a PICO question that you can use to help guide your search for evidence to help make a decision about providing dental hygiene treatment today.

2. After talking to Christopher and his mother, you determine that his habit of drinking juice all day long is a health-related behavior that needs to be changed in order to reduce the risk for additional dental caries. However, Mrs. Michaels insists that he really enjoys drinking the juice and that she gives him at least five containers each day because she believes that juice is a healthy way for him to drink lots of liquids when he is active. Write a short paragraph reflecting on a patient education approach that may begin help her move toward a willingness to change both her and Christopher's behavior. Is simply providing information enough?

3. Core values in dental hygiene practice include autonomy and respect. An example of this value is that you, as the dental hygienist, must respect your patients' right to refuse dental hygiene recommendations or treatment, even when your professional opinion is that doing so may cause deterioration of their oral health status.

   Select another one of the core values in dental hygiene practice and give an example to illustrate it. Discuss your example with student colleagues.

4. Identify an expression, gesture, or movement that you commonly make (see Table 3-3 in Chapter 3 for some ideas). Explain how your action can have unintended meaning or be the cause of a misunderstanding that will have a negative effect on the relationship you are developing with a patient of cultural background that is different than your own.

5. Explain why systematic reviews and meta-analysis articles are considered to constitute the highest level of evidence to support the selection of dental hygiene interventions for patient care.

 DISCOVERY EXERCISES

1. Obtain a copy of the rules or laws that govern the practice of dental hygiene in your state or country. Answer the following questions.
   - *What specific services are the dental hygienists in your state or area licensed to provide?*
   - *What type of supervision must dental hygienists have when they provide care for the patients?*
   - *Does your state have any provisions that allow dental hygienists to provide care in a collaborative practice or under reduced supervision to provide direct access care for underserved populations or in any specific kinds of public health or alternative practice settings?*
   - *What are continuing education requirements for dental hygienists who practice in your state or country?*

2. Find a contact person for the dental hygiene professional association nearest to you and ask questions about membership, continuing education, and leadership opportunities.

3. Initiate a PubMed search to identify recent articles related to cultural competence in health care and then narrow the search to see what you can find related specifically to oral health care.

4. Explore the Internet to find additional resources related to cultural competence in health care.

5. Initiate a PubMed search to find recent articles related to dental hygiene practice in alternative settings.

 FOR YOUR PORTFOLIO

Use the basic information from the four chapters in Section I of the **textbook** to write a personal philosophy of dental hygiene practice statement. Describe how you believe yourself to be as a dental hygiene professional. Identify characteristics that describe the way you will provide dental hygiene care. Do this at the beginning of your training just after you complete these chapter and section exercises, and then do it again just before you graduate (don't peek at what you wrote the first time, please). Finally, write a summary of how these two documents reveal your personal growth during your training as a professional.

SECTION I CROSSWORD PUZZLE

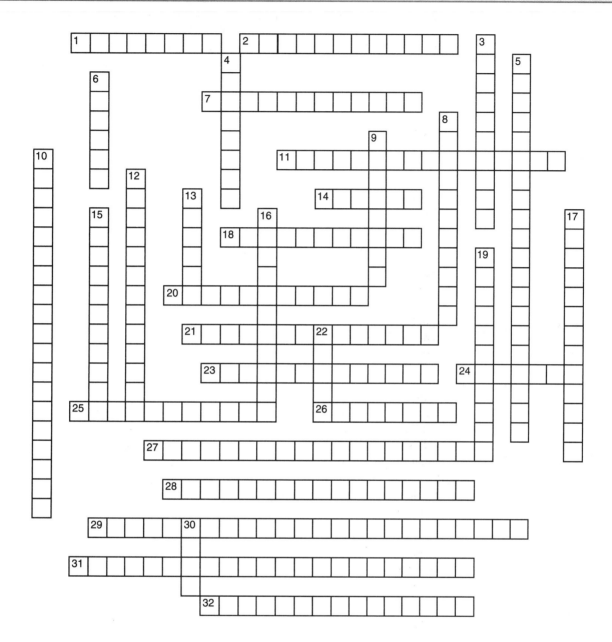

Puzzle Clues

Across

1. Research significance that indicates practical or observed difference expected in patient care outcomes.

2. Allows a dental hygienist to initiate dental hygiene treatment based on assessment of the patient's needs and without the specific authorization or presence of a dentist (two words).

7. Approaches that has consistently shown results (outcomes) superior to those achieved with other means (two words).

11. Summary and critical analysis of published sources on a particular topic (two words).

14. A sense of moral obligation.

18. The dental hygienist who coordinates efforts with the dentist and the patient to attain and maintain oral health of the patient.

20. Type of research study that uses numbers to describe the main features or characteristics of a particular person, event, or group; determine the frequency with which something occurs; or categorize information.

21. The ability of a patient to obtain, process, understand, and respond to measures that promote and maintain good health (two words).

23. A framework of activities for delivering quality dental hygiene care (three words).

24. An ethical problem that involves two morally correct choices or courses of action.

25. Type of study that collects numerical data designed to allow generalization from a sample to a population.

26. Source of information used to support, determine, or demonstrate the truth of a statement.

27. Making an effort to understand the language, culture, and behaviors of diverse individuals and groups (two words).

28. Integrated preventive and treatment services administered by a dental hygienist (three words).

29. A patient-centered communication approach to changing health behaviors (two words).

31. Identification of oral health problem that a dental hygienist is qualified and licensed to treat (three words).

32. Process of adequately explaining research to prospective patients and ensuring that they understand what will happen to them, especially associated risks and benefits (two words).

Down

3. Possessing skills, understanding, and values necessary for beginning professional practice.

4. The receiver's direct response to a communicated message.

5. Inability to perform one or more ADL without help (two words).

6. State of physical, mental, and social well-being, not only the absence of disease.

8. Attitudes or judgments (either positive or negative) made about people.

9. Ability to measure what was intended.

10. Post-licensure short-term educational experiences (two words).

12. Relationship of dental hygienist who is working with a consulting dentist under general supervision.

13. The statistical notation for probability value.

15. A legal relationship between dentist and dental team members in practice.

16. The significance of research findings as identified by the "p-value" notation.

17. Process of defining the meaning of a message shared between a sender and one or more intended recipients.

19. Ability of a measurement instrument or test to get the same results repeatedly.

22. Ethical problem for which a solution is readily grounded in the governing practice act, recognized laws, or acceptable standards of care.

30. A dental hygiene-based alternative workforce model proposed by the American Dental Hygienists' Association (acronym).

EVERYDAY ETHICS

Surf health-related websites, government websites, online health literature databases, or any other online resource to find information related to ethics in healthcare, research, or public health. In particular, topics such as informed consent, HIPAA, public health access, licensure, and so on, provide good topics to investigate on the Internet. Identify a URL that others can use to locate the website or resource you discover, and then annotate the citation by writing a brief description, provide an overview of the contents, and explain how the resource might be helpful for the study of professional ethics.

Combine what you discover with ethics-related materials identified by other student colleagues to develop an annotated bibliography of online resources everyone can use to help further explore the Everyday Ethics scenarios throughout the **textbook**.

(**Annotate:** *to provide a critical or explanatory description.*)

DIAGNOSE
Problem
identification

PLAN
Selection of
interventions

ASSESS
Data
collection

IMPLEMENT
Activating
the plan

DOCUMENT
Comprehensive
record-keeping

EVALUATE
Feedback on
effectiveness

Preparation for Dental Hygiene Practice

Chapters 5–9

SECTION II LEARNING OBJECTIVES

Completing the exercises in this section of the workbook will prepare you to:

1. Apply concepts of infection/exposure control to protect the safety of self and patient during the dental hygiene appointment.

2. Position self, patient, and equipment to promote comfort, safety, and efficiency during the dental hygiene appointment.

3. Prevent and respond to emergency situations during patient care.

COMPETENCIES FOR THE DENTAL HYGIENIST (APPENDIX A)

Competencies supported by the learning in Section II

    Core Competencies: C1, C2, C3, C4, C5, C6, C9, C11, C12, C14

    Health Promotion and Disease Prevention: HP2, HP4, HP6

    Patient/Client Care: PC2, PC3, PC4, PC5

Infection Control: Transmissible Diseases

KNOWLEDGE EXERCISES

Also refer to Sections I, II, and IX-K in the CDC Guidelines for Infection Control in Dental Healthcare Settings (Appendix V in the **textbook**) as you complete the exercises for this chapter.

Infomaps 5-1 to 5-3 in Chapter 5 of the **textbook** provide an excellent summary of details related to a variety of infectious agents that are of special concern for healthcare providers. You should study these tables carefully. Ask your instructor to tell you how thoroughly (or to what level of detail) you will need to study the information in these tables at this point in your dental hygiene program.

Write your answers for each question in the space provided.

1. Standard precautions apply regarding direct contact with:

2. List additional precautions that the healthcare providers are required to address.

3. In your own words, define *cross-contamination*.

4. List six factors that are necessary for transmission of disease.

5. Preventing disease from infectious agents requires breaking the chain of transmission. The use of standard precautions during patient care breaks the chain at every point. Identify additional ways that the dental team can break the chain and prevent transmission of infection.

_____

_____

_____

_____

6. Identify items in the dental setting that can serve as reservoirs for infectious agents.

_____

_____

_____

7. Identify three ways infectious particles can be airborne in the dental setting.

_____

_____

_____

8. Identify ways of controlling airborne transmission of infection in the dental setting.

_____

_____

_____

_____

_____

9. Both Chapter 2 and Section IX-K of the CDC guidelines (see **textbook** Appendix V) mention tuberculosis as an infectious disease that is of concern for dental healthcare providers. Identify the microorganism that causes tuberculosis.

_____

10. In what way is tuberculosis infection most commonly transmitted?

_____

_____

11. Describe XDR-TB.

_____

_____

_____

12. What course of action does CDC guidelines recommend if a patient with symptoms or history suggestive of tuberculosis presents for elective dental services, such as dental hygiene care?

_____

_____

_____

INFOMAP 5-1	HEPATITIS INFECTIONS		
HEPATITIS TYPE	VIRUS	MODE OF TRANSMISSION	METHOD FOR PREVENTION
"Infectious" hepatitis			
"Serum hepatitis"			
Type C hepatitis			
Delta hepatitis			
Type E hepatitis			

Note: Use information from Table 5-1 and the **textbook** information about viral hepatitis to compare modes of transmission and methods for preventing transmission of each type in the dental office setting.

13. What is the significance of HbsAg?

_____

_____

_____

_____

14. What is the significance of anti-HBs?

_____

_____

_____

15. Which type of virus can be found in periodontitis pockets with relatively high prevalence?

_____

16. Which of the herpesviruses can establish a latent infection in the trigeminal nerve ganglion that can reactivate and erupt in a surface lesion later?

_____

17. Which type of virus is associated with lesions on hands and eyes?

_____

_____

18. What clinical management protocol applies for a patient with an active HSV-1 lesion?

_____

_____

_____

19. AIDS is associated with infection by the _____ virus.

20. List the ways the HIV can be transmitted from one individual to another.

_____

_____

_____

_____

_____

INFOMAP 5-2	HUMAN HERPESVIRUS INFECTIONS		
VIRUS	ACRONYM	MODE OF TRANSMISSION	ASSOCIATED OROFACIAL CONDITIONS
Herpes simplex virus type 1			
Herpes simplex virus type 2			
Varicella–zoster virus			
Epstein–Barr virus			
Cytomegalovirus			
Herpes lymphotropic virus			
Human herpesvirus 7			
Kaposi sarcoma–related virus			

Note: Many herpesvirus infections are associated with intraoral findings. Use the information in Tables 5-1 and 5-3 as well as the **textbook** information to complete the Infomap 5-2. Include the acronym, mode of transmission, and associated orofacial conditions for each herpesvirus listed.

21. A count of which serologic marker is most often used to evaluate and monitor the progression of HIV infection.

_____

_____

22. In HIV disease, the number of CD4+ T lymphocytes _____ as the infection and symptoms become more severe.

23. At what level does the CD4+ T cell count indicate late-stage disease or AIDS infection?

_____

24. As the count of indicator cells decreases, the symptoms of disease and the incidence of oral infections or oral lesions related to the HIV infection _____.

25. What are the most common oral lesions associated with HIV infection?

_____

_____

_____

_____

_____

_____

_____

26. Describe the appearance of linear gingival erythema.

_____

_____

_____

_____

27. What does the abbreviation HAART stand for?

_____

_____

_____

28. Describe how HAART has influenced HIV-related oral lesions.

_____

_____

_____

29. How is MRSA spread?

_____

_____

30. List the risk factors for becoming infected with MRSA.

_____

_____

_____

_____

31. There are numerous prescribed HIV medications. Match the category of drug to the generic name of the drug. Some drug categories are used more than once.

Drug Category	Generic Name
A. Nucleoside reverse transcriptase inhibitors (NRTIs)	_____ Dolutegravir
	_____ Atazanavir
B. Non-nucleoside reverse transcriptase inhibitors (NNRTIs)	_____ Zidovudine
	_____ Maraviroc
C. Fusion inhibitor	_____ Cobicistat
D. CCR5 antagonists	_____ Efavirenz
E. Protease inhibitors (PIs)	_____ Ritonavir
F. Integrase strand transfer inhibitors (INSTIs)	_____ Enfuvirtide
	_____ Emtricitabine
G. Pharmacokinetic (PK) enhancer	_____ Fosamprenavir
	_____ Elvitegravir
	_____ Rilpivirine
	_____ Nevirapine
	_____ Tenofovir alafenamide

✓ COMPETENCY EXERCISES

Apply information from the chapter and use critical thinking skills to complete the competency exercises. Write responses on a paper or create electronic documents to submit your answers.

1. The very first section of CDC Guidelines for Infection Control in Dental Health Care Settings (see **textbook** Appendix V), which is titled Recommendations, provides a description of the evidence-based categories used to support each recommendation made in the report. Discuss, in your own words, what each of the recommendation categories means.

2. In your own words, write a paragraph or two summarizing the recommendations (in Section II of CDC guidelines) for preventing transmission of blood-borne pathogens. In general, indicate the category of evidence that supports these recommendations.

3. In your own words, identify clinical management procedures to follow if your patient's medical history raises concerns about tuberculosis infection (Section IV-K of the CDC guidelines can provide guidance).

EVERYDAY ETHICS

Before completing the learning exercises below, reread and reflect on the Everyday Ethics Scenario and Questions for Consideration in this chapter of the **textbook**. It may also be useful to review the Dental Hygiene Ethics discussion in Chapter 1, the Ethical Applications in the introduction pages for each section in the **textbook**, as well as the Codes of Ethics in **textbook** Appendices I–IV.

Individual Learning Activity

Imagine the scenario from the patient's perspective. How might the patient's response to the questions following the scenario be different from those of the dental hygienist involved?

Discovery Activity

Ask a dental hygienist who has been practicing for a year or more to read the scenario. Provide them with a copy of the Code of Ethics as well. Share the responses you have made to answer each question and ask that person to discuss the situation with you. What insights did you have or what did you learn during this discussion?

Factors to Teach the Patient

This scenario is related to the following factors listed in this chapter of the **textbook**:

▷ Reasons for postponing an appointment when a herpes lesion (fever blister or cold sore) is present on the lip or in the oral cavity.

▷ Importance of not touching or scratching the lesion because of self-infection to the fingers or eyes, for example.

▷ How the viruses can survive on objects and transfer infection to other people.

Your patient, Ms. Janette Whitlow, arrives just on time for her dental hygiene appointment, and you greet her cheerfully. As you update her health history, she mentions that she is grumpy because she is getting another cold sore and her lip itches and burns. You look closely and observe a reddened, slightly swollen area on her lower lip that is just beginning to get small bumps. As she talks, Janette slowly rubs her hand up across her face and eyes and up into her hair.

Write the outline that contains the main points you will cover in a conversation explaining to Janette why you recommend postponing her appointment until another day. Also explain why she should not touch or scratch the sore area on her lip.

Ask a student colleague or dental hygiene instructor to give feedback on the conversation you create, and then modify the conversation based on what you learned from the feedback.

MeSH TERMS

Use a combination of MeSH terms and other key words to develop an effective and efficient PubMed literature search strategy.

Communicable diseases	Herpes labialis
Hepatitis	Herpesvirus 1, human
Hepatitis, viral, human	Herpesvirus 2, human
HIV	Herpesvirus 3, human
Tuberculosis	Herpesvirus 4, human
Methicillin-resistant	Herpesvirus 6, human
Staphylococcus aureus	Herpesvirus 7, human
Herpes simplex	Herpesvirus 8, human

CHAPTER 5 CROSSWORD PUZZLE

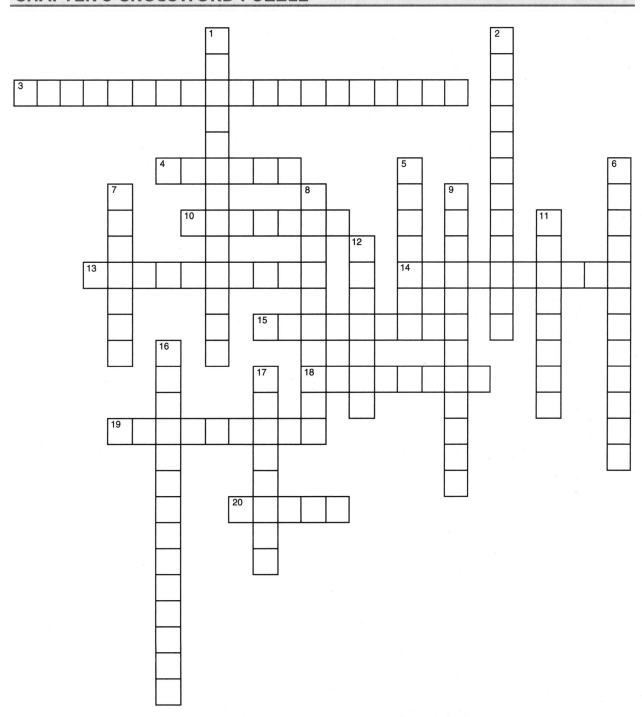

Puzzle Clues

Across

3. An infection control approach that protects both healthcare providers and patients from pathogens (two words).

4. The type of infection in which the causative agent remains inactive for a period of time within certain body cells.

10. A substance that induces an immune response.

13. Dead bone tissue.

14. The period of time between initial contact with an infectious agent and the appearance of clinical symptoms of the disease.

15. A latent viral infection that reactivates at a later date.

18. The presence of a virus in certain body secretions, excretions, or surface lesions.

19. Early or premonitory symptom (adjective).

20. A genetic entity that contains either DNA or RNA, or both; replicates inside living cells.

Down

1. A pathogen that causes infection only when the host's resistance is lowered.

2. An infectious agent may be transferred directly or indirectly from an infected person to another person.

5. The type of immunity that is transferred from the mother or acquired by inoculation of protective antibodies.

6. A mode of transmission of some forms of hepatitis.

7. Constant presence of a disease within a geographic area.

8. A path of entry through a mucous membrane.

9. An entry through the skin.

11. Produced and secreted by body cells in response to, and able to bind to, a specific antigen.

12. Someone who harbors a specific infectious agent but shows no clinical signs of disease.

16. After exposure, the serum marker for the disease changes.

17. A natural or an acquired resistance against disease.

Exposure Control: Barriers for Patient and Clinician

LEARNING OBJECTIVES

Upon successful completion of these exercises, you will be able to:

1. Identify and define the key terms and concepts related to exposure control, clinical barriers, and latex allergies.

2. Apply and remove clinical barrier materials without cross-contamination.

3. Identify and explain the rationale for handwashing and other exposure-control techniques used during patient care.

4. Identify the criteria for selecting appropriate protective barrier materials.

 KNOWLEDGE EXERCISES

Write your answers for each question in the space provided. Also refer to Sections III, IV, and V in the CDC Guidelines for Infection Control in Dental Healthcare Settings (Appendix V) as you complete the exercises for this chapter.

1. An organized system for exposure control that treats body fluids of all patients as though they were infectious is a description of _____.

2. Identify the term or concept related to each of the following statements.
    - Physically blocks exposure to bodily fluids to prevent disease transmission.

    _____

    - A specific, potentially health-threatening bodily contact with infectious material while you are providing dental hygiene care.

    _____

    - Contact with infectious material that is reasonable to expect as a component of providing dental hygiene care.

    _____

3. List three purposes for having a written exposure control plan.

    _____

    _____

    _____

4. Define the following terms in your own words.
    - *Immunization*

    _____

    - *Contamination*

    _____

    _____

    - *Antiseptic*

    _____

    _____

    _____

- *Cross-contamination*

  _____

  _____

- *Occupational exposure*

  _____

  _____

- *DHCP*

  _____

  _____

5. Explain what respiratory hygiene is and why it is implemented in the dental care setting.

6. List the basic immunizations recommended for DHCP.

   _____

   _____

   _____

7. List the factors that describe an appropriate clinic gown or uniform.

   _____

   _____

   _____

   _____

   _____

   _____

8. During patient care, long hair should be fastened back and facial hair should be covered by _____ _____.

9. List the essential characteristics of an ideal face mask.

   _____

   _____

   _____

   _____

10. Particles in aerosols smaller than _____ can remain suspended up to 24 hours.

11. What size particle can penetrate to the alveoli of lungs when inhaled?

    _____

12. What size are the tuberculosis-causing bacterium particles?

    _____

    _____

13. When should a clinician wear a face shield over a regular mask?

    _____

    _____

14. How is a contaminated mask removed from your face?

    _____

    _____

15. Who wears protective eyewear during dental hygiene care?

    _____

    _____

16. List the types of eyewear appropriate for wear during patient care.

    _____

    _____

    _____

    _____

    _____

17. List the features of acceptable eyewear.

    _____

    _____

    _____

    _____

18. List three steps you can use to disinfect and provide care for eyewear worn during patient care.

    _____

    _____

    _____

    _____

    _____

19. List glove safety factors that are important for both the patient and the dental hygienist during dental hygiene care.

    _____

    _____

    _____

_____

_____

20. When you are selecting the type of gloves to use during patient care, which glove factor is important for clinician comfort?

_____

_____

21. The cuffs of your gloves should _____ the cuffs of your long-sleeved clinic wear to provide a complete barrier to contamination.

22. After positioning your gloves before patient care, you should touch only:

_____

_____

23. List factors that can affect the ability of gloves to provide a complete aseptic barrier.

_____

_____

_____

_____

_____

_____

24. When are heavy-duty utility gloves used?

_____

_____

25. During clinical practice, you will wash your hands many, many times each day. List the indications for washing your hands.

_____

_____

_____

_____

_____

26. In your own words, describe the characteristics of an ideal sink for handwashing before patient care.

_____

_____

_____

_____

27. List the sequence of steps used for the antiseptic handwashing procedure you will perform before patient care.

_____

_____

_____

_____

_____

_____

_____

28. Match each term with the correct description. Write the letter of the appropriate description in the space next to the term it refers to.

Term	Description
____ Standard mask filtration	A. Relatively stable on skin; reduced by washing
____ Surgical soap	B. Blocks particles with greater than 95% efficiency
____ Antiseptic handwash	C. Used before patient care
____ Handwashing	D. Most important in preventing cross-contamination
____ Wide-coverage eyewear	E. Never at the sink used for patient care handwashing
____ Resident bacteria	F. Used by both clinician and patient
____ Transient bacteria	G. Contains antimicrobial agent
____ Skin integrity	H. Contaminates skin if contacted; reduced by washing
____ Gloves	I. Available in nonsterile and presterilized forms
____ Glove integrity	J. Affected by many things, including length of time worn
____ Eyewash station	K. Can be protected by covering abrasions with a liquid bandage

29. In your own words, define the following terms related to a latex allergic response.

- *Allergen*

  _____

  _____

- *Urticaria*

  _____

  _____

- *Aeroallergen*

  _____

  _____

- *Type I hypersensitivity reaction*

  _____

  _____

  _____

  _____

- *Type IV hypersensitivity reaction*

  _____

  _____

  _____

30. List five pieces of equipment used when providing dental hygiene care (other than gloves) that may contain latex.

_____

_____

_____

_____

_____

_____

_____

_____

_____

31. List factors that increase risk for latex sensitivity.

_____

_____

_____

_____

32. What actions, taken prior to patient care for an at-risk patient, can reduce the risk of a latex allergy-related emergency?

_____

_____

_____

_____

_____

_____

33. Refer to **textbook** Appendix V (CDC Guidelines for Infection Control in Dental Healthcare Settings) as you answer the following questions.

- In the CDC 2003 guidelines, Section III, an alternative hand hygiene method for hands that are not visibly soiled, is given the highest category (IA) recommendation. What is the method recommended for hands that are not visibly soiled?

  _____

  _____

- What is the recommendation included in the CDC 2003 guidelines regarding hand jewelry and what does the category II and the numbers (in parentheses at the end of the statement) included in the recommendation mean?

  _____

  _____

  _____

  _____

  _____

  _____

  _____

- If your gloves become torn, cut, or punctured during patient care, what should you do?

  _____

  _____

  _____

  _____

- The CDC guidelines recommend changing a mask between patients or during patient care if the mask becomes _____.
- If your protective covering (clinic gown) becomes visibly soiled during patient care, what should you do?

_____

_____

_____

_____

_____

 COMPETENCY EXERCISES

Apply information from the chapter and use critical thinking skills to complete the competency exercises. Write responses on paper or create electronic documents to submit your answers.

1. Use the information in Chapter 6 to develop a step-by-step checklist, in proper sequence, for getting ready to provide patient care. Consider the sequence for handwashing as well as applying all of the personal protective barriers that you use in your clinic. Pay careful attention to creating a detailed system that minimizes the possibility of cross-contamination.
2. Compare your checklist to the lists that other student colleagues have created or to one provided by your instructor. Refine your list and use it as part of your own personal written exposure control plan.
3. Describe at least three ways you can prevent cross-contamination during handwashing in the clinic at your school.
4. Practice removing gloves using the system illustrated in Figure 6-4 in the **textbook**. Explain how this procedure will prevent cross-contamination.

5. Explain why it is necessary to document a latex allergy on the patient's permanent record. Identify how that information is recorded in the patient records at your school.

? QUESTIONS PATIENTS ASK

What sources of information can you identify to help you answer your patient's questions in this scenario?

How do I know this room was cleaned after the last patient was in here? Did you wash your hands? Is everything you use brand new for each patient? How do I know that I won't be exposed to an infectious disease during my dental hygiene treatment?

 Factors to Teach the Patient

This scenario is related to the following factors listed in this chapter of the **textbook**:

▷ Purposes for use of barriers (face mask, protective eyewear, and gloves) by the clinician for the benefit of the patient.
▷ Importance of eye protection.

Mrs. Johnson is bringing her 3-year-old son, Jimmy, in for his first dental hygiene appointment. She states that he is frightened by the mask and asks you not to wear it during the appointment. She is also concerned because she has never been asked to wear glasses during previous dental hygiene appointments at another dental office. She states that Jimmy will probably protest at having to wear the child-size glasses you have ready.

Write a paragraph you will use to explain to Mrs. Johnson the importance of, and the rationale for, using these barriers. Include some comments that will help explain their use to Jimmy.

INFOMAP 6-1

METHOD	PREPARATION	LATHERING METHOD	SITUATION IN WHICH THE TECHNIQUE IS RECOMMENDED
Routine handwash			
Antiseptic handwash			
Surgical antisepsis			
Antiseptic hand rub			

Instructions: Fill out to compare the methods of handwashing. Then use the information in the Infomap to verbally describe the differences between the methods to a fellow student or a patient.

EVERYDAY ETHICS

Before completing the learning exercises below, reread and reflect on the Everyday Ethics Scenario and Questions for Consideration in this chapter of the **textbook**. It may also be useful to review the Dental Hygiene Ethics discussion in Chapter 1, the Ethical Applications in the introduction pages for each section in the **textbook**, as well as the Codes of Ethics in **textbook** Appendices I–IV.

Individual Learning Activity

Imagine that you are the dental hygienist in this scenario. Answer each of the questions for consideration at the end of the scenario.

Collaborative Learning Activity

Work with a small group to develop a 2–5-minute role-play that introduces the everyday ethics scenario described in the chapter (a great idea is to video record your role-play activity). Then develop separate 2-minute role-play scenarios that provide at least two alternative approaches/solutions to resolving the situation. Ask classmates to view the solutions, ask questions, and discuss the ethical approach used in each. Ask for a vote on which solution classmates determine to be the "best."

 MeSH TERMS

Use a combination of MeSH terms and other key words to develop an effective and efficient PubMed literature search strategy.

Communicable disease control
- Hand hygiene
- Hand disinfection
- Infection control
- Universal precautions

Masks
Aerosols
Gloves, protective
Gloves, surgical
Hypersensitivity
- Hypersensitivity, delayed
- Hypersensitivity, immediate
- Latex hypersensitivity

Infection Control: Clinical Procedures

 KNOWLEDGE EXERCISES

Write your answers for each question in the space provided.

1. Define *asepsis* in your own words.

_____

_____

_____

_____

2. What does *infection control* mean?

_____

_____

_____

_____

3. What is the purpose of maintaining proper infection control when you are providing dental hygiene care.

_____

_____

_____

_____

4. List three infection-control components that are all necessary for preventing transmission of infection and eliminating cross-infection.

_____

_____

_____

5. What objects or features of a dental hygiene treatment room are important to consider when discussing infection control measures?

_____

_____

_____

_____

_____

_____

6. In your own words, describe the two processing steps to implement before sterilizing instruments used for patient care.

_____

_____

_____

_____

_____

_____

7. List the three basic methods for precleaning instruments prior to sterilization.

_____

_____

_____

8. What procedures will protect you and others during manual scrubbing of instruments?

_____

_____

_____

_____

_____

9. Identify three approved sterilization methods and list the time requirement that ensures adequate sterilization for each method.

_____

_____

_____

10. Which method of sterilization processes instruments at the highest temperature?

_____

11. List three types of tests used to determine whether sterilization has been achieved.

_____

_____

_____

12. Describe a type of chemical indicator used each time on packaging to identify instruments that have been processed.

_____

_____

13. What microorganism is used as a biologic monitor for a steam autoclave system.

_____

_____

14. How frequently is biologic monitoring of sterilization procedures recommended in the dental office setting?

_____

15. List the two types of autoclave systems and their temperatures for sterilization.

_____

_____

_____

_____

16. Which type of autoclave sterilizes instruments the fastest?

_____

17. Identify contraindications or special considerations to think about before using steam autoclaving as a method for sterilization.

_____

_____

_____

_____

_____

18. What is the effect of pressure generated by an autoclave sterilizer?

_____

_____

19. List actions that can enhance the penetrability of the steam during an autoclave cycle.

_____

_____

_____

_____

_____

_____

_____

_____

20. During a dry heat sterilization cycle, a temperature of _____ is maintained for 2 hours.

21. List two disadvantages of the dry-heat method of sterilization.

_____

_____

_____

_____

22. Chemical vapor sterilization cannot be used for materials and objects that _____; it also cannot be used for heavy, tightly wrapped packages that _____.

23. Chemical vapor sterilization systems should not be used in a small room because _____ is required for safe use.

24. A chemical vapor sterilization system is tested weekly with biologic indicator strips containing _____.

25. When is spore testing done?

_____

_____

_____

_____

26. Briefly describe a system for remembering to regularly monitor sterilization effectiveness.

_____

_____

_____

_____

27. To keep your instruments contamination free after sterilizing, you can store them in the _____.

28. List three uses for chemical disinfectants.

_____

_____

_____

29. Describe the three levels of chemical disinfectants.

_____

_____

_____

_____

_____

_____

30. List the factors you will consider when selecting a chemical disinfectant for use in your dental hygiene treatment room.

_____

_____

_____

_____

_____

_____

_____

_____

31. What information on a product label tells you about the effectiveness of the chemical agent you use for disinfection?

_____

_____

_____

_____

32. List the product label items to look for when you prepare and use a chemical disinfectant.

_____

_____

_____

_____

_____

33. Define each of the following types of waste.
    * _Infectious waste_

    _____

    * _Contaminated waste_

    _____

    * _Hazardous waste_

    _____

    * _Regulated waste_

    _____

34. Items such as needles are disposed of in a _____ .

35. Correctly number the sequence of steps for disinfecting environmental surfaces in the treatment room by placing the numbers 1–4 in the space provided.

Order	Description of Step
_____	Spray surfaces and allow to air-dry
_____	Put on PPE, including heavy-duty household gloves
_____	Scrub surfaces with gauze sponges or paper towels
_____	Spray all surfaces liberally and completely

36. According to CDC recommendations, water lines should be flushed for _____ at the beginning of the day and for _____ between patients to reduce microbial counts.

37. Identify two oral procedures that can reduce microbial counts before dental hygiene treatment.

_____

_____

_____

_____

_____

38. What additional patient-related factors can be included as standard procedures that will help manage infection control during treatment?

_____

_____

_____

_____

_____

_____

_____

39. Describe how a permucosal exposure to blood or other body fluids might occur.

_____

_____

_____

40. What basic procedures are followed when a clinician experiences a percutaneous exposure to blood or contaminated body fluids?

_____

_____

_____

_____

_____

_____

_____

_____

41. Why is it important to clean the exposed parts of your face regularly during your clinical day?

_____

_____

_____

42. What two components regarding infection control are included in an office policy manual?

_____

_____

_____

_____

_____

_____

_____

43. Refer to **textbook** Appendix V (CDC Guidelines for Infection Control in Dental Healthcare Settings) as you answer the following questions.

- CDC 1. Section VI-A of the CDC guideline recommend that you use only FDA-cleared medical devices and that you follow manufacturer's instructions for sterilization. The category for this recommendation is IB. What does IB recommendation mean?

_____

_____

_____

- CDC 2. What procedure does Section VI-F of the CDC guidelines recommend in the case of a positive spoor-monitoring test?

_____

_____

_____

- CDC 3. The CDC guidelines, Section VII, recommends the use of _____-level chemical disinfectants of clinical contact surfaces that are visibly contaminated with blood.

 COMPETENCY EXERCISES

Apply information from the chapter and use critical thinking skills to complete the competency exercises. Write responses on paper or create electronic documents to submit your answers.

1. _Putting it all together:_ Review both Chapters 6 and 7 to answer this question. Write brief statements or lists to summarize all of the procedures you can follow every day to maintain the chain of asepsis and prevent disease transmission in each of the following categories.
   - You and your colleagues
   - Your patient
   - The clinic
   - During treatment
   - Posttreatment

2. Explain the difference between decontamination, disinfection, and sterilization.

3. Identify specific ways planning ahead prior to seating a patient in the dental chair can ensure you will maintain asepsis and eliminate cross-contamination during patient treatment.

4. The **textbook** describes features of dental treatment room equipment that facilitate optimum infection control. Describe the features in your school clinic that meet these criteria.

MeSH TERMS

Use a combination of MeSH terms and other key words to develop an effective and efficient PubMed literature search strategy.

Infection control, dental   Sterilization
Universal precautions   Dental waste

 EVERYDAY ETHICS

Before completing the learning exercises below, reread and reflect on the Everyday Ethics Scenario and Questions for Consideration in this chapter of the **textbook**. It may also be useful to review the Dental Hygiene Ethics discussion in Chapter 1, the Ethical Applications in the introduction pages for each section in the **textbook**, as well as the Codes of Ethics in **textbook** Appendices I–IV.

Individual Learning Activity

Imagine that you are the dental hygienist in this scenario. Answer each of the questions for consideration at the end of the scenario.

Collaborative Learning Activity

Ask a dental hygienist who has been practicing for a year or more to read the scenario. Share the responses you have made to answer each question and ask that person to discuss the situation with you. What insights did you have or what did you learn during this discussion?

Factors to Teach the Patient

This scenario is related to the following factors listed in this chapter of the **textbook**:

▷ The meaning of *standard precautions* and what is included under the term; how these precautions protect the patient and the dental team members.

▷ Methods for sterilization of instruments, including hand pieces, and how the autoclave or other sterilizer is tested daily or weekly.

Mrs. Norton is on the telephone again. She recently made a first dental appointment for Daniella, her 3-year-old daughter, and she is clearly nervous about it. This is the second time she has called in with questions. This time, she wants to be assured that her daughter will not be exposed to any infectious diseases during dental hygiene treatment.

Using the information you learned in Chapters 6 and 7 of the **textbook**, write a statement explaining infection control procedures and reassuring Mrs. Norton.

Patient Reception and Ergonomic Practice

8

KNOWLEDGE EXERCISES

Write your answers for each question in the space provided.

1. Identify the treatment room factors you will prepare before your patient arrives for the dental hygiene appointment.

2. List two factors to include when you are welcoming your patient to the dental hygiene treatment room.

3. The more attention you pay to ergonomics, the more likely you are to avoid cumulative trauma injuries during your dental hygiene career. In your own words, define the following terms.

   • *Ergonomics*

   • *Safe work practices*

   • *Cumulative trauma*

4. The main objectives in preferred patient positioning discussed in this chapter are that both you and your patient are as _____ as possible during dental hygiene treatment and that visibility and access during care are enhanced.

5. List the four main patient positions used during dental hygiene care.

6. Describe the supine position.

_____

_____

_____

_____

7. List three contraindications for placing a patient in the supine position.

_____

_____

_____

8. Your patient is positioned in the dental chair with her brain lower than her heart and her legs and feet raised. What is this position called?

_____

9. In your own words, describe the characteristics of an ideal dental chair.

_____

_____

_____

_____

_____

10. Explain how the dental chair is arranged before each patient is seated when he or she arrives for treatment.

_____

_____

_____

_____

11. List the proper sequence of steps you would use to adjust the dental chair and patient to the final working position after the patient is seated.

_____

_____

_____

12. After completing dental hygiene treatment and raising the dental chair to an upright position, what important step is included to ensure patient safety?

_____

_____

_____

13. What is postural hypotension?

_____

_____

_____

14. List ergonomic factors that put the dental hygiene clinician at risk for musculoskeletal disorders.

_____

_____

_____

_____

_____

15. Identify the ergonomic positioning errors often observed during clinical practice that can cause each of the following musculoskeletal disorders.

Carpal tunnel syndrome

_____

Tendonitis

_____

Thoracic outlet syndrome

_____

16. Identify components of neutral seated position for the dental hygiene clinician.

_____

_____

_____

_____

_____

_____

_____

_____

_____

_____

17. Identify characteristics of an acceptable clinician's stool.

_____

_____

_____

_____

_____

_____

_____

_____

18. When both you and your patient are in the correct position during dental hygiene treatment, your relaxed elbows are at the same level as _____, and the distance between your eyes and your patient's mouth is about _____.

19. Clock-hour positioning for the dental hygiene clinician is associated with enhanced access to:

_____

20. Flexibility of both the clinician's and patient's positioning during dental hygiene care can increase both _____ and _____ to oral structures for the dental hygienist.

21. Identify two ways to enhance the clinician's visual access to the oral cavity while providing dental hygiene care.

_____

_____

22. List the characteristics of a good dental light.

_____

_____

_____

23. List the characteristics of an ergonomically designed handpiece or power instrument.

_____

_____

_____

_____

_____

24. Identify the major components of ergonomic dental hygiene practice and self-care principles for health and well-being.

_____

_____

_____

_____

_____

_____

_____

✓ COMPETENCY EXERCISES

Apply information from the chapter and use critical thinking skills to complete the competency exercises. Write responses on paper or create electronic documents to submit your answers.

1. Practice each of the daily functional exercises found in **workbook** Appendix F. (Doesn't that feel good? Let's do it again!)

2. Explain how ergonomically designed power-driven equipment can help prevent physical occupational disorders.

3. Describe any characteristics in the clinical work area at your school's clinic that might contribute to negative health outcomes for the clinician. Develop a plan to maintain appropriate ergonomic positioning while working in the clinic.

4. A treatment room that is completely prepared when each patient arrives demonstrates professionalism and inspires patient confidence. The dental hygiene instruments are arranged for each patient, with the sterile packaging sealed until the patient is seated and the appointment has started. Explain how your body language can affect a patient's impression of your professionalism as you welcome him or her into your treatment room.

5. Mrs. Virginia Weatherbee, a 50-year-old with a charming smile, has been a patient in your clinic for many years. In a previous appointment with you, Mrs. Weatherbee has said that you may call her Ginny. Right after you get your patient settled in the dental chair, Samantha, who is in her first year of college and working for the summer as the dental hygiene assistant, peeks in to ask you a question. Discuss several reasons why it might be important to introduce your patient to Samantha as "Mrs. Weatherbee" prior to, or even instead of, explaining that she has asked you to call her Ginny.

DISCOVERY EXERCISES

Ask a student colleague to observe you periodically as you provide care for a patient or practice instrumentation during your preclinic labs. What risk factors for physical occupational disorders does your colleague identify in the way you are positioning yourself during instrumentation? What steps will you need to take to help maintain personal wellness throughout your career?

Factors to Teach the Patient

This scenario is related to the following factors listed in this chapter of the **textbook**:

▷ How patient cooperation makes it possible for the dental hygienist to practice with less stress and strain to prevent musculoskeletal discomfort and pain, and deliver better patient care.

The patient in your chair today is a curious and very fidgety 10-year-old boy named Nathan. Even before you get him seated in the dental chair, he starts asking you questions about how things work and the function of each button and switch. He just can't seem to sit still.

Use the motivational interviewing approach (see **workbook** Appendix D) to write a statement explaining the dental chair and how it helps keep both Nathan and you safe and comfortable. Use the conversation you create to role-play this situation with a fellow student. If you are the patient in the role-play, be sure to ask questions. If you are the dental hygienist in the role-play, try to anticipate questions and answer them in your explanation—and remember as you talk that Nathan is only 10 years old.

EVERYDAY ETHICS

Before completing the learning exercises below, reread and reflect on the Everyday Ethics Scenario and Questions for Consideration in this chapter of the **textbook**. It may also be useful to review the Dental Hygiene Ethics discussion in Chapter 1, the Ethical Applications in the introduction pages for each section in the **textbook**, as well as the Codes of Ethics in **textbook** Appendices I–IV.

Individual Learning Activity

Imagine that you are the dental hygienist in this scenario. Answer each of the questions for consideration at the end of the scenario.

Discovery Activity

Ask a dental hygienist who has been practicing for a year or more to read the scenario. Provide them with a copy of the Code of Ethics as well. Share the responses you have made to answer each question and ask that person to discuss the situation with you. What insights did you have or what did you learn during this discussion?

MeSH TERMS

Use a combination of MeSH terms and other key words to develop an effective and efficient PubMed literature search strategy.

Bursitis
Carpal tunnel syndrome
Cumulative trauma
   disorders
Head-down tilt

Orthostatic hypotension
Supine position
Tendinopathy
Thoracic outlet syndrome

Emergency Care

 KNOWLEDGE EXERCISES

Write your answers for each question in the space provided.

1. Identify the patient assessment components that will help you know enough about your patient to help prevent an emergency during dental hygiene treatment.

2. Identify five patient-related factors that contribute to increased risk for medical emergency in a dental setting. (*Hint*: These are identified in several places throughout Chapter 9 in the **textbook**; some are psychosocial and some are specific to patient health status.)

3. Identify at least two dental treatment–related factors that contribute to greater risk for emergencies.

4. Recognizing the signs of patient stress is one important way to prevent medical emergencies. Identify ways by which you can reduce your patient's stress during dental hygiene treatment.

5. Where in the patient's dental record is medical information indicating that the patient is predisposed to medical emergencies listed?

_____

_____

6. What additional information should you document in the patient record about your patient's risk for medical emergency?

_____

_____

_____

_____

7. What information must be clearly posted by the telephone in a dental clinic?

_____

_____

8. What does EMS stand for?

_____

_____

9. When a medical emergency happens in the dental setting, it is essential to document all pertinent information as well as everything that happens during the event and as well as in the patient's record after the event. Why?

_____

_____

_____

_____

_____

10. In a medical emergency, your patient is "compensating" if the vital signs are:

_____

_____

11. In your own words, describe what happens if your patient goes into shock.

_____

_____

12. When a patient is in shock, he or she is often placed in the Trendelenburg position. What does this mean?

_____

_____

13. If an emergency situation occurs, you will first quickly _____ the situation and then _____ promptly but not hastily to provide basic life support as indicated.

14. Define *dyspnea.*

_____

_____

15. Describe the actions of a patient with a "mild" airway obstruction.

_____

_____

16. What are the signs of a "severe" airway obstruction?

_____

_____

17. If your patient is in distress and coughing but he or she appears to have good air exchange, what should you do?

_____

_____

18. Describe the difference between hypoxia and hypoxemia?

_____

_____

_____

19. Direct delivery of oxygen is useful in most emergencies, but it is contraindicated in which two situations?

_____

_____

_____

20. If your patient is not breathing, _____ oxygen delivery is indicated, and a bag mask or _____ is used to deliver _____ percent oxygen.

21. If a regular face mask oxygen delivery system is used, _____ L per minute and _____ percent oxygen is delivered to the patient.

22. If the patient is breathing and needs only low levels of oxygen, the use of a _____ device is indicated. Supplemental oxygen is started at _____ L per minute.

23. If a bag mask device is used, the bag is compressed at _____ second intervals for an adult and _____ second intervals for a child.

24. What will you do if your patient's chest does not rise and fall after applying an oxygen delivery system?

_____

_____

25. Place the steps for turning on an oxygen tank and using an oxygen delivery system in the correct order by placing numbers 1–4 in the space beside each step.

Order	Description of Step
_____	Attach delivery system to the patient
_____	Attach the delivery system to the tank
_____	Read and adjust the flow (turning knob in direction the arrow indicates)
_____	Turn the key counterclockwise

COMPETENCY EXERCISES

Apply information from the chapter and use critical thinking skills to complete the competency exercises. Write responses on paper or create electronic documents to submit your answers.

1. The only real way to become competent in responding to emergencies in the dental setting is to practice, practice, practice, and then practice some more. This exercise should be ongoing and include everyone in your dental clinic.

First, all students, faculty, and support personnel should study Tables 9-3 and 9-4 in the **textbook** and be able to list the procedure to follow in each emergency. Next, refer to Figure 9-3 in the **textbook** and write the list of duties assigned to each emergency team member on three small cards. (Or use your school's already established emergency protocols and procedures instead.) Finally, write the signs and symptoms of each emergency health situation listed in Tables 9-3 and 9-4 on a 3 × 5 inch card. If you'd like, write the list of procedures to follow for each emergency on the back of each signs and symptoms card so that you will have a handy reference for evaluating everyone's response to that situation.

When everything is ready, randomly give three people one of the three emergency team member cards and one person one of the emergency situation cards. The person who receives the emergency situation card is the patient and acts out the signs and symptoms listed. The emergency team must respond appropriately to the situation.

It is a great idea to practice this in your clinic setting, if possible. Try to initiate a round of this game when it is not expected, to add to the reality of the situation. When you and your colleagues become proficient at responding, try doing this role-play when patients are in the clinic receiving treatment. If you do this, talk quietly to each patient and make sure he or she knows what is going on; you will find that the patients are delighted to see you are practicing your emergency response. Some of them might even be willing to participate by pretending to be the patient who is experiencing the emergency!

DISCOVERY EXERCISE

1. Locate the emergency cart or kit in your school clinic. Use the emergency equipment list in Table 9-1 in the **textbook** to identify what items are included in the kit.

2. Does your school have a written plan for medical emergencies in the dental clinic? Is the procedure outlined similar to or different from the example in Figure 9-3 in the **textbook**? In what ways is your school's emergency report form similar to or different from Figure 9-2 in the **textbook**?

3. Determine how emergency medical services are activated in your school and/or in your community.

Factors to Teach the Patient

This scenario is related to the following factors listed in this chapter of the **textbook**:

▷ Stress minimization to prevent emergencies.

It is clear that Mr. Montgomery is an extremely anxious dental patient. He is scheduled with you today for presentation of the dental hygiene care plan you have developed. His health history indicates that he has type-2 diabetes, hypertension, and angina. He has a past history of alcohol abuse, and he still uses tobacco.

Mr. Montgomery is extremely overweight and has trouble catching his breath after walking from the reception area to your treatment room. His periodontal status is poor, and he will require multiple appointments for scaling and root planing. In your dental hygiene care plan, there are several dental hygiene diagnosis statements that address his risk for medical emergencies during treatment.

To minimize the risk of a medical emergency, you plan to educate Mr. Montgomery carefully about how his treatment will proceed. Use a motivational interviewing approach as a guide to develop a conversation to use when you are talking to Mr. Montgomery about ways to reduce his stress during his dental hygiene treatment.

EVERYDAY ETHICS

Before completing the learning exercises below, reread and reflect on the Everyday Ethics Scenario and Questions for Consideration in this chapter of the **textbook**. It may also be useful to review the Dental Hygiene Ethics discussion in Chapter 1, the Ethical Applications in the introduction pages for each section in the **textbook**, as well as the Codes of Ethics in **textbook** Appendices I–IV.

Individual Learning Activities

Imagine that you are the dental hygienist in this scenario. Answer each of the questions for consideration at the end of the scenario.

Identify a situation you have experienced that presents a similar ethical dilemma. Write about you would do differently now than you did at the time the incident happened—support your discussion with concepts from the dental hygiene codes of ethics.

MeSH TERMS

Use a combination of MeSH terms and other key words to develop an effective and efficient PubMed literature search strategy.

Advanced cardiac life support
Cardiopulmonary resuscitation
Defibrillators
Airway management
Heimlich maneuver
Emergency medical service communication systems

Preparation for Dental Hygiene Practice

Chapters 5–9

 COMPETENCY EXERCISES

Apply information from the chapter and use critical thinking skills to complete the competency exercises. Write responses on paper or create electronic documents to submit your answers.

1. Prior to seating the patient, you are handed the information in the Assessment Summary, received during a preappointment telephone call. This is a first-ever dental appointment for young Jean Luc Aristide who has recently arrived in this country from Haiti to live with a foster family while he receives treatment for his disease. He speaks very little English, but his bright smile and curious gaze capture your attention and make you smile back at him. Marge Black, a social worker who is arranging access to healthcare services, accompanies him to the dental appointment. What questions will you need to ask his guardian in order to determine Jean Luc's health status before providing dental hygiene care?

2. What steps will you take to protect both Jean Luc and yourself while you collecting the rest of your assessment data and providing oral hygiene instructions during this first appointment?

3. Identify any potential for emergency situations that could happen during Jean Luc's dental visit. What would be your response to any situation you have identified?

4. Examine the personal protective barrier equipment (protective eyewear, masks, gloves, etc.) you have selected for your own use in clinic and describe how they meet the characteristics of acceptable exposure-control barriers.

5. Locate the eyewash station in your clinic that is nearest to your treatment area. Practice using the eyewash.

6. Plan and initiate an Emergency Situation Practice Session such as that outlined in Competency Exercise #1 in Chapter 9 of this **workbook**.

 DISCOVERY EXERCISES

1. Search online or in the library to discover the purpose and function of each of the following federal, state, and local government organizations and discuss how they relate to the practice of dental hygiene.
   - CDC
   - EPA
   - FDA
   - OSAP
   - OSHA
   - Department of Community Health

2. The CDC Guidelines for Infection Control in Dental Healthcare Settings that you will find in Appendix V in the **textbook** contains only the outlined recommendations, not the full text of the report. You can access the complete report in your library by looking for the Centers for Disease Control and Prevention's *Guidelines for Infection Control in Dental Health Settings—2003 (MMWR 2003;52, no. RR-17)* or online at http://www.cdc.gov/mmwr/preview/mmwrhtml/rr5217a1.htm. Scroll down to explore the full report to find and read the section titled "Contact Dermatitis and Latex Hypersensitivity." Write a brief summary of what you learned. When you have time, explore the information in other sections of the report.

3. Investigate the sterilization methods and procedures used at your school clinic.

4. Investigate to determine your school clinic's protocol for procedures to follow if you experience a percutaneous or permucosal exposure to blood or other bodily fluids in the clinic.

5. Imagine that you have been asked to select a new handwashing soap that will be used in your clinic. Search for scientific evidence of effectiveness of antibacterial agents commonly used in handwashing soaps that are available for use by dental hygienists. Select the best alternative, and explain why you made your selection. (*Hint:* Check the soap currently in use in your clinic as well as some dental supplier catalogs to find the most commonly used antibacterial agents, and then develop a PICO question to help you review the scientific literature for research evidence of effectiveness.)

6. Investigate dental supply catalogs to determine the types of gloves available for use in dental clinics and the cost of each type. What scientific evidence is available to help you determine which type of glove provides the most effective barrier to microorganisms you are likely to encounter during patient care?

 FOR YOUR PORTFOLIO

1. Develop a personal, written exposure-control plan. Don't forget to include an appropriate reference list to indicate that you have based your personal plan on scientific evidence. Consider making the plan in a format that could be easily updated and adapted to any setting later on when you are a practicing dental hygienist.

2. List your personal selections/recommendations for handwashing soap, gloves, and any other infection-control supplies used in dental hygiene care. Support each recommendation with a brief written summary of product characteristics and how the product meets criteria for acceptability.

3. Develop a personal, written long-term plan to avoid cumulative trauma injuries related to dental hygiene practice. Update this plan yearly as you learn more about working conditions that compromise your comfort and effectiveness when you are providing dental hygiene care.

4. Compile a personal immunization log. Identify any missing immunizations and make arrangements to receive them.

SECTION II—PATIENT ASSESSMENT SUMMARY

Patient Name: *Jean Luc Aristide*	Age: *11*	Gender: F	☑ Initial Therapy
			☐ Maintenance
Provider Name: *D.H. Student*	Date: *Today*		☐ Re-evaluation

Chief Complaint:

According to a preappointment telephone conversation with a social worker, there are no immediate dental problems. The social worker is trying to help the foster family provide the child with dental care.

Assessment Findings

Health History

- HIV positive status

Social and Dental History

- Pt is newly emigrated to the United States and has never been to the dentist

At Risk For:

- Risk status is unclear without further medical information

At Risk For:

SECTION II SUMMARY CROSSWORD PUZZLE

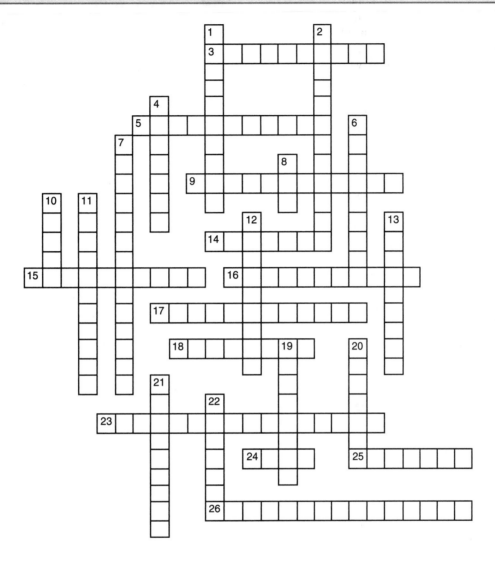

Puzzle Clues

Across

3. Refers to the people, equipment, and other materials identified as a link in the chain of disease transmission.

5. A state that can occur if a patient is suddenly brought upright after being in a supine position for a long period of time.

9. Involuntary muscular contraction; in the heart muscle can be a cause of cardiac arrest.

14. Temporary loss of consciousness caused by sudden fall in blood pressure.

15. Agent that can be used to reduce surface pathogens on mucosa or skin.

16. Repetitive movements, use of a forceful grasp, and vibration are commonly recognized ergonomic _____ (two words).

17. Refers to exposure to disease that may result from the performance of one's usual duties.

18. A virus, microorganism, or other substance that causes disease or infection.

23. Eye, mouth, mucous membrane, nonintact skin, or parenteral contact with blood or other potentially infectious material (two words).

24. Useful for protecting face and respiratory system from aerosols when providing dental hygiene treatment.

25. Particles suspended in air.

26. Carpal tunnel syndrome is a _____ disorder that commonly affects dental hygienists.

Down

1. Abnormal heartbeat rhythm.

2. Refers to the period of time when an infectious agent can be transferred from an infected person to another person.

4. Diminished oxygen in body tissues.

6. To apply substances that destroy most (but not all) infective organisms onto an inanimate object.

7. Position in which the patient is supine on an inclined surface with heart higher than the head.

8. Emergency cardiac care that supports ventilation and maintains blood flow (acronym).

10. Wiping, scrubbing, or other process that reduces bioburden, but does not completely eliminate contamination on clinical instruments or surfaces.

11. Process of introducing a substance into the body to produce immunity to a specific disease.

12. A chemical _____ is used to change the color of a marker on autoclave tape to indicate that the package has been brought to a specific temperature.

13. Kill all forms of life, as with an autoclave.

19. A preventive, functional-movement strategy that, performed daily, can help reduce the dental hygienist's risk for musculoskeletal injury and prevent pain.

20. Labored or difficult breathing.

21. A substance contaminated with biomaterial that has the potential to transmit infection.

22. A type of dental hygiene practice that includes attention to equipment, work layout, and work processes that decrease strain and fatigue and protect the functional health and well-being of both the clinician and the patient.

Documentation

SECTION III LEARNING OBJECTIVES

Completing the exercises in this section of the workbook will prepare you to:

1. Document all aspects of dental hygiene care.

COMPETENCIES FOR THE DENTAL HYGIENIST (APPENDIX A)

Competencies supported by the learning in Section III

    Core Competencies: C2, C5, C11

    Patient/Client Care: PC1, PC13

Documentation for Dental Hygiene Care

KNOWLEDGE EXERCISES

Write your answers for each question in the space provided.

1. Why do dental professionals document patient care activities and maintain a permanent, comprehensive patient record?

_____

_____

_____

_____

_____

2. What actions regarding a patient record are essential to ensure accurate documentation of patient care in case the record is needed during a legal action?

_____

_____

_____

_____

_____

_____

3. List five types of documentation discussed in this chapter that comprise a permanent, comprehensive patient record.

_____

_____

_____

_____

_____

4. List types of information that are never included in a patient record.

_____

_____

_____

_____

5. Identify the important components of the patient record.

_____

_____

_____

_____

_____

_____

6. Handwritten records are recorded legibly and written in _____.

7. What does the acronym HIPAA stand for?

_____

_____

_____

8. What are the components of the current HIPAA law?

_____

_____

_____

_____

9. List patient rights that are protected by HIPAA.

_____

_____

_____

_____

_____

_____

_____

_____

_____

10. List HIPAA-designated responsibilities of healthcare providers, employers, and facilities.

_____

_____

_____

_____

_____

_____

_____

_____

11. Identify the purposes for maintaining complete and accurate periodontal and dental records for each patient.

_____

_____

_____

_____

12. Identify the types of chart forms that can be used to record your patient's dental charting.

_____

_____

_____

_____

13. Define _systematic procedure_ as it relates to dental charting.

_____

_____

_____

14. In your own words, briefly describe the following clinical observations included in your patient's periodontal charting.

- _Gingival changes_

_____

_____

- _Items charted_

_____

_____

_____

- *Deposits*

_____

_____

_____

_____

- *Factors related to occlusion*

_____

_____

_____

- *Radiographic findings*

_____

_____

_____

_____

_____

_____

15. What items are documented in a dental charting record?

_____

_____

_____

_____

_____

_____

_____

16. What factors are included in a patient progress note?

_____

_____

_____

_____

_____

17. Briefly describe each of the components in the SOAP note method for documenting patient visits.

_____

_____

_____

_____

18. Because different tooth numbering systems are used in dental offices and clinics, it is necessary for you to be familiar with all of them. Refer to Figures 10-1 to 10-3 in the **textbook** to provide guidance as you complete Infomap 10-1. Completing this exercise will help you compare the three types of tooth numbering systems.

INFOMAP 10-1					
TOOTH NUMBERING SYSTEM	ORGANIZATION (ARCHES OR QUADRANTS)	PERMANENT DENTITION	PRIMARY DENTITION	ADDITIONAL FEATURES	EXAMPLE: MAXILLARY RIGHT CENTRAL INCISOR
Palmer Notation System					
International tooth numbering (FDI)					
Universal Coding System (American Dental Association)					

COMPETENCY EXERCISES

Apply information from the chapter and use critical thinking skills to complete the competency exercises. Write responses on paper or create electronic documents to submit your answers.

1. Caroline Lacy arrives for your 10:00 am appointment. She is 3 years old. Identify the correct tooth number for the two teeth listed below using each of the tooth numbering systems.

	Mandibular Left Primary First Molar	Molar Maxillary Left Primary First Molar
Palmer system tooth numbering		
Fédération Dentaire Internationale (FDI)		
Universal tooth numbering		

2. The dental practice where you work has decided to change from a charting system that uses anatomic drawings of the complete teeth to one that contains only geometric diagrams. The plan is to chart both restorative and periodontal findings on the new form. You are asked for your opinion at the staff meeting. What is your response? Make sure to state your opinion of the benefits and limitations of each type of form.

MeSH TERMS

Use a combination of MeSH terms and other key words to develop an effective and efficient PubMed literature search strategy.

Dental records	Confidentiality
Health records, personal	Informed consent
Electronic health records	Patient access to records

EVERYDAY ETHICS

Before completing the learning exercises below, reread and reflect on the Everyday Ethics Scenario and Questions for Consideration in this chapter of the **textbook**. It may also be useful to review the Dental Hygiene Ethics discussion in Chapter 1, the Ethical Applications in the introduction pages for each section in the **textbook**, as well as the Codes of Ethics in **textbook** Appendices I–IV.

Discovery Activities

Ask a dental hygienist who has been practicing for a year or more to read the scenario. Provide a copy of the Code of Ethics as well. Share the responses you have made to answer each question and ask that person to discuss the situation with you. What insights did you have or what did you learn during this discussion?

Ask a friend or relative who is not involved in health care to read the scenario and discuss it with you from the perspective of a "patient" who receives services within the healthcare system. Discuss what you learned from the concerns, insights, or difference in perspective that person expressed.

Factors to Teach the Patient

This scenario is related to the following factors listed in this chapter of the **textbook**:
▷ Interpretation of all recordings; meaning of all numbers used, such as for probing depths.

You have just completed the periodontal and dental charting during a patient's initial appointment. The patient asks you to explain all those numbers and letters you were calling out to the dental assistant who was writing everything down for you.

List the main points you would want to cover in a conversation that explains the all of the kinds of numbers and letters that are used to document periodontal and dental conditions.

Documentation

Chapter 10

 COMPETENCY EXERCISE

1. Examine the past progress notes from a patient chart in your school clinic. Analyze each to determine whether the SOAP components have been included in each entry. Infomap 10-1 and Box 10-2 in the **textbook** chapter should provide some guidance for this exercise. What, if any, information missing from any of the progress notes you sample?

 DISCOVERY EXERCISE

1. Examine the HIPAA (or the Canadian PIPEDA) documents provided for each patient in your school clinic. Interview several patients who have just received the documents to determine their level of understanding about their rights related to their medical records. What questions did patient have related to their right to confidentiality and privacy of their patient records? What questions did they have about their right to access their own information? What questions did they have related to security of their health information? Explain how this exercise might change your approach to presenting these documents to patients in the future.

SECTION III SUMMARY WORD SEARCH PUZZLE

Do you know the ADA abbreviations for the following terms used to document patient information? Appendix VIII in the **textbook** may help you find the answers in the puzzle.

```
X   Z   P   X   X   T   K   F   D   D   H   R   P   T   U   O   L
B   M   K   O   C   C   L   J   O   T   C   I   F   U   R   C   S
V   A   S   O   Q   L   C   S   U   T   W   V   H   P   Q   P   C
E   N   S   B   M   A   N   D   R   I   L   R   Q   Y   H   F   J
X   V   B   O   V   Q   Z   Q   V   Y   F   U   F   K   Y   C   D
Y   M   B   P   M   Y   I   E   G   L   N   B   W   H   P   C   O
L   M   O   N   K   A   M   T   I   B   W   U   J   K   S   B   K
O   M   U   C   H   K   R   S   N   V   V   T   S   T   J   T   X
R   A   X   L   A   L   I   Q   U   A   D   Q   A   I   C   B   W
I   X   E   V   T   V   V   A   R   R   Q   X   T   D   V   N   N
Q   B   D   Q   X   R   E   A   P   P   T   U   A   O   W   L   L
H   Y   G   V   D   S   L   F   C   C   L   B   P   K   S   B   P
W   Q   V   H   S   K   S   L   T   A   R   R   F   Q   A   B   R
S   W   S   U   D   F   Q   F   I   L   F   B   H   T   I   W   P
R   H   U   X   T   O   H   I   G   T   K   D   E   N   N   X   A
P   E   B   U   Q   E   S   U   P   R   A   S   K   E   T   H   X
M   H   H   H   Q   E   S   U   P   R   A   S   K   E   Q   I   K
```

Puzzle Clues

1. Clinical attachment level
2. Bleeding on probing
3. Bite wing radiograph
4. Check or observe
5. Dental history
6. Evaluate
7. Examination
8. Acidulated phosphate fluoride
9. Furcation
10. Gingival
11. Health history
12. Hypertension
13. Dental hygiene
14. Lidocaine
15. Xylocaine
16. Vasoconstrictor
17. Mandibular
18. Maxillary
19. No known allergies
20. Next visit
21. Occlusal or occlusion
22. Oral hygiene instruction
23. Over the counter
24. Prognosis
25. Patient
26. Quadrant
27. Lower right quadrant
28. Re-appoint
29. Scaling and root planing
30. Prescription
31. Immediately
32. Subgingival
33. Supragingival
34. Toothbrush
35. Treatment
36. Varnish
37. Within normal limits
38. Systolic blood pressure

Assessment

Chapters 11–21

SECTION IV LEARNING OBJECTIVES

Completing the exercises in this section of the workbook will **prepare you to:**

1. Identify the components of a complete patient assessment.

2. Apply a variety of assessment methods to gather data and document the patient's health status.

3. Determine the individual and community oral health status using a variety of dental indices.

4. Document assessment findings.

COMPETENCIES FOR THE DENTAL HYGIENIST (APPENDIX A)

Competencies supported by the learning in Section IV

    Core Competencies: C5, C10, C12, C13

    Health Promotion and Disease Prevention: HP2, HP3, HP4, HP5, HP6

    Community Involvement: CM1, CM2, CM6

    Patient/Client Care: PC1, PC2, PC3, PC4

11

Medical, Dental, and Psychosocial Histories

LEARNING OBJECTIVES

Upon successful completion of these exercises, you will be able to:

1. Identify and define the key terms and concepts related to preparing patient histories.

2. Discuss the purposes of the personal, medical, and dental histories.

3. List and discuss the types, systems, forms used, question types, and styles used to collect patient-history data.

4. Recognize considerations for patient care that are identified by various items recorded on the patient history.

 KNOWLEDGE EXERCISES

Write your answers for each question in the space provided.

1. In your own words, explain why taking a complete and accurate patient history is necessary prior to providing dental hygiene care.

   _____

   _____

   _____

2. In your own words, list the purposes of taking personal, medical, and dental histories during patient assessment.

   _____

   _____

   _____

   _____

   _____

   _____

   _____

   _____

3. List and briefly describe each of the systems for obtaining the patient's history.

   _____

   _____

   _____

   _____

   _____

   _____

   _____

4. List the characteristics of an adequate patient-history form.

   _____

   _____

   _____

   _____

   _____

5. What factors can affect the accuracy of a patient history?

_____

_____

_____

_____

_____

6. List factors that can contribute to success in gaining patient cooperation during the history interview.

_____

_____

_____

_____

_____

7. Describe each type of patient-history questionnaires in your own words.
   • *System-oriented*

   _____

   _____

   • *Disease-oriented*

   _____

   _____

   • *Symptom-oriented*

   _____

   _____

   • *Culture-oriented*

   _____

   _____

8. Identify the advantages associated with each method of collecting patient data. Each answer may be used more than one time.

Methods of Data Collection	Advantage
A. Questionnaire	_____ Legal written record with patient's signature
B. Interview	_____ Consistent
	_____ Development of rapport
	_____ Time-saving
	_____ Flexibility for individual needs

9. Why is it important to record contact information for the patient's physician in the personal history?

_____

_____

_____

10. List three types of medical consultation related to the development of the patient history.

_____

_____

11. Which medical conditions require that a patient receive antibiotic premedication prior to some dental and dental hygiene procedures?

_____

_____

_____

12. Dental hygiene procedures that require antibiotic premedication for a patient at risk for endocarditis include those involving _____ of gingival tissue or _____ of oral mucosa.

13. State the standard antibiotic premedication regimen prescribed for at-risk adult patients prior to dental procedures.

_____

_____

_____

COMPETENCY EXERCISES

Apply information from the chapter and use critical thinking skills to complete the competency exercises. Write responses on paper or create electronic documents to submit your answers.

Review the patient-history questionnaire forms used in your practice setting (either your dental hygiene program clinic or the dental practice where you receive care). Use the information in the "Considerations for Appointment Procedures" column of Tables 11-1 to 11-3 to identify the reason for including each of the items included on the form.

Compare the patient-history form used in your practice or school clinic with the medical, dental, and psychosocial forms included in the **textbook** chapter. What are the similarities and differences between the forms?

Using the format required in your dental hygiene program clinic, document an imaginary patient appointment during which personal, dental, and medical histories are obtained.

DISCOVERY EXERCISE

Search online to find patient health history questionnaires in languages other than English.

EVERYDAY ETHICS

Before completing the learning exercises below, reread and reflect on the Everyday Ethics Scenario and Questions for Consideration in this chapter of the **textbook**. It may also be useful to review the Dental Hygiene Ethics discussion in Chapter 1, the Ethical Applications in the introduction pages for each section in the **textbook**, as well as the Codes of Ethics in **textbook** Appendices I–IV.

Individual Learning Activity

Imagine that you are the dental hygienist in this scenario. Answer each of the questions for consideration at the end of the scenario.

Discovery Activity

Ask a dental hygienist who has been practicing for a year or more to read the scenario. Provide a copy of the Code of Ethics as well. Share the responses you have made to answer each question and ask that person to discuss the situation with you. What insights did you have or what did you learn during this discussion?

Factors to Teach the Patient

This scenario is related to the following factors listed in this chapter of the **textbook**:

▷ The need for obtaining the personal, medical, and dental history before performing dental and dental hygiene procedures and the need for keeping the histories up-to-date.

▷ The assurance that recorded histories are kept in strict professional confidence.

▷ The relationship between oral health and general physical health.

▷ The interrelationship of medical and dental care.

You are just starting to treat Jon Wojeckick, who is 37 years old. You begin to ask questions about his medical history. You notice that he has stopped making eye contact and is hesitating over some of

the answers. You have a feeling that he is not giving you accurate information, and you want to be sure you are obtaining all the data you need to provide optimum safe care. You know from studying Tables 11-1 to 11-3 in the **textbook** that items from the patient history have a connection to how you provide dental hygiene care for your patient.

Use the Motivational Interviewing approach (see **workbook** Appendix D) as a guide to write a statement explaining the relationship between oral health and physical health. Explain the need for accurate information to facilitate treatment planning. Include at least three examples of appointment considerations that are linked to items in the patient history. Be sure to assure Mr. Wojeckick that recorded histories are kept in strict professional confidence.

MeSH TERMS

Use a combination of MeSH terms and other key words to develop an effective and efficient PubMed literature search strategy.

Dental records	Electronic medical records
History-taking	Medical history-taking
Health records, personal	Antibiotic prophylaxis

Vital Signs

LEARNING OBJECTIVES

Upon successful completion of these exercises, you will be able to:

1. Identify and define the key terms and concepts related to recording vital signs.

2. Identify four vital signs and describe the range of expected values.

3. Describe the procedures for determining and recording a patient's temperature, pulse, respiration, and blood pressure.

4. Discuss the importance of regular determination of vital signs for a patient receiving dental hygiene care.

 KNOWLEDGE EXERCISES

Write your answers for each question in the space provided.

1. Describe how you will position your patient to explain and record vital signs.

_____

_____

_____

_____

2. If your patient's vital signs are not within the normal range, what should you do?

_____

_____

3. What are the normal adult ranges for each of the vital signs?

_____

_____

_____

_____

4. What factors should you consider when you decide to take your patient's temperature?

_____

_____

_____

5. The normal average temperature varies among individuals, but in general, the average temperature of an adult over 70 years is slightly _____ than the adult average, and the temperature of a child under 5 years may be slightly_____.

6. List the factors that can increase the body temperature.

_____

_____

_____

_____

7. The most common location for taking a temperature is the mouth. What contraindications would lead you to select another method?

_____

_____

8. What emergency situations may cause your patient to exhibit an increased pulse rate? (*Hint*: See Table 9-3 in the Emergency Care chapter of the **textbook**.)

_____

_____

_____

_____

_____

_____

_____

9. In your own words, describe how to obtain and record your patient's pulse.

_____

_____

_____

_____

10. Define a respiration.

_____

11. Describe the factors to observe while you are counting your patient's respiration rate.

_____

_____

_____

_____

12. The count of respirations is taken immediately after counting the pulse. The fingers used to count the pulse remain positioned. Why is this procedure followed?

_____

_____

_____

_____

_____

_____

13. What emergency situations can cause a change in your patient's respiration?

_____

_____

_____

_____

_____

_____

_____

14. What physical factors determine the maintenance of blood pressure?

_____

_____

_____

15. Emergencies such as fainting, blood loss, and shock will cause blood pressure to _____.

16. What action should you take if your patient's blood pressure is at a prehypertension level or above?

_____

_____

17. How frequently should your patient's blood pressure be taken and recorded?

_____

_____

_____

COMPETENCY EXERCISES

Apply information from the chapter and use critical thinking skills to complete the competency exercises. Write responses on paper or create electronic documents to submit your answers.

1. You have just seated Maura Kennedy in the dental chair for her dental hygiene maintenance appointment. You read in her patient record that she is 33 years old, has no remarkable health problems, and is taking no medications. She reports that the only change in her health history is that she has had a sinus infection for the last 2 weeks. She reports that she started taking antibiotics the day before yesterday and is feeling a bit better, but her nasal passages are still all stuffed up. Write a brief statement that you will use to inform Maura that you are going to determine and record her vital signs.

2. When you take Maura's temperature, you find that it is normal. Her pulse rate is 70 beats per minute; while you still have your fingers on her wrist, you count her respirations. Her respiration is slightly fast, 20 per minute, and you note that she takes several shallow breaths, followed by one or two gulps of air and that she wheezes a bit when she exhales. However, you note that her color is good, so she must not be having any real problem with air exchange, and her breathing problems may just be the result of her stuffy nose. You wrap the blood pressure cuff around her right arm, pump it up, and place the stethoscope. You hear the sounds begin at the 122 mark on the manometer, and

the last sound you hear is at 83. After a discussion with Maura and with Dr. Ichero, you all decide to reschedule Maura for her maintenance visit in a couple of weeks when her sinus infection is gone.

Using your institution's guidelines for writing in patient records, document that you assessed Maura's vital signs at this appointment and rescheduled her appointment for a future date.

3. Create a brief step-by-step guide for determining and recording all of the vital signs on a 3 × 5-inch card (this is sometimes called a "job aid"). If you can laminate your job aid, you will be able to disinfect it to use during patient care. Practice using your step-by-step guide to determine and record vital signs for family members, friends, or student colleagues. If you practice with a dental hygiene instructor as your patient, you can receive valuable feedback on your techniques!

🖥 MeSH TERMS

Use a combination of MeSH terms and other key words to develop an effective and efficient PubMed literature search strategy.

Vital signs	Respiration
Blood pressure	Blood pressure
Body temperature	determination
Heart rate	Sphygmomanometer
Respiratory rate	Stethoscopes
Pulse	Auscultation

EVERYDAY ETHICS

Before completing the learning exercises below, reread and reflect on the Everyday Ethics Scenario and Questions for Consideration in this chapter of the **textbook**. It may also be useful to review the Dental Hygiene Ethics discussion in Chapter 1, the Ethical Applications in the introduction pages for each section in the **textbook**, as well as the Codes of Ethics in **textbook** Appendices I–IV.

Individual Learning Activity

Identify a situation you have experienced that presents a similar ethical dilemma. What did you

learn from how the situation was (or was not) resolved at the time it happened?

Collaborative Learning Activity

Answer each of the questions for consideration at the end of the scenario in the **textbook**. Compare what you wrote with answers developed by another classmate and discuss differences/similarities.

Factors to Teach the Patient

This scenario is related to the following factors listed in this chapter of the **textbook**:

▷ How vital signs can influence dental and dental hygiene appointments.

▷ The importance of having a blood pressure determination at regular intervals.

Mr. Borman Gorbachov, the CEO of a large manufacturing firm, is always in a hurry. He simply cannot seem to sit still for his whole appointment and is always chiding you that you should work faster so that he can be done and get back to work. Today he sighs heavily and then protests loudly when you tell him that you are going to take and record his vital signs. He states that he just had his blood pressure taken a month or so ago at his doctor's office and there is nothing wrong with him. You look in his patient record to discover that the previous blood pressure, taken almost 2 years ago, was normal.

Use a motivational interviewing approach as a guide to prepare a conversation you can use to educate Mr. Gorbachov about the reasons you determine a patient's vital signs at each appointment. Use the conversation you create to educate a patient or friend, and then modify it based on what you learned from the interaction.

CHAPTER 12 WORD SEARCH PUZZLE

```
V H U O Q S E O P E N Y N Z K R H
A C A R O T I D W S O O S Q S T C
B J U Y B A V J S Z R Q P I Y Y I
D Y S E A F P G O U M F H E S M H
T G C H P P D N T M O V Y B T P Y
Y Y U Y H U N K B W T T G R O A P
E Q L P B Z L E U A E A M A L N O
A A T E B I D S A R N C O C E I T
H A A R R B I X E H S H M H K C H
A P T T A K A V C Y I Y A I K C E
N Y I E D R S I K T V C N A S J R
O R O N Y F T T O H E A O L W B M
X E N S C E O A R M Q R M J R Y I
I X V I A D L L O M K D E A S Q A
A I O O R D E S T E P I T C S D G
Z A K N D X Y I K R C A E R T U K
T R A D I A L G O C N G R K I C C
S G L Z A M K N F U I Y C U F F Y
E F I D T J N S F R X T R E B P O
S I Z G E M Q B F Y L B J S T Z E
```

Puzzle Clues

1. Specific measurements of a patient's essential bodily functions (two words).
2. Artery in the neck that is the site for taking a pulse during cardiopulmonary resuscitation.
3. Device for determining blood pressure.
4. A contraction of the heart ventricles during which blood is forced into the aorta and the pulmonary artery.
5. Element used in a device that records blood pressure.
6. Fever; temperature values greater than 37.5°C or 99.5°F.
7. Heartbeat at a rate greater than 100 beats per minute.
8. Inflatable component of a sphygmomanometer that wraps around the patient's arm during recording of a blood pressure.
9. Listening for sounds produced within the body.
10. The lower number in a recorded blood pressure fraction; marks the pressure at the last distinct tap heard on the sphygmomanometer.
11. Lower-than-normal body temperature; values below 35.5°C or 96.0°F.
12. Normal tension or tone; pertaining to having normal blood pressure.
13. Noted along with volume and strength when counting the pulse rate.
14. Oxygen deficiency.
15. A count of heartbeats; can also refer to the pressure that is the difference between systolic and diastolic blood pressure.
16. Pulse taken using fingertips placed at the wrist.
17. The site used to find the pulse for an infant.
18. Sounds originating within the blood passing through the vessel or produced by vibratory motion of the arterial wall.
19. A systolic blood pressure of 130 mmHg or greater and diastolic blood pressure of 80 mmHg or greater.
20. Temporary cessation of spontaneous respirations.
21. A type of thermometer that is gently inserted into the ear canal.
22. Unusually slow heartbeat and pulse; below 50 beats per minute.

13

Extraoral and Intraoral Examination

 KNOWLEDGE EXERCISES

Write your answers for each question in the space provided.

1. In your own words, explain the purpose of performing an intraoral and extraoral examination for each patient.

_____

_____

2. Before you get ready to perform an examination for your patient, you first need to:

• *Review:*

_____

_____

• *Examine:*

_____

_____

_____

• *Explain:*

_____

_____

3. In your own words, explain the advantages of using a systematic sequence for the patient examination.

_____

_____

_____

4. List and briefly describe the types of intraoral/extraoral examinations.

_____

_____

_____

_____

_____

5. Identify the anatomical landmarks shown in Figures 13-1, 13-2, and 13-3 by writing the appropriate term on each line.

Figure 13-1

Figure 13-2

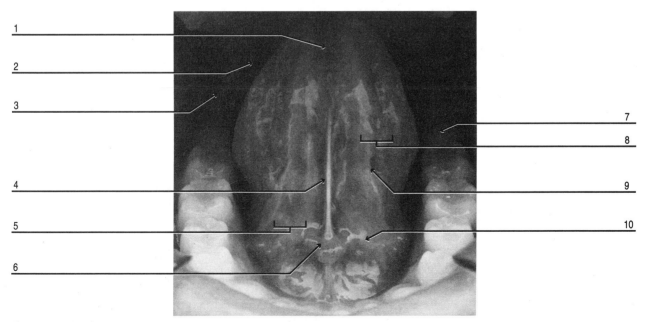

Figure 13-3

6. List the methods used to accomplish the extraoral and intraoral examinations.

_____

_____

_____

_____

_____

_____

7. What is auscultation?

_____

8. Match the types of palpation with the appropriate definition and description. There are two answers for each type of palpation.

Types of Palpation	Definition/Description
Digital: ____ and ____	A. Use of finger or fingers and thumb from each hand applied simultaneously in coordination
Bimanual: ____ and ____	B. Use of a finger C. Two hands used at the same time to examine corresponding structures on opposite sides of the body
Bilateral: ____ and ____	D. Use of finger and thumb of the same hand E. Palpation of the lips
Bidigital: ____ and ____	F. Index finger applied to the inner border of the mandible beneath the canine–premolar area to determine the presence of a torus mandibularis
	G. Index finger of one hand palpates the floor of the mouth inside, while a finger or fingers from the other hand press on the same area from under the chin externally
	H. Fingers placed beneath the chin to palpate the submandibular lymph nodes

9. In your own words, explain where lymph nodes in the cervical chain are located.

_____

_____

_____

_____

10. Describe the difference in the location of the submental and submandibular lymph nodes.

_____

_____

_____

11. In your own words, define the following types of documentation recorded for each oral lesion.

• History:

_____

_____

_____

_____

_____

_____

_____

• Location and extent:

_____

_____

_____

• Physical characteristics:

_____

_____

_____

_____

_____

_____

_____

_____

_____

12. Identify the characteristics you would expect to observe for each of the following types of oral lesions.

• Indurated:

_____

• Blisterform:

_____

- *Pustule:*

  _____

- *Plaque:*

  _____

- *Ulcer:*

  _____

- *Erythema:*

  _____

- *Torus:*

  _____

- *Papillary:*

  _____

13. Early oral cancer takes many forms. Write a brief description of the characteristics you might observe for each of the five basic forms listed below.

- *White areas:*

  _____

  _____

  _____

  _____

  _____

- *Red areas:*

  _____

  _____

  _____

  _____

- *Ulcers:*

  _____

  _____

- *Masses:*

  _____

  _____

  _____

- *Pigmentation:*

  _____

  _____

14. What characteristics indicate that a lesion should be biopsied?

  _____

  _____

  _____

  _____

  _____

  _____

  _____

15. In your own words, explain the rationale for conducting adjunctive cytologic testing.

  _____

  _____

16. List three methods of adjunctive cytologic testing.

  _____

  _____

  _____

17. What is the difference between excisional biopsy and incisional biopsy?

  _____

  _____

  _____

18. Match each pathology report with its descriptor.

Pathology Report Category	Description
___ HSIL	A. Normal; benign
___ IFN	B. Specific type of cancer
___ SCC	C. Mild-to-moderate dysplasia
___ NILM	D. Undetermined
___ LSIL	E. Severe dysplasia

INFOMAP 13-1		
OBSERVATION		**INDICATION AND INFLUENCES ON THE APPOINTMENT**
Overall appraisal of patient	Labored breathing	
Face	Evidence of fear or apprehension	
Skin	Multiple light-brown macules	
Eyes	Eyeglasses (corrective)	
Nodes—submental; submandibular	Lymphadenopathy; induration	
Temporomandibular joint	Tenderness; sensitivity; noises (clicking, popping, grating)	
Lips	Blisters, ulcers	
Breath odor	Cigarette odor	
Labial and buccal mucosa	Multiple red nodules on left buccal mucosa	
Tongue	Coating	
Floor of mouth	Limitation or freedom of movement of tongue	
Saliva	Evidences of dry mouth; lip wetting	
Hard palate	Tori	
Soft palate, uvula	Large uvula	
Tonsillar region, throat	Large tonsils	

19. Using the information in Box 13-2 and Table 13-1 in the **textbook**, imagine that your patient presents with the conditions listed in Infomap 13-1 in the **workbook**. Complete the infomap by identifying the indications and influences on the appointment associated with each observation.

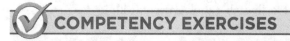 **COMPETENCY EXERCISES**

Apply information from the chapter and use critical thinking skills to complete the competency exercises. Write responses on paper or create electronic documents to submit your answers.

1. In your own words, explain the importance of careful description and documentation of any abnormality discovered during an intraoral and extraoral examination.

2. In your own words, describe the sequence of steps you will follow to provide a systematic and comprehensive extraoral and intraoral examination for your patient.

3. Your patient, Kurt Bachleim, age 23 years, presents with localized, coalescing multiple lesions on the right buccal mucosa. Mr. Bachleim also has an exostosis extending from tooth 12 to tooth 15 and trismus. Describe what you would expect to see and any possible adaptations you will need to make for the appointment.

4. Your patient, Yoon Chang, presents with a tiny (about 1 mm) bluish-black lesion on the top right half of her tongue. She said that it wasn't bothering her at all. You palpate the lesion, but do not feel anything unusual. Ms. Chang reports that the same thing had come up on her palate a few weeks ago. As you continue to

question her, she mentions that she has had a broken blood vessel or two on her fingers in the past. She had actually forgotten about it until you started asking questions. Dr. Pine is not in the office today, so you document the lesion in the patient record in order to discuss it with him tomorrow and decide appropriate follow-up procedures.

Use your institution's guidelines for writing in the patient record and the information in Chapter 12 to describe the lesion on Ms. Chang's tongue.

MeSH TERMS

Use a combination of MeSH terms and other key words to develop an effective and efficient PubMed literature search strategy.

Diagnosis, oral
Anatomic landmarks
Mouth
Palpation

Auscultation
Self-examination
Lymph nodes
Oral ulcer

EVERYDAY ETHICS

Before completing the learning exercises below, reread and reflect on the Everyday Ethics Scenario and Questions for Consideration in this chapter of the **textbook**. It may also be useful to review the Dental Hygiene Ethics discussion in Chapter 1, the Ethical Applications in the introduction pages for each section in the **textbook**, as well as the Codes of Ethics in **textbook** Appendices I–IV.

Collaborative Learning Activity

Note: The Everyday Ethics Scenario in this chapter contains two different ethical components for the dental hygienist: providing information for her patient and approaching her coworkers to change office policies. Work with a group of students to provide alternate approaches for each of the two ethical concerns in the scenario.

Work with a small group to develop a 2- to 5-minute role-play that introduces the Everyday Ethics Scenario described in the chapter (a great idea is to video record your role-play activity). Then develop separate 2-minute role-play scenarios that provide at least two alternative approaches/solutions to resolving the situation. Ask classmates to view the solutions, ask questions, and discuss the ethical approach used in each. Ask for a vote on which solution classmates determine to be the "best."

Factors to Teach the Patient

This scenario is related to the following factors listed in this chapter of the **textbook**:

▷ The reasons for a careful extraoral and intraoral examination at each maintenance appointment.

▷ A method for self-examination. (The examination should include the face, neck, lips, gingiva, cheeks, tongue, palate, and throat. Any changes should be reported to the dentist and the dental hygienist.)

▷ The warning signs of oral cancer.

Aishia Williams presents with an oral lesion that may be malignant. She has previously been treated for a precancerous oral lesion and is at risk for recurrence. She has not been reevaluated for 18 months.

Use the motivational interviewing approach (see **workbook** Appendix D) as a guide to write a statement explaining the need for careful follow-up and frequent evaluation by a dental professional as well as the need for Ms. Williams to perform a regular oral self-examination and to be aware of the warning signs of oral cancer.

Use the conversation you create to role-play this situation with a fellow student. If you are the patient in the role-play, be sure to ask questions. If you are the dental hygienist, try to anticipate questions and answer them in your explanation.

14

Family Violence

LEARNING OBJECTIVES

Upon successful completion of these exercises, you will be able to:

1. Identify and define the key terms and concepts related to family abuse and neglect.

2. Describe the various types of family violence.

3. Recognize and document the physical, behavioral, and intraoral signs of abuse.

4. Describe the dental hygienist's role in recognizing and reporting abuse and neglect.

 KNOWLEDGE EXERCISES

Write your answers for each question in the space provided.

1. Define *forensic dentistry*.

_____

_____

2. Identify three programs that can provide training to help you learn more about how to assess and respond to suspected abuse and neglect during a patient/provider interaction.

_____

_____

_____

The factors involved in the recognition and management of suspected maltreatment of children, the elderly, people with disabilities, and women are similar. When answering the following questions, be sure to take all of these potential at-risk groups into consideration, unless the question specifies a particular group or groups.

3. List the four major types of maltreatment that can occur in families.

_____

_____

_____

_____

4. In your own words, describe Munchausen Syndrome by Proxy (MSBP).

_____

_____

5. In your own words, define *dental neglect*.

_____

_____

_____

6. When a child patient mentions that there is no one at their house to help them brush their teeth, what

additional indicators might lead you to suspect that your patient is neglected?

_____

_____

_____

_____

_____

_____

_____

7. Identify the signs of lice infestation.

_____

_____

_____

8. Identify personal appearance factors that might lead you to suspect that an individual is being physically abused.

_____

_____

_____

_____

_____

9. In your own words, describe the raccoon sign.

_____

10. What is an area of baldness that is caused by pulling out hair by the roots?

_____

11. What is the medical term used to identify a bruise?

_____

12. Describe what you might notice about site of an accidental injury versus the common sites you might notice if the injuries are inflicted or deliberate.

_____

_____

_____

_____

_____

13. List some potential intraoral signs of physical abuse.

_____

_____

_____

_____

_____

_____

14. Identify general signs that may indicate physical abuse in a child patient.

_____

_____

_____

_____

_____

_____

15. In what way do these general signs compare with what you might notice if an adult patient is experiencing family violence?

_____

_____

_____

_____

16. Extremely aggressive behavior by a child when you try to examine his or her mouth can be a behavioral indicator for _____ as well as for physical abuse.

17. Identify intraoral signs of sexual abuse.

_____

_____

_____

_____

18. List nonabuse-related conditions that can mimic the physical signs of abuse.

_____

_____

_____

19. One important role for the dental hygienist in cases of suspected abuse is to document the observable facts in the patient's record. What information is necessary to have available when you are reporting abuse to state authorities?

_____

_____

_____

_____

20. Briefly describe human trafficking.

_____

_____

_____

_____

 COMPETENCY EXERCISES

Apply information from the chapter and use critical thinking skills to complete the competency exercises. Write responses on paper or create electronic documents to submit your answers.

1. Read the information in the Everyday Ethics case study for this **workbook** chapter. Using your institution's guidelines for writing in patient records, document your findings regarding Mrs. Kelly. Important note: write your progress note entry so that it includes only factual, objective information about the dental hygienist's observations and no subjective statements or personal opinions.

2. Outline the thought process you will use when making a decision to report suspected child abuse to state authorities. Discuss your outline with a small group of your student colleagues. Use the results of this discussion to write an office protocol for reporting suspected abuse.

 DISCOVERY EXERCISES

1. Investigate the laws and the processes for reporting child, elder, or spouse abuse in your state.

2. Investigate the agencies in your area where abused elders or battered spouses can obtain help or emergency assistance.

3. Investigate the PANDA program, the AVDR Tutorial for Dentists, or project RADAR to learn more about recognizing and reporting family abuse and neglect.

 EVERYDAY ETHICS

Before completing the learning exercises below, reread and reflect on the Everyday Ethics Scenario and Questions for Consideration in this chapter of the **textbook**. It may also be useful to review the Dental Hygiene Ethics discussion in Chapter 1, the Ethical Applications in the introduction pages for each section in the **textbook**, as well as the Codes of Ethics in **textbook** Appendices I–IV.

Collaborative Learning Activities

Identify a situation in which you have resolved an ethical dilemma and share the story with a classmate. Discuss how that person might have acted differently to resolve the situation.

Work with a small group to develop a 2- to 5-minute role-play that introduces the everyday ethics scenario described in the chapter (a great idea is to video record your role-play activity). Then develop separate 2-minute role-play scenarios that provide at least two alternative approaches/solutions to resolving the situation. Ask classmates to view the solutions, ask questions, and discuss the ethical approach used in each. Ask for a vote on which solution classmates determine to be the "best."

Factors to Teach the Patient

This scenario is related to the following factors listed in this chapter of the **textbook**:

▷ The value of oral hygiene with age-appropriate materials.

▷ What the bacterial biofilm is on teeth, using a disclosing agent.

▷ How to use the new toothbrush the child just received.

▷ Why it is especially important to brush the teeth and tongue just before going to sleep.

Johnny is 8 years old. This is his first dental hygiene visit with you, and his dental history indicates that he has not seen a dentist since the HeadStart program required a dental examination when he was 3 years old. His parents scheduled this dental appointment as a result of a directive from state authorities after a report by his teacher.

   Johnny is very shy, but after he gets to know you a bit during his appointment, he seems interested in what you are doing and asks all kinds of questions. You note during your intraoral examination that his teeth are completely covered with dental biofilm. Johnny states he doesn't really have a very good toothbrush. He obviously is not performing daily self-care, and you suspect that his parents are not helping or encouraging him in any way. Fortunately, there are no carious lesions, but his gingival tissue is red and bleeds easily when you touch it.

   Use the principles of motivational interviewing (see **workbook** Appendix D) as a guide, and use language appropriate for a child to explain to Johnny why he needs to brush his teeth every day.

MeSH TERMS

Use a combination of MeSH terms and other key words to develop an effective and efficient PubMed literature search strategy.

Child abuse	Elder abuse
Child abuse, sexual	Mandibular injuries
Battered child syndrome	Maxillofacial injuries
Spouse abuse	Mandatory reporting

15

Dental Radiographic Imaging

LEARNING OBJECTIVES

Upon successful completion of these exercises, you will be able to:

1. Identify and define the key terms, abbreviations, and concepts related to exposing and processing dental radiographs.

2. Describe the procedures for producing and processing radiographic films and digital radiographic images.

3. Identify the measures to protect yourself and your patient from ionizing radiation.

4. Select image receptor size and type, image receptor–holding devices, and clinical radiographic techniques for patient surveys.

5. Describe the positioning of individual intraoral image receptors based on area of the mouth and clinical technique.

6. Use guidelines to determine the indication for exposure of dental radiographs.

7. Identify the probable causes of common radiographic inadequacies.

 KNOWLEDGE EXERCISES

Write your answers for each question in the space provided.

Exposing and Processing Radiographs

1. In your own words, state two important objectives of dental radiology.

_____

_____

_____

_____

_____

2. Using the diagrams and descriptions in the **textbook** as a reference, describe in your own words how X-rays are produced after the power switch on the X-ray machine is activated.

_____

_____

_____

_____

3. Collimation refers to:

_____

_____

_____

_____

4. How does a change in mA affect the final radiographic image?

_____

_____

_____

_____

_____

_____

_____

_____

5. Identify how increasing the kilovoltage affects the image density.

_____

_____

_____

6. How is image contrast affected by increasing the kilovoltage?

_____

_____

7. List two advantages of high kVp.

_____

_____

8. List three advantages of lengthening the target-to-image receptor distance during exposure of patient radiographs.

_____

_____

_____

_____

_____

9. How is the target-to-image receptor distance lengthened on an individual X-ray unit?

_____

_____

_____

_____

10. Which film speed will most effectively reduce radiation exposure for the patient?

_____

_____

_____

11. What are the advantages of using digital radiography?

_____

_____

_____

_____

_____

_____

_____

_____

_____

_____

12. Correctly sequence the following steps in producing an _indirect_ digital radiograph, numbering them from 1 to 5 (1 = first step; 5 = final step).

_____ Electronic charge activates the sensor

_____ Image is scanned using a laser scanner

_____ Image stored on the PSP plate

_____ Sensor placed in patient's mouth

_____ Image displayed on computer

13. What type of digital imaging uses a sensor with a cord attached?

_____

14. List the four types of image receptors.

_____

_____

_____

_____

Radiation Safety

1. Identify three factors that influence the biologic effects of radiation on cells.

_____

_____

_____

2. List human tissues and organs that are highly radiosensitive.

_____

_____

_____

3. List three ways to protect yourself from primary and leakage radiation while making patient radiographs.

_____

_____

4. Relative to your patient's head, where can you best stand to protect yourself from secondary radiation?

_____

_____

_____

_____

5. List the ways you can protect your patient during exposure of dental radiographs.

_____

_____

_____

_____

_____

_____

_____

Clinical Techniques

1. Describe a complete dental radiographic survey.

_____

_____

2. When a rectangular PID is used for beam collimation while exposing dental radiographs, how do you adjust the X-ray machine to accommodate both horizontal and vertical film/sensor positioning?

_____

_____

_____

_____

_____

_____

3. Match the area of the mouth or teeth listed below with the radiographic film or sensor size most frequently used.

Intraoral Area	Film/Sensor Size
____ Overlapping anterior teeth	A. Size no. 0
____ Permanent dentition bitewings	B. Size no. 1
____ Primary teeth	C. Size no. 2
____ Adult posterior (periapical view)	
____ Child maxillary (occlusal view)	

4. When exposing a periapical image receptor of tooth 12, directing the central ray with too much vertical angle will produce an image of the tooth with roots that appear to be very _____.

5. Identify three reasons why the paralleling technique usually produces better images with increased patient safety compared to the bisecting-angle technique.

_____

_____

_____

_____

_____

6. When positioning the film inside the patient's mouth, the stippled or colored side of the film packet is placed:

_____

7. To maintain a visually open contact on a bitewing radiograph, the horizontal angle of the central beam is directed:

_____

_____

_____

8. How do you position the patient's head when you are making an occlusal survey image of the mandibular teeth?

_____

_____

9. If the patient's head is tilted to the side or the occlusal plane is not parallel with the floor, the angle of the PID must be altered to adapt the central ray to the patient's position. List two conditions that must be met when you are using the paralleling technique to expose periapical radiographs.

_____

_____

_____

_____

10. List the reasons why images of oral structures on a panoramic radiograph may have poor detail or be distorted even if you are very careful to use proper techniques when exposing the radiograph.

_____

_____

_____

_____

11. Identify one reason a panoramic image may be ordered instead of or in addition to periapical images for an individual patient.

_____

_____

In and Out of the Darkroom

1. Exposure to radiation changes the silver halide crystals coating traditional X-ray film to _____ and _____ ions.

2. After developing the film, only the amount of _____ corresponding to radiolucency and radiopacity remains.

3. The fixer solution removes the _____ crystals that were not exposed to radiation.

4. What type of lighting is safe for use as darkroom lighting?

_____

_____

5. When are handheld X-ray devices commonly used in dentistry.

_____

_____

6. Match the image inadequacy commonly found on dental radiographs (first column) with the most probable cause of the problem (second column).

Image Inadequacy	Probable Cause
_____ Dark lines across film	A. Extreme increase in vertical angle
_____ Double image	B. Film exposed twice
_____ Foreshortening	C. Bent film
_____ Large dark stain on one end of the film safelight	D. Unsafe safelight
	E. Sudden temperature change in processing solutions
_____ Light image with a pattern overlaying the image	F. Static electricity
_____ Puckered surface	G. Film placed backward in mouth
_____ Stretched appearance of images	H. Overlap of film in developer
_____ Whole film too dark	

7. List anatomic landmarks (besides the teeth) you might observe on a radiograph of your patient's mandibular incisor area.

_____

_____

_____

8. Name a mandibular structure that could appear on a maxillary third molar radiograph.

_____

_____

9. Identify the factors that will enhance interpretation of images on patient radiographs.

_____

_____

_____

_____

_____

_____

_____

_____

COMPETENCY EXERCISES

Apply information from the chapter and use critical thinking skills to complete the competency exercises. Write responses on paper or create electronic documents to submit your answers.

1. In your own words, explain the relationship between the tooth, the image receptor, and the central beam of radiation when using the paralleling technique. (*Hint:* Use your hands as a three-dimensional way to "draw" the images so you can visualize them as you try to explain.)

2. Mrs. Honey Davis, age 42, presents in your clinic for her initial appointment. She states she has come because she needs her teeth cleaned and because a tooth on the upper left side of her mouth has been bothering her. She has not been to visit a dentist for 2 years. She states that she had a lot of X-rays taken when she was last examined by her previous dentist just before she moved to your town but that she did not bring them with her today.

   When collecting your initial assessment data, you identify no positive clinical signs/symptoms of periodontal disease and no clinical evidence of active dental caries. She has six small amalgam restorations in her posterior teeth; only tooth 19 has a restoration on a proximal surface. However, Mrs. Davis reports intermittent use of mint candy to combat a feeling of dry mouth caused by a medication she takes. You also note an accumulation of biofilm on proximal tooth surfaces.

   You are planning to ask Dr. Gray, your employer, to examine Mrs. Davis. You know that he will probably order some X-rays. Using Tables 15-4 and 15-5 in the **textbook**, determine which X-rays would be recommended for Mrs. Davis and why.

3. You plan to expose a periapical radiograph of Mrs. Davis's tooth 15 using the paralleling technique. Explain the following:
   - Where the front edge of the image receptor should be positioned.
   - How the image receptor is placed relative to the long axis of tooth 15 and the mesial/distal line of that tooth.
   - How the central beam of radiation is directed relative to the long axis of tooth 15.
   - Where the lingual cusp of tooth 15 should rest in a disposable styrofoam film/sensor holder.

4. After you take all of the images prescribed for Mrs. Davis and place the films in a paper cup, you will go into the darkroom to process the films. Write out a step-by-step procedure for infection control and processing the films. For comparison, describe the infection control procedures for processing an indirect digital image.

5. In spite of your attempts to reassure him of the appropriateness and safety of the bitewing X-rays prescribed by the dentist, your patient, Jeff Darlington, has refused to have any X-rays taken at his recall appointment. Using your institution's guidelines for writing in patient records, document that he has refused the recommended exposures.

6. Gather a variety of dental radiographs taken in your clinic that are currently not being used for patient care. Place them in X-ray mounts for easy viewing. Evaluate the radiographs using Table 15-6 in the **textbook**.

   Identify any errors in technique or processing and describe possible causes and corrections you can make to eliminate the problem. Compare your evaluation of the images with those made by one or two of your student colleagues. Discuss any differences in the way you each evaluated the same image or the corrective measure you described for an error.

DISCOVERY EXERCISE

Gather a variety of dental radiographs taken in your clinic and identify as many anatomical landmarks as you can. What additional resources will help you to identify the landmarks visible on each film?

MeSH TERMS

Use a combination of MeSH terms and other key words to develop an effective and efficient PubMed literature search strategy.

Radiography, dental	Tomography scanners,
Radiography, dental, digital	X-ray computed
Radiography, panoramic	Radiation, ionizing
Radiography, bitewing	Scattering, radiation
X-ray film	Electromagnetic radiation
X-ray intensifying screens	Film dosimetry
Radiation equipment and	Gamma rays
supplies	

EVERYDAY ETHICS

Before completing the learning exercises below, reread and reflect on the Everyday Ethics Scenario and Questions for Consideration in this chapter of the **textbook**. It may also be useful to review the Dental Hygiene Ethics discussion in Chapter 1, the Ethical Applications in the introduction pages for each section in the **textbook**, as well as the Codes of Ethics in **textbook** Appendices I–IV.

Individual Learning Activity

Imagine that you are the dental hygienist in this scenario. Answer each of the questions for consideration at the end of the scenario.

Discovery Activity

Ask a friend or relative who is not involved in health care to read the scenario and discuss it with you from the perspective of a "patient" who receives services within the healthcare system. Discuss what you learned from the concerns, insights, or difference in perspective that person expressed.

Factors to Teach the Patient

This scenario is related to the following factors listed in this chapter of the **textbook**:

▷ When the patient asks about the safety of radiation

As you talk with Mr. Glazier, you realize that not only is he concerned about why additional X-rays are necessary, but he is also extremely concerned about the safety and negative effects of the additional dose of radiation he will receive. Using a motivational interviewing approach as a guide, write a statement explaining all of the safety factors in place in your clinic to protect him from excessive exposure to radiation.

Use the conversation you create to role-play this situation with a fellow student. If you are the patient in the role-play, be sure to ask questions. If you are the dental hygienist, try to anticipate questions and answer them in your explanation.

CHAPTER 15 CROSSWORD PUZZLE

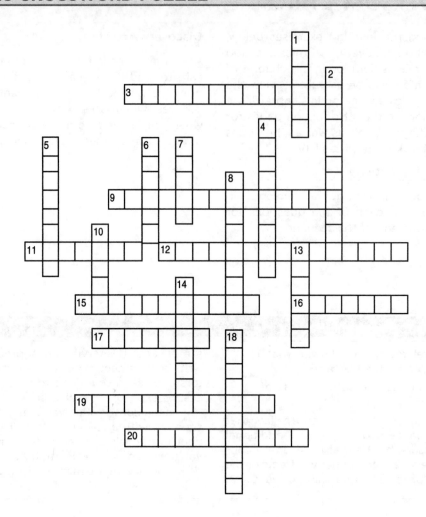

Puzzle Clues

Across

3. Refers to traditional film and/or digital sensor.
9. The product of absorbed dose and modifying factors; the unit is the Sievert (Sv).
11. Radiation that comes directly from the target of the anode of an X-ray tube.
12. Forms of radiation energy propagated by wave motion as photons.
15. Deflected radiation.
16. Radiation that escapes through the protective shielding of the X-ray unit tube head.
17. A measure of film exposure time.
19. Energy imparted by ionizing radiation to a specific exposure point; the unit is the gray (Gy).
20. The art and science of making radiographs.

Down

1. A finite bundle of energy of visible light or electromagnetic radiation.
2. Exposure to radiation.
4. The emission and propagation of energy in the form of waves or particles.
5. The blurred margin of an image detail (geometric unsharpness).
6. The CCD, CMOS, or PSP that is placed intraorally to capture a radiographic image.
7. The smallest discrete component of an electronic image.
8. To convert an image into a digital form.
10. Short-wavelength, high-energy electromagnetic radiation of nuclear origin.
13. Continuous and variable representation of an image as opposed to digital.
14. Container in which X-ray image receptors are placed.
18. The visible image created by exposure of an image receptor to ionizing radiation.

16

Hard Tissue Examination of the Dentition

LEARNING OBJECTIVES

Upon successful completion of these exercises, you will be able to:

1. Identify the three divisions of the human dentition.

2. Recognize and explain developmental and noncarious dental lesions.

3. Describe the types of dental injuries and tooth fractures.

4. Describe the G.V. Black and the International Caries Detection and Assessment System classifications of dental carious lesions.

5. Explain the initiation and development of early childhood caries (ECC).

6. Compare the methods for determining the vitality of the pulp of a tooth.

7. List the factors to be observed and recorded during a complete dental charting with a new patient.

8. Explain the basic principles of occlusion.

9. Classify occlusion according to Angle's classification and describe facial profile associated with each classification.

10. Describe the functional and parafunctional contacts.

11. Explain the effects of occlusal trauma on oral structures.

12. Explain the purposes and uses of study models.

 ## KNOWLEDGE EXERCISES

Write your answers for each question in the space provided.

1. List the three divisions of the human dentition.

2. List the causes of various types of hypoplasia.

3. In your own words, describe the difference between hypomineralization and hypomaturation.

4. Describe the appearance of a tooth with defects in dentin.

_____

_____

5. What is the difference between amelogenesis imperfecta and dentinogenesis imperfecta?

_____

_____

_____

6. List three types of injury to teeth caused by trauma.

_____

_____

_____

7. Match the term to the correct definition.

Term	Definition
___ Abrasion	A. Loss of tooth substance by a chemical process that does not involve bacterial action
___ Attrition	
___ Avulsion	B. Dislocation of a tooth within its socket
___ Erosion	C. Mechanical wearing away of tooth substance by forces other than mastication
___ Abfraction	
___ Luxation	D. Microfractures in enamel or dentin
	E. Complete displacement of a tooth from its socket
	F. Wearing away of a tooth as a result of tooth-to-tooth contact

8. Complete each section of the infomap below to help you differentiate among attrition, erosion, abrasion, and abfraction.

Defect	Location	Etiology	Appearance
Attrition			
Erosion			
Abrasion			
Abfraction			

9. What is cavitation?

_____

_____

_____

10. Match the description of types of dental caries with the correct term. Each term is used only once.

Terminology	Description
A. Simple	____ Involves MOD surfaces
B. Compound	____ Involves two surfaces
C. Complex	____ Begins in minute fault where closure of enamel plates in imperfect
D. Pit and fissure	
E. Smooth surface	____ Occurs where there is no initial groove or other defect
	____ Involves only one surface of a tooth

11. Match the description of types of dental caries with the correct term. Each term is used only once.

Terminology	Description
A. Primary	____ Adjacent to a previous restoration
B. Recurrent	
C. Arrested	____ Early sign, no breakthrough of enamel
D. Rampant	
E. ECC	____ Hard, stained, stationary surface
F. Root caries	____ Common cause is use of nursing bottle at bedtime
G. Incipient	____ Tends to spread laterally
	____ Rapidly spreading, multiple lesions
	____ Initial caries

12. Match each description with the correct Dr. G.V. Black classification. Each classification is used only once.

G.V. Black Classifications	Descriptions
A. Class I	____ In pits and fissures
B. Class II	____ Proximal surface/involves incisal angle
C. Class III	
D. Class IV	____ Cervical 1/3
E. Class V	____ Proximal surfaces of premolar or molar
F. Class VI	____ Incisal edge or cusp tip
	____ Proximal surfaces only of incisor or canine

13. Match each description with the correct ICCMS code classification. Each classification is used only once.

ICCMS Code	Descriptions
A. Code 0	_____ Opacity and/or visible discoloration of the surface enamel only
B. Code 1 or 2	
C. Code 3	_____ Opaque or discolored enamel with visible dentin
D. Code 4	
E. Code 5 or 6	_____ Enamel breakdown with underlying dentin shadow
	_____ Localized enamel breakdown with no visible dentin exposure
	_____ No questionable changes after air-drying

14. List three microbes associated with early childhood caries.

_____

_____

15. List the relevant result for each response during an electric pulp test.

Patient Response	Result
No response	
Exaggerated/lingering response after removal of stimulus	
Pain subsides promptly	

16. Label each figure with the correct facial profile.

_____   _____   _____

17. Complete each section of the infomap below and on the next page to describe and compare types of occlusion in permanent dentition.

Occlusion	Facial Profile	Molar Relationship	Canine Relationship	Potential Additional Considerations
Normal				
Class I				
Class II				
Class II Division 1				

Occlusion	Facial Profile	Molar Relationship	Canine Relationship	Potential Additional Considerations
Class II Division 2				
Class III				

18. Briefly describe the following malrelations of groups of teeth.

Type of Malrelation	Description
Crossbite	
Edge-to-edge	
End-to-end	
Open bite	
Overjet	
Underjet	
Overbite	

19. What is the location of primal spaces in a primary dentition?

20. What is the effect of a first molar terminal step?

21. List some negative effects of parafunctional contacts or trauma from occlusion.

22. What is fremitus?

23. List two reasons for making a bite registration during making of study models.

COMPETENCY EXERCISES

Apply information from the chapter and use critical thinking skills to complete the competency exercises. Write responses on paper or create electronic documents to submit your answers.

1. During an initial examination, you inform your patient, Cindy Markowitz, that you will be making impressions for study models. She protests because having impressions made always makes her gag, and she asks you why you need to make those models of her teeth. Explain the purpose and uses of study models for your patient.

2. Your patient, Oliver Summerlin, uses a hard toothbrush and an abrasive nonfluoride-containing dentifrice. He wears a partial denture on the mandible and takes a medication that causes xerostomia. You note abrasion in all four quadrants and root caries on the facial surfaces of teeth 27–30. Differentiate abrasion from root caries and develop a Motivational Interviewing strategy to discuss the prevention of both root caries and abrasion with your patient.

3. Your patient at 3:00 pm is Paulo Jacoby. He is 16 years old, is an avid basketball player, and never wears a mouthguard. Describe potential oral injuries.

4. Use Table 16-1 in the **textbook** to inform your responses to the following three patients.
   a. Clive Williams is 10 years old. He wants to know if he will get "more grown-up teeth." Explain to him the formative stages that his remaining teeth are in and the age at which most children can expect more permanent teeth to erupt.

b. Clive's cousin Jamal is 5 years old. He and Clive have a bet as to who still has the most teeth to erupt. Who will win the bet and why?

c. Jamal's sister wants to get in on the bet. She is 15 years old and says she will not have any more teeth erupt because all of her teeth are in and she is a grown-up. She has never had any teeth extracted. Who will win the bet and why?

5. You are performing an examination and attempting to determine whether your patient has an overbite or an overjet. Describe the strategies you will use and explain how you will describe your findings to your patient.

6. The best way to become competent in doing an oral hard tissue examination and assessment is to practice. Get together with several classmates and study a copy of Table 16-2 from the **textbook**. Use forms available at your school for hard tissue examination and work in pairs to examine a classmate's hard tissues and discuss the results.

7. Practice classifying any active dental caries lesions you detect during a patient examination using each of the classification methods described in the chapter (G.V. Black, ADA Caries Classification, and International Caries Detection and Assessment System).

 DISCOVERY EXERCISE

Review the data collection forms that are used in your dental hygiene program. What forms will you need to use to document each of the examination features that are listed in Table 16-2 in the **textbook**? How do you need to document in the daily progress notes following the patient's visit that you have performed a complete hard tissue exam?

 EVERYDAY ETHICS

Before completing the learning exercises below, reread and reflect on the Everyday Ethics Scenario and Questions for Consideration in this chapter of the **textbook**. It may also be useful to review the Dental Hygiene Ethics discussion in Chapter 1, the Ethical Applications in the introduction pages for each section in the **textbook**, as well as the Codes of Ethics in **textbook** Appendices I–IV.

Individual Learning Activity

Imagine that you are the dental hygienist in this scenario. Answer each of the questions for consideration at the end of the scenario.

Discovery Activity

Ask a dental hygienist friend who has been practicing for a year or more to read the scenario. Provide a copy of the Code of Ethics as well. Share the responses you have made to answer each question, and ask that person to discuss the situation with you. Alternatively, ask a friend or relative who is not involved in health care to read the scenario and discuss it with you from the perspective of a "patient" who receives services within the healthcare system. What insights did you have or what did you learn from these discussions?

Factors to Teach the Patient

This scenario is related to the following factors listed in this chapter of the **textbook**:

▷ The cause and process of enamel or root caries formation and development for the patients at risk.

▷ Methods for prevention of dental caries, such as fluorides, biofilm prevention and control, and control of cariogenic foods in the diet.

▷ Methods for prevention of early childhood caries. (Nothing but plain water should be used in bedtime or nap-time nursing bottles. Avoid the use of a sweetener on a pacifier. Use of a cup for milk or juice by the baby's first birthday.)

Andrea Carfagno has arrived in the reception area of the clinic. She is holding her 26-month-old daughter, Nicole, and her 9-month-old twin boys are in a stroller. Nicole is your patient today. The girl is holding a baby bottle filled with fruit juice. She is a happy, attentive youngster who is anxious to please.

Use the motivational interviewing (see **workbook** Appendix D) as a guide to write a dialogue explaining the need to have Nicole switch from a bottle to a cup. Be sure to address the use of fruit juices in a bottle and to explain early childhood caries. These issues pertain to both Nicole and her brothers.

Use the conversation you create to role-play this situation with a fellow student. If you are the patient in the role-play, be sure to ask questions. If you are the dental hygienist, try to anticipate questions and answer them in your explanation.

MeSH TERMS

Use a combination of MeSH terms and other key words to develop an effective and efficient PubMed literature search strategy.

Dentition, mixed	Dental occlusion
Dentition, permanent	Tooth demineralization
Dentition, primary	Tooth abrasion
Dental caries	Tooth attrition
Dental impression materials	Tooth erosion
Dental impression technique	Tooth exfoliation
	Tooth abnormalities
	Malocclusion

17

Dental Soft Deposits, Biofilm, Calculus, and Stains

LEARNING OBJECTIVES

Upon successful completion of these exercises, you will be able to:

1. Identify and define the key terms and concepts related to biofilm, calculus, and stains.

2. Describe biofilm, calculus, and stains in terms of type, location, distribution, occurrence, appearance, and consistency.

3. Differentiate dental biofilm from pellicle, materia alba, and food debris in terms of composition, significance, and detection.

4. Describe biofilm and calculus formation, composition, and attachment.

5. Discuss the implications of dental biofilm, calculus, and stains in terms of periodontal disease and caries.

6. Classify various stains as to their location and source.

KNOWLEDGE EXERCISES

Write your answers for each question in the space provided.

1. In your own words, describe each of the four types of nonmineralized tooth deposits listed below

- *Acquired pellicle:*

- *Dental biofilm:*

- *Materia alba:*

- *Food debris:*

2. Why is acquired pellicle significant?

_____

_____

_____

_____

_____

3. Acquired pellicle is composed primarily of

_____

_____

_____

_____

4. _____ pellicle can become embedded in the tooth structure, particularly where the tooth surface is partially demineralized.

5. What is the role of EPS in biofilm formation?

_____

_____

_____

_____

_____

_____

_____

6. In your own words, describe *quorum sensing* and why it is significant in biofilm formation.

_____

_____

_____

_____

_____

7. Make a drawing of the shape of each of these types of bacteria.

Bacillus

Staphylococci

Streptococci

Spirella

Vibrios

8. In the left hand column, identify the microorganisms present in biofilm in the graphic below. In the right hand column, indicate the timeframe for the development of the observed changes in the bacteria over time when the teeth are not cleaned.

Accumulative Changes in Biofilm Bacteria at the Gingival Margin

9. How does the dental hygienist detect biofilm during patient assessment?

_____

_____

_____

_____

10. The interactions involved in the formation of biofilm are listed below. Number the list in the correct order (1 = first interaction; 5 = last interaction).

_____ Secretion of extracellular matrix

_____ Bacteria adhere to pellicle

_____ Biofilm growth

_____ Bacteria multiply and colonize

_____ Release of cells to spread and colonize other areas

11. Gingivitis is clinically evident within _____ when biofilm is left undisturbed on tooth surfaces.

12. Match the following descriptions of biofilm with the correct type. Each type is used more than once.

Type of Biofilm	Description
A. Supragingival biofilm B. Subgingival biofilm	_____ Shape and size are affected by the friction of tongue, cheeks, and lips
	_____ The main source of nutrients for bacterial proliferation is gingival crevicular fluid
	_____ Coronal to the margin of the free gingiva
	_____ May become thicker as the diseased pocket wall becomes less tight
	_____ Heaviest collection on areas not cleaned daily by patient
	_____ Found most often on the cervical third, especially facial surfaces, the lingual mandibular molars, and proximal surfaces
	_____ Down growth of bacteria from supragingival biofilm
	_____ Diseased pocket; primarily gram-negative, motile, spirochetes, rods
	_____ Sources of nutrients for bacterial proliferation are saliva and ingested food
	_____ Made up of three layers
	_____ The structure is an adherent, densely packed microbial layer over pellicle on the tooth surface

13. List the microorganisms in each layer of subgingival biofilm.
- *Initial layer:*

  _____

- *Intermediate layer:*

  _____

  _____

- *Top layer:*

  _____

  _____

14. What three minerals are more concentrated in biofilm than in saliva?

_____

_____

_____

15. List the patient self-care interventions that can increase the amount of fluoride in dental biofilm.

_____

_____

_____

16. Carbohydrate intake can contribute to the _____ of biofilm microorganisms to each other and the teeth.

17. Explain the significance of the two types of cariogenic microorganisms in biofilm.

_____

_____

_____

18. What is the typical pH level in dental biofilm prior to eating?

_____

_____

19. What happens to the pH level of dental biofilm immediately following the intake of sucrose?

_____

20. Explain the significance of the change in pH level of biofilm following intake of sucrose.

_____

_____

_____

21. Calculus is mineralized _____.

22. List the major inorganic compounds that are the primary components of mature calculus.

_____

_____

_____

_____

_____

_____

_____

23. Dental calculus is classified by its location on a tooth surface in relation to the _____.

24. Match the description with the type of calculus deposit. Each type of deposit is used more than once.

Classification of Calculus Deposit	Description
A. Supragingival calculus	_____ Light to dark brown, dark green, or black
B. Subgingival calculus	_____ May be stained by tobacco, food, or other pigments
	_____ Crusty, spiny, or nodular
	_____ Shape of calculus mass is determined by the anatomy of teeth; contour of gingival margin; and pressure of tongue, lips, and cheeks
	_____ Calcium-to-phosphorus ratio is lower
	_____ Thin, smooth veneers
	_____ Amorphous, bulky
	_____ Increased amount in tobacco smokers
	_____ Newest deposits near bottom of pocket are less dense and hard
	_____ White, creamy yellow, or gray
	_____ Brittle, flintlike
	_____ Finger- and fernlike
	_____ Slight deposits may be invisible until dried with compressed air
	_____ Flattened to conform with pressure from the pocket wall
	_____ Moderately hard
	_____ Stains derived from blood pigments from diseased pocket
	_____ Newer deposits less dense and hard

25. List the three basic steps in calculus formation.

_____

_____

_____

26. What is the range of formation time required for the primary biofilm deposit to change to mature mineralized calculus?

_____

_____

27. List three ways to prevent or control calculus formation.

_____

_____

_____

28. What is the main objective for dental hygiene interventions that remove calculus from the surfaces of teeth?

_____

_____

_____

29. List the agents that can be used as active ingredients in mouthrinses and dentifrices that inhibit mineralization of calculus.

_____

_____

_____

30. Fill in the blanks as you learn about supragingival calculus.

Supragingival calculus is located on the _____ crown of the tooth, _____ to the margin of the gingiva. The heaviest deposits of supragingival calculus are often related to the openings of _____, especially those located near the facial surface of maxillary molars and the lingual surface of mandibular anterior teeth. Calculus can also be found on surfaces of _____ and barbells worn in tongue piercings.

31. What is the source of elements for mineralization of supragingival calculus?

32. Fill in the blanks in the statements below as you read about subgingival calculus.

Subgingival calculus is located apical to the _____ of the gingiva. It extends nearly to the _____ of the pocket. As the pocket is deepened by _____, calculus forms on the exposed root surface. This deposit may be _____ on a group of teeth or_____ on a single tooth. Heaviest deposits are often found on the _____ surfaces.

33. What is the source of minerals for subgingival calculus formation?

_____

_____

34. Why is subgingival calculus considered a predisposing factor in pocket development?

_____

_____

_____

35. True or False (circle the correct answer). Small amounts of calculus that have not been stained are frequently more visible when they are wet with saliva.

36. Identify some strategies that will help you find both supragingival and subgingival calculus in your patient's mouth.

_____

_____

_____

_____

_____

37. The ease or difficulty of calculus removal can be related to the manner of _____ of the calculus to the tooth surface.

38. List three means of attachment of calculus to the tooth.

_____

_____

_____

39. The concentration of fluoride in calculus varies and is influenced by:

_____

_____

_____

40. Match each term with its definition.

Terms Related to Calculus	Definition
_____ Pyrophosphate	A. Forms on a dental prosthesis
_____ Amorphous	B. Without definite shape or visible differentiation in structure
_____ Germ-free	
_____ Matrix	C. Intercellular or intermicrobial substance of a tissue or the tissue from which a structure develops, gains support, and is held together
_____ Calculus	
_____ Nidus	
_____ Apatite	D. Nucleus; focus; point of origin
_____ Incremental lines	E. Free from microorganisms
	F. Crystalline mineral component of bones and teeth that contains calcium and phosphate
_____ Denture calculus	
_____ Supersaturated	G. Mineralized biofilm composed of inorganic and organic content
_____ Mineralization	
	H. Examples are pulp stones, denticles, and salivary calculi
	I. Addition of mineral elements, such as calcium and phosphorus, to the body or a part thereof with resulting hardening of the tissue
	J. Inhibitor of calcification that occurs in parotid saliva of humans in variable amounts; anticalculus component of tartar-control dentifrices
	K. Evidence that calculus grows through apposition of new layers

41. Match the following terms with the correct definition.

Term	Definition
A. Chlorophyll	_____ Incomplete development or underdevelopment of an organ or a tissue
B. Endogenous	
C. Chronologic	_____ Producing color or pigment
D. Chromogenic	_____ Imperfect formation of enamel; hereditary condition in which the ameloblasts fail to lay down the enamel matrix properly or at all
E. Dentinogenesis imperfecta	
F. Amelogenesis imperfecta	
G. Hypoplasia	_____ Originating outside or caused by factors outside
H. Intrinsic	_____ Hereditary disorder of dentin formation in which the odontoblasts lay down an abnormal matrix; can occur in both primary and permanent dentitions
I. Exogenous	
J. Extrinsic	
	_____ Produced within or caused by factors within
	_____ Situated entirely within
	_____ Green plant pigment essential to photosynthesis
	_____ Arranged in order of time
	_____ Derived from or situated on the outside; external

42. Stains are classified by location and source.

  • List examples of extrinsic exogenous stains.

_____

_____

_____

_____

_____

  • List examples of intrinsic endogenous stains.

_____

_____

_____

_____

_____

  • List examples of intrinsic exogenous stains.

_____

_____

_____

_____

_____

_____

43. Your patient presents with a stained pulpless tooth. Describe the clinical appearance of the stain and explain how it was formed. The patient is scheduled for endodontic treatment on another tooth and wants to know if that tooth will also stain. What would you tell this patient?

_____

_____

_____

_____

_____

_____

_____

_____

44. Clinically you observe enamel that is partially or completely missing because of a generalized disturbance of

the ameloblasts. Teeth are yellowish-brown or gray-brown. What is this condition called?

_____

45. Your patient was born with erythroblastosis fetalis (Rh incompatibility). This condition may a leave the teeth with a _____ hue.

46. Which drugs are associated with dental stains?

_____

_____

47. Which drug may stain teeth after eruption?

_____

_____

48. Complete Infomap 17-1 to help you organize information about extrinsic stains.

☑ COMPETENCY EXERCISES

Apply information from the chapter and use critical thinking skills to complete the competency exercises. Write responses on paper or create electronic documents to submit your answers.

1. As you evaluate Mrs. Eltheia Shore, you note that she presents with a significant amount of supragingival, subgingival, gingival, and fissure biofilm. Educate her

INFOMAP 17-1					
TYPE OF STAIN	APPEARANCE	DISTRIBUTION	OCCURRENCE	CAUSE/ORIGIN	CLINICAL ISSUES
Yellow					
Green					
Other green					
Black line					
Tobacco					
Other brown					
Orange and red					
Metallic-industrial					
Metallic-drugs					

about the factors that can contribute to biofilm accumulation and the surfaces most commonly affected. Describe the strategies used for detection of biofilm.

2. You are providing patient education for Alison Alverez and her 10-year-old son, Juan. Juan has multiple carious lesions, and his mother is very interested in preventing more from occurring. Juan drinks soda daily. He purchases a 32-oz. bottle on his way to school and sips the soda every chance he gets. Juan's mother remembers hearing something about acids in the mouth and wants to know more about this. Describe your patient education approach.

3. Your patient, John Weston, is wondering about calculus formation. He is trying to understand the exact time frame of the process. Help him understand calculus formation by defining pellicle, biofilm, and calculus and discussing the influencing factors. Make a list or draw a picture that describes calculus formation in terms of minutes, hours, and days.

4. While scaling in the mandibular right quadrant, you are having varying degrees of difficulty detecting and removing the calculus. Describe the three modes of calculus attachment. Explain how each mode affects detection and removal.

5. Your 1:30 patient, Fawez Sadarage, 47 years old, presents with a stain on all the second and third molars caused by tetracycline. Describe the stain that you might see and list some follow-up questions you will ask Mr. Sadarage. Indicate why you would ask the questions.

6. The patient in the scenario posed in Question 1 presented with generalized gray-brown stain on second and third molars. Why weren't all teeth affected?

7. At what age do you think the patient took the antibiotic?

8. Several strategies will help you recognize and identify stains that you observe during assessment of the oral cavity. Explain the types of stains (color and cause) that can be identified using each of the strategies listed below.
   - *Medical history*
   - *Questions about industrial occupation*
   - *Questions about dietary habits*
   - *Dental history*
   - *Dental charting (e.g., endodontic therapy, restorative materials)*

 MeSH TERMS

Use a combination of MeSH terms and other key words to develop an effective and efficient PubMed literature search strategy.

Amelogenesis imperfecta	Dentin dysplasia
Bacterial processes	Dentinogenesis
Biofilms	imperfecta
Dental deposits	Fluorosis, dental
Dental enamel hypoplasia	Gram-negative bacteria
Dental pellicle	Gram-positive bacteria
Dental plaque	Minerals
Dental polishing	Odontodysplasia
Dental prophylaxis	Tetracyclines
Dental scaling	Tooth bleaching

 EVERYDAY ETHICS

Before completing the learning exercises below, reread and reflect on the Everyday Ethics Scenario and Questions for Consideration in this chapter of the **textbook**. It may also be useful to review the Dental Hygiene Ethics discussion in Chapter 1, the Ethical Applications in the introduction pages for each section in the **textbook**, as well as the Codes of Ethics in **textbook** Appendices I–IV.

Individual Learning Activity

Imagine that you are the dental hygienist in this scenario. Answer each of the questions for consideration at the end of the scenario.

Collaborative Learning Activity

Work with another student colleague to role-play the scenario. The goal of this exercise is for you and your colleague to work though the alternative actions in order to come to consensus on a solution or response that is acceptable to both of you.

Factors to Teach the Patient

This scenario is related to the following factors listed in this chapter of the **textbook**:

▷ Location, composition, and properties of dental biofilm and calculus with emphasis on its role in dental caries and periodontal infections.

▷ Effects of personal oral care procedures in the prevention of dental biofilm, calculus, and stain.

▷ What calculus is and how it forms from dental biofilm.

▷ Select products with an American Dental Association or Canadian Dental Association Seal of Acceptance.

Louisa Gregory, a 53-year-old first-grade teacher, is busy with her two daughters, aged 12 and 14. She does not take time for herself and has come to the dental hygiene clinic after a 5-year absence. She uses any type of toothpaste that is on sale, and her current dentifrice is in a decorative dispenser; she does not know anything else about it, except that it matches her bathroom perfectly! As you examine Louisa's mouth, you see generalized moderate to heavy biofilm and heavy supragingival and subgingival calculus. She wants to know what to do about "all this hard stuff" on her teeth.

Use a motivational interviewing approach (see **workbook** Appendix D) to create a conversation to educate Louisa about the impact of good oral hygiene and frequent professional care for complete scaling on the levels of supragingival and subgingival calculus. Be sure to address product selection criteria and the need for the use of an anticalculus toothpaste.

Use the conversation you create to role-play this situation with a fellow student. If you are the patient in the role-play, be sure to ask questions. If you are the dental hygienist, try to anticipate questions and answer them in your explanation.

The Periodontium

 KNOWLEDGE EXERCISES

Write your answers for each question in the space provided.

1. Use the following terms to label the following figure with each of the components of the gingiva and periodontium.
   - Alveolar bone
   - Alveolar mucosa
   - Attached gingiva
   - Cementoenamel junction
   - Enamel
   - Free gingiva
   - Free gingival groove
   - Gingival margin
   - Gingival sulcus
   - Junctional epithelium
   - Mucogingival junction

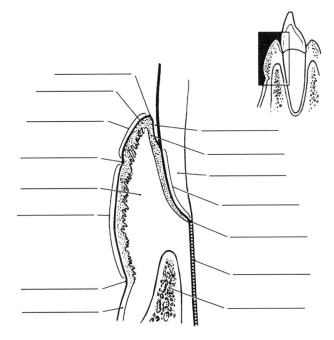

2. Draw the following gingival fibers in their correct position on the following figure. Use colored pencils to help differentiate.
   - *Alveologingival fibers*
   - *Circumferential fibers*
   - *Dentogingival fibers*
   - *Dentoperiosteal fibers*

3. Draw and label the periodontal ligament in the correct position on the same diagram.

4. Match each term with the appropriate definition.

Terms Related to the Gingiva	Definition
_____ Generalized	A. A change that is confined to the free or marginal gingiva
_____ Marginal	
_____ Edematous	B. The gingiva is involved about all or nearly all of the teeth throughout the mouth
_____ Clinical crown	
_____ Papillary	
_____ Embrasure	C. A change that involves a papilla but not the rest of the free gingiva around a tooth
_____ Anatomic root	
_____ Diffuse	D. Spread out, dispersed; affects the gingival margin, attached gingiva, and interdental papillae; may extend into alveolar mucosa
_____ Anatomic crown	
_____ Localized	
_____ Clinical root	E. Indicates the gingiva around a single tooth or a specific group of teeth

F. The part of the tooth above the attached periodontal tissues; can be considered the part of the tooth where clinical treatment procedures are applied

G. The part of the tooth below the base of the gingival sulcus or periodontal pocket; the part of the root to which periodontal fibers are attached

H. The part of the tooth covered by enamel

I. The part of the tooth covered by cementum

J. The space below the contact area of two adjacent teeth

K. Enlargement caused by fluids in inflamed tissue

5. Define the following terms in your own words. (*Hint:* You may want to think about location as you define each term.)
   - *Masticatory mucosa*

   _____

   _____

   - *Lining mucosa*

   _____

   _____

   _____

   _____

   - *Cementum*

   _____

   _____

   _____

   _____

   - *Alveolar bone*

   _____

   _____

   _____

   _____

• *Free gingival groove*

_____

_____

• *Gingival sulcus (crevice)*

_____

_____

_____

_____

• *Interdental gingiva*

_____

_____

• *Col*

_____

_____

_____

6. Use the following terms to label the following diagram of teeth and gingiva.

• *Alveolar mucosa*
• *Attached gingiva*
• *Free gingiva*
• *Interdental papilla*
• *Mandibular labial frenum*
• *Maxillary labial frenum*
• *Mucogingival junction*

7. Describe the difference between friable gingiva and bulbous gingiva.

_____

_____

_____

8. Match the gingival fiber group with the correct location and purpose.

Gingival Fiber Group	Location and Purpose
_____ Dentogingival fibers	A. From the cervical area of one tooth across to an adjacent tooth (on the mesial or distal side only) to provide resistance to separation of teeth
_____ Transseptal fibers	
_____ Dentoperiosteal fibers	B. From the cementum in the cervical region into the free gingiva to give support to the gingiva
_____ Apical fibers	
_____ Interradicular fibers	C. From the root apex to adjacent surrounding bone to resist vertical forces
_____ Circumferential fibers	
_____ Oblique fibers	D. From the root above the apical fibers obliquely toward the occlusal to resist vertical and unexpected strong forces
_____ Alveolar crest fibers	
_____ Alveologingival fibers	E. From the alveolar crest into the free and attached gingiva to provide support
_____ Horizontal fibers	
	F. From the cervical cementum over the alveolar crest to blend with fibers of the periosteum of the bone
	G. From the cementum in the middle of each root to the adjacent alveolar bone to resist tipping of the tooth
	H. From the alveolar crest to the cementum just below the cementoenamel junction to resist intrusive forces
	I. Continuous around the neck of the tooth to help maintain the tooth in position
	J. From the cementum between the roots of multirooted teeth to the adjacent bone to resist vertical and lateral forces

9. To complete this exercise using the following figure, you will need red, blue, and green pencils.

- On the left-hand side of the drawing, color the interdental papilla in both the maxillary and mandibular arch in red.
- On the right-hand side of the drawing, color the free gingiva in blue.
- On the right-hand side of the drawing, color the attached gingiva in green.

10. You are getting ready to do an examination of Patrice Davis, who is a professional ice-skater and is curious about everything. She wants to know exactly how you are going to check her "gum tissues," and she does not want you to "skate over anything." She really wants to have a nice smile for the competitions! Explain the purpose of the examination to Patrice and list the markers you will use to describe the appearance of her oral tissues.

_____

✓ COMPETENCY EXERCISES

Apply information from the chapter and use critical thinking skills to complete the competency exercises. Write responses on paper or create electronic documents to submit your answers.

1. Your patient, Tucker McLeimgreen, presents with clinically normal-appearing gingiva. Describe in your own words what you expect to observe as you examine Tucker's gingival tissues both visually and with a probe.

2. Your patient, Xin Singer, is very concerned about the areas of localized, wide, shallow recession she has on teeth 6 and 7 and the narrow, deep (with missing attached gingiva) recession she has on teeth 24 and 25. Using the figures in the **textbook** chapter as a guide, draw a sketch of the recession that is described here. Then identify the points you will discuss with Xin.

3. Your patient, Frank Catty, presents with gingiva that looks like the tissue pictured in Figure 18-13B in the **textbook**. On the basis of your understanding of this condition, describe Frank's gingival tissue using the following markers: color, size, shape, consistency, surface texture, position of the gingival margin, and bleeding.

_____

_____

_____

4. You are providing care for Kathleen Gallagher. She is a research scientist particularly interested in inflammation. You have just completed the gingival examination and are planning to discuss the information you have gathered and the causes for the oral changes you have documented. Kathleen has not received dental care for 5 years, and she is worried about her "bleeding gums" and wants to know exactly why these changes are occurring. Refer to Table 18-1 in the **textbook** to help you collect your thoughts and then explain the reasons for each change listed below.

- *Color: bright red*
- *Size: enlarged*
- *Shape: bulbous papillae*
- *Consistency: soft, spongy (dents readily when pressed with probe)*
- *Surface texture: smooth, shiny gingiva*
- *Position of gingival margin: enlarged; higher on the tooth, above normal; pocket deepened*
- *Position of junctional epithelium: probing is within normal limits*
- *Bleeding: spontaneous*
- *Exudate: none on pressure*

5. For some types of patient records, you will need to describe a patient's condition in sentence form. In the space provided, document a brief gingival description that you will include in Kathleen Gallagher's record.

MeSH TERMS

Use a combination of MeSH terms and other key words to develop an effective and efficient PubMed literature search strategy.

Periodontium	Gingiva
Alveolar process	Periapical tissue
Dental cementum	Periodontal ligament
Epithelial attachment	Hemidesmosomes

EVERYDAY ETHICS

Before completing the learning exercises below, reread and reflect on the Everyday Ethics Scenario and Questions for Consideration in this chapter of the **textbook**. It may also be useful to review the Dental Hygiene Ethics discussion in Chapter 1, the Ethical Applications in the introduction pages for each section in the **textbook**, as well as the Codes of Ethics in **textbook** Appendices I–IV.

Individual Learning Activities

Identify a situation you have experienced that presents a similar ethical dilemma. Write about what you would do differently now than you did at the time the incident happened—support your discussion with concepts from the dental hygiene codes of ethics.

Discovery Activity

Summarize this scenario for faculty member at your school and ask them to consider the questions that are included. Is their perspective different than yours or similar? Explain.

Factors to Teach the Patient

This scenario is related to the following factors listed in this chapter of the **textbook**:

▷ Characteristics of normal healthy gingiva.

▷ The significance of bleeding; healthy tissue does not bleed.

▷ Relationship of findings during a gingival examination to the personal daily care procedures for infection control.

You have just seen Kathleen Gallagher, the patient described in Competency Exercise 4. She is very anxious now that you have told her about all the implications of your findings from the gingival examination.

Working with the data you have collected and the causative factors you have identified, and using the principles of motivational interviewing (see **workbook** Appendix D) as a guide, write a dialogue explaining what type of tissue changes you would like to see at Kathleen's next appointment.

Use the conversation you create to role-play this situation with a fellow student. If you are the patient in the role-play, be sure to ask questions. If you are the dental hygienist, try to anticipate questions and answer them in your explanation.

CHAPTER 18 CROSSWORD PUZZLE

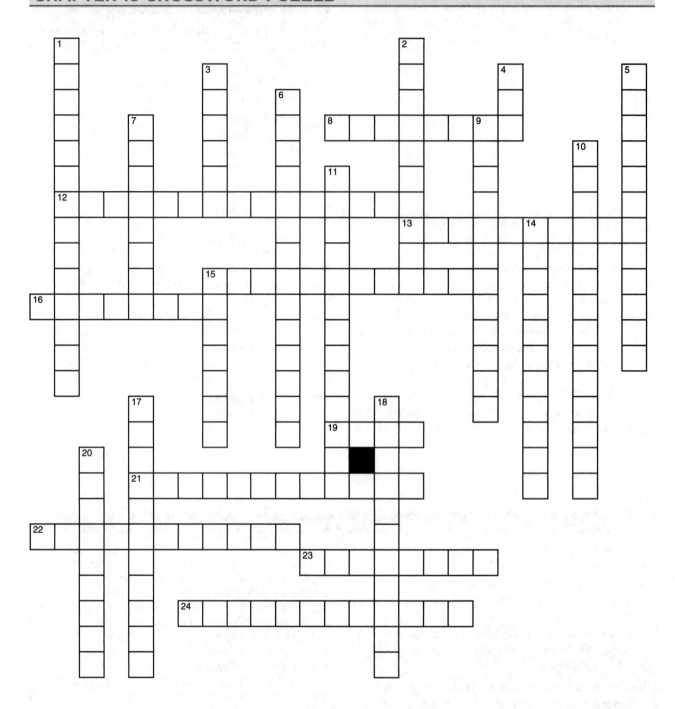

Puzzle Clues

Across

8. A fibrous change of the mucous membrane as a result of chronic inflammation.

12. Measured from the CEJ to the base of the sulcus or pocket (two words).

13. Base of the sulcus; formed by cementum, periodontal ligament, and the alveolar bone.

15. Tissue that surrounds and supports the teeth.

16. A space between two natural teeth.

19. The type of epithelial tissue that serves as a liner for the intraoral mucosal surfaces.

21. The distance from the gingival margin to periodontal attachment at the base of the pocket (two words).

22. Increase in size of tissue or organ caused by an increase in size of its constituent cells.

23. The type of epithelium that is composed of a layer of flat, scalelike cells, or may be stratified.

24. Junction between the attached gingiva and the alveolar mucosa.

Down

1. The type of mucosal lining in which the stratified squamous epithelial cells retain their nuclei and cytoplasm.

2. Fiber-producing cell of the connective tissue.

3. Narrow fold of mucous membrane that passes from a more fixed to a more movable area of the oral mucosa.

4. Contains leukocytes, degenerated tissue elements, tissue fluids, and microorganisms.

5. Variation in gingival color related to complexion or race.

6. The development of a horny layer of flattened epithelial cells.

7. Fibrous connective tissue that surrounds and attaches the roots of teeth to the alveolar bone.

9. Characterized by increased blood flow, increased permeability of capillaries, and increased collection of defense cells and tissue fluid/ usually produces alterations in color, size, shape, and consistency of tissue.

10. Abnormal thickening of the keratin layer (stratum corneum) of the epithelium.

11. One of two structures that together create a cell junction and form an attachment between junctional epithelial cells and the tooth surface.

14. Abnormal increase in volume of a tissue or organ caused by formation and growth of new normal cells.

15. Fills the interproximal area between two teeth.

17. Formation of pus.

18. The act of chewing.

20. The pitted, orange-peel appearance frequently seen on the surface of the attached gingiva.

19

Periodontal Disease Development

LEARNING OBJECTIVES

Upon successful completion of these exercises, you will be able to:

1. Identify and define the key terms and concepts related to the development of periodontal disease.

2. Identify and define the key terms and concepts related to periodontal staging and grading.

3. Classify and describe periodontal diseases and conditions.

4. Discuss the development of gingival and periodontal infections.

5. Identify the risk factors for development of periodontal disease.

 KNOWLEDGE EXERCISES

Write your answers for each question in the space provided.

1. Does periodontitis cause cardiovascular disease? Explain your answer.

_____

_____

_____

_____

_____

_____

2. List four reasons for conducting a periodontal risk assessment.

_____

_____

_____

_____

_____

_____

_____

_____

3. List the common modifiable risk factors for periodontal disease.

_____

_____

_____

_____

4. What percentage of risk is genetic for periodontal disease?

_____

5. List the signs associated with perfect periodontal health.

_____

_____

_____

_____

_____

6. What are the clinical signs of gingivitis?

_____

_____

_____

_____

7. What is the primary cause of gingivitis?

_____

_____

8. List the types of medications commonly associated with drug-induced gingivitis.

_____

_____

_____

_____

9. Define the term *microbiome.*

_____

_____

_____

_____

10. What is the difference between the microbiome of gingivitis compared to the microbiome of periodontitis?

_____

_____

_____

_____

11. Name the systemic diseases and conditions that can influence the occurrence and severity of periodontitis.

_____

_____

_____

_____

_____

12. Periodontitis can be associated with genetic disorders. Name the types of conditions associated with periodontitis.

_____

_____

_____

13. Describe the tissue appearance of necrotizing periodontal disease.

_____

_____

_____

14. List the dental factors that modify or predispose the area to biofilm-induced gingival diseases/periodontitis. Provide an example of each factor.

_____

_____

_____

_____

_____

15. Describe the term *mucogingival involvement.*

_____

_____

_____

_____

16. Match each descriptive statement with the appropriate stage of development of gingivitis and periodontal disease. Each answer may be used more than once.

Developmental Stage	Description
A. Initial lesion	_____ Inflammatory response to biofilm occurs within 2–4 days
B. Early lesion	_____ The gingivitis is reversible when biofilm is controlled and inflammation is reduced; healthy tissue may be restored
	_____ Migration and infiltration of white blood cells into the junctional epithelium and gingival sulcus
	_____ Signs of gingivitis become apparent with slight gingival enlargement
	_____ No clinical evidence of change
	_____ Infiltration of fluid, lymphocytes, and neutrophils with a few plasma cells into the connective tissue
	_____ Biofilm becomes older and thicker (7–14 days; time reflects individual differences)
	_____ Increased flow of gingival sulcus fluid

17. Match each descriptive statement with the appropriate stage of development of gingivitis and periodontal disease. Each answer may be used more than once.

Developmental Stage	Description
C. Established lesion	_____ Alveolar bone resorption and collagen breakdown occurs
	_____ Plasma and B-lymphocyte migration into connective tissues increase
D. Advanced lesion	_____ Exposed cementum where Sharpey fibers were attached becomes altered by inflammatory products of bacteria and the sulcus fluid
	_____ Clear evidence of inflammation is present, with marginal redness, bleeding on probing, and spongy marginal gingiva; later, chronic fibrosis develops
	_____ Proliferation of the junctional and sulcular epithelium continues in an attempt to wall out the inflammation
	_____ Periods of disease activity alternating with periods of activity
	_____ Connective tissue fibers below the junctional epithelium are destroyed; the epithelium migrates along the root surface
	_____ Coronal portion of junctional epithelium becomes detached
	_____ Diseased cementum contains a thin superficial layer of endotoxins from the bacterial breakdown
	_____ Formation of pocket epithelium

18. In your own words, define and describe a periodontal pocket. Include the following in your description:
- *What distinguishes a pocket from a sulcus?*
- *Describe the walls and the base of a pocket.*
- *Compare the histology of a healthy pocket and the histopathology of a diseased pocket.*

_____

_____

_____

_____

_____

_____

_____

_____

_____

_____

_____

_____

19. Use the following terms to label the following figure, which illustrates types of periodontal pockets.

A   B   C   D

- *Normal relationship*
- *Gingival pocket*
- *Periodontal pocket*
- *Suprabony*
- *Intrabony*
- *Cementoenamel junction*
- *Alveolar bone*
- *Gingival tissue*
- *Calculus*

A. _____

B. _____

C. _____

D. _____

20. In your own words, describe a pseudopocket.

_____

_____

_____

_____

_____

_____

_____

_____

21. When a pocket is identified as an infrabony pocket, where is the base of the pocket?

_____

_____

22. What is the main factor considered when classifying periodontitis?

_____

_____

23. When the extent and distribution of bone loss is limited to the incisor and molar areas, what might this suggest to the clinician?

_____

_____

24. Match each of the following definitions with the correct term.

Factor	Definition
A. Etiologic factor	_____ A factor that lends assistance to, supplements, or adds to a condition or disease
B. Predisposing factor	
C. Risk factor	_____ A factor that results from or is influenced by a general physical or mental disease or condition
D. Contributing factor	
E. Local factor	_____ A factor that is the actual cause of a disease or condition
F. Systemic factor	
	_____ A factor in the immediate environment of the oral cavity or specifically in the environment of the teeth or periodontium
	_____ A factor that renders a person susceptible to a disease or condition
	_____ An exposure that increases the probability that disease will occur

25. List the types of information/data collected during a basic periodontal examination.

_____

_____

_____

_____

_____

_____

_____

_____

_____

_____

26. List the symptoms of periodontal disease that a patient may notice or feel.

_____

_____

_____

_____

_____

_____

27. Match the term to the description of periodontal disease.

Term	Description
___ Severity	A. More than 30% of the gingiva is involved
___ Marginal	B. Spread out, dispersed, affects multiple tissues
___ Papillary	
___ Generalized	C. Change confined to free gingiva
___ Diffuse	D. Involvement around a single tooth or specific group of teeth
___ Localized	
	E. Quantity of clinical attachment loss
	F. The tissue change does not involve the free gingiva

28. Use the information from the Flow Chart for Grading Periodontitis (Figure 19-16 in the **textbook**) to answer the following questions

a. What risk factors are used to help determine the periodontitis grade?

_____

_____

b. When the loss of periodontal tissues is in proportion to the amount of biofilm deposit, what is the rate of periodontitis progression?

_____

_____

c. List two examples of direct evidence.

_____

_____

d. How are the risk factors used to grade periodontitis?

_____

_____

29. Use the information from the Flow Chart for Periodontitis Staging (Figure 19-15 in the **textbook**) to answer the following questions.

a. What type of bone loss is evident in stage II periodontitis?

_____

_____

b. If the CAL is 1–2 mm, what is the stage of the periodontitis?

_____

_____

c. What stage of periodontitis is associated with 6 mm or more probing depths?

_____

_____

d. If seven teeth have been lost due to periodontitis, what is the periodontal stage?

_____

_____

30. Match the grading and staging term to the description of the action by the clinician. Terms may be used more than once.

Term	Action by Clinician
A. Initial assessment	_____ Assess extent and distribution of disease and factors impacting complexity
B. Staging	_____ Assess rate of progress by diving RBL (radiographic bone loss) by age
C. Grading	_____ Conduct risk assessment
	_____ Assess risk factors such as smoking and diabetes control
	_____ Identify areas of interdental clinical attachment loss (CAL)
	_____ Complete patient history, radiographs, and periodontal examination
	_____ Evaluate the extent and distribution of disease and factors impacting complexity
	_____ Determine the rate of bone loss, either CAL or RBL, over time based on past records
	_____ Evaluate extent of RBL and maximum CAL
	_____ Rule out nonperiodontal causes for loss of attachment
	_____ Evaluate attachment loss in relationship to the amount of biofilm present
	_____ Identify type of bone loss and furcation involvement

COMPETENCY EXERCISES

Apply information from the chapter and use critical thinking skills to complete the competency exercises. Write responses on paper or create electronic documents to submit your answers.

1. After probing, you determine that disease is limited to the gingiva. Discuss the care planning objectives and some questions you may have for your patient.

2. Your next patient presents with interproximal apical positioning of the periodontal attachment, with alveolar bone loss and other indications of periodontitis. Identify some questions, concerns, and general guidelines you will consider as you start to plan treatment for this patient.

3. As you assess your patient Chu His, you observe that clear evidence of inflammation is present, with marginal redness, bleeding on probing, and spongy marginal gingival. He has poorly contoured restorations and a history of diabetes and candidiasis infections. Describe the disease classification you would use for this patient.

4. You detect a Class II furcation on tooth 30 and a Class III furcation involvement on tooth 31 as you collect data for your 10:00 am patient, Woody Green. Woody asks many questions and wants to understand what these terms mean. Explain the terms to him, and use drawings of the teeth to help describe the conditions.

5. You are asked to develop patient education materials for the practice you are in. You decide to focus on local contributing factors in disease development. Develop a checklist that can be filled out during a patient education session to identify specific factors relevant for each individual patient.

EVERYDAY ETHICS

Before completing the learning exercises below, reread and reflect on the Everyday Ethics Scenario and Questions for Consideration in this chapter of the **textbook**. It may also be useful to review the Dental Hygiene Ethics discussion in Chapter 1, the Ethical Applications in the introduction pages for each section in the **textbook**, as well as the Codes of Ethics in **textbook** Appendices I–IV.

Discovery Activity

Ask a dental hygienist who has been practicing for a year or more to read the scenario. Provide a copy of the Code of Ethics as well. Share the responses you have made to answer each question and ask that person to discuss the situation with you. What

insights did you have or what did you learn during this discussion?

Collaborative Learning Activity

Work with a small group to develop a 2–5-minute role-play that introduces the everyday ethics scenario described in the chapter (a great idea is to video record your role-play activity). Then develop separate 2-minute role-play scenarios that provide at least two alternative approaches/solutions to resolving the situation. Ask classmates to view the solutions, ask questions, and discuss the ethical approach used in each. Ask for a vote on which solution classmates determine to be the "best."

Factors to Teach the Patient

This scenario is related to the following factors listed in this chapter of the **textbook**:

▷ Factors that contribute to disease development and progression.

▷ What a risk factor is and the importance of planning personal and professional care to include risk factor problems.

During data collection for your patient Maria Manuela Rodriguez, you note the following information:

▷ She smokes two packs of cigarettes per day.

▷ She takes 10 mg Fosamax (alendronate) per day to prevent/control osteoporosis.

▷ There is a family history of diabetes.

▷ She is overweight.

▷ She takes 10 mg Procardia three times a day to treat her high blood pressure and ventricular arrhythmia (this is nifedipine, which is a calcium channel blocker).

▷ She tends to have a soft diet.

Use the principles of motivational interviewing as a guide to write a dialogue explaining Maria's risk factors for periodontal disease. Use the ideas from this written dialogue to role-play a counseling session with a student colleague.

MeSH TERMS

Use a combination of MeSH terms and other key words to develop an effective and efficient PubMed literature search strategy.

Periodontal diseases   Gingivitis
Periodontitis   Gingival pocket
Periodontal pocket   Gingival recession
Gingival diseases   Gingival hyperplasia

CHAPTER 19 WORD SEARCH PUZZLE

```
L P E W I M O O E K S R I B R L D R L S D Y Y I
D Y M Z P C J A R H W S L Q N F V X K Y T R U I
P L Y X N X V L N S N G U S U H D J N C J O M T
I F Z M C M I X C N E U Y Z Z A Y M X I B P J U
L H N P I C C Y O O Z T V W K T O S U T A U S J
H X E A O G R W L B F F Y D P W Y A V C I I I J
S P E T B U U K L Y S I B C E X E Z T E T A A I
A E J H V B M I A X E V A H O D Y I Z I J J N I
U R K O K M C A G K T T I T E K O Q V B M N H H
C I I G L W F C E W J A E M R N U I H F S O O W
K O Q E U N I P N H F I A I S O G E T B S N O E
T D B N Z I W X Z A X G H S Z N G S L T F F P X
D O L E G X I Y M D D D N C I Q Q E R F W W A J
W N X S Q O O A E I D W V G E N J E N W Q N K P
U T V I N T L I E A M Z C P O Z S A E I P I A V
Y I O S S U Q M V S E N L A O P T N R E C S J Y
C T A F M L M O P T J L T R O L A H X Z K F C E
G I L F L M L T E E N N B N M E C X X K S B Y V
F S G U Z F M S Q M Q O S A Z V O R W G P V E W
E S H C H O W O R A F E I G E L O U L V V B J K
K T O Q N C S R N P O Y G S G M Z Z V Q H H A Y
R O J G R U I E A Y U F S C E Z R E N K D U G V
P N A T Y C A X N N V G W W D L T E Z Y K L D G
O D B A N O I T A M A U Q S E D Y N P P D R Y Z
```

Puzzle Clues

1. Refers to wounds, sores, ulcers, tumors, or any other tissue damage.
2. The numbers of these increase inside the diseased pocket as inflammation increases.
3. White fibers of the connective tissue.
4. Poison; protein produced by certain animals, higher plants, and pathogenic bacteria.
5. Shedding of the outer epithelial layer of the stratified squamous epithelium of skin or mucosa.
6. Accumulation of excessive fluid in cells or tissues.
7. Forceful wedging of food into the periodontium by occlusal forces.
8. Inflammation of the gingiva.
9. Natural open contact.
10. Inflammation of the periodontium.
11. Protein secreted by body cells that acts as a catalyst to induce chemical changes in other substances.
12. Permitting passage of a fluid.
13. Dryness of the mouth from a lack of normal secretions.
14. Process by which a disease develops and progresses.
15. The way in which an individual's immune response interacts with microorganisms (two words).
16. Resulting from treatment by a professional person.

20

Periodontal Examination

 KNOWLEDGE EXERCISES

Write your answers for each question in the space provided.

1. List the basic instruments used for the periodontal examination.

_____

_____

_____

_____

2. Describe the purposes and uses of mouth mirrors.

_____

_____

_____

_____

_____

_____

_____

_____

3. Match each term with the correct definition (see continuation of this question on the next page).

Examination Procedures Term	Definition
_____ Horizontal bone loss	A. A slender instrument, usually round in diameter with a rounded tip, designed for examination of the teeth and soft tissues
_____ Clinical attachment level	
_____ Explorer	B. Probing depth as measured from the cementoenamel junction (or other fixed point) to the location of the probe tip at the coronal level of attached periodontal tissues
_____ Bifurcation	
_____ Fremitus	C. Determination of the accuracy of an instrument by measurement of its variation from a standard
_____ Tactile	
_____ Explorer tip	D. The distance from the gingival margin to the location of the periodontal probe tip at the coronal border of attached periodontal tissues
_____ Calibration	

Examination Procedures Term	Definition
_____ Probe _____ Probing depth _____ Tactile discrimination	E. A slender stainless-steel instrument with a fine, flexible, sharp point used for examination of the surfaces of the teeth to detect irregularities F. A vibration perceptible by palpation G. Pertaining to touch H. The ability to distinguish relative degrees of roughness and smoothness I. Two roots J. Slender, wirelike, circular in cross section, and tapering to a fine, sharp point K. When the crest of the bone is parallel with a line between the cementoenamel junctions of two adjacent teeth

4. How does the application of air improve assessment procedures?

_____

_____

_____

_____

_____

_____

5. List the purposes of using an explorer.

_____

_____

_____

_____

_____

6. List the parts of an explorer.

_____

_____

_____

7. List two sensory stimuli engaged through use of an explorer.

_____

_____

8. What operator techniques will contribute to increased tactile sensitivity?

_____

_____

_____

9. What information is learned by the dental hygienist through auditory stimuli when using an explorer?

_____

_____

_____

10. Why is it important to not remove the explorer from the pocket after each stroke?

_____

_____

11. What action will prevent damage to the tissue by the tip and point of the explorer during subgingival exploring?

_____

12. What are the purposes of using a periodontal probe?

_____

_____

_____

_____

_____

_____

_____

_____

_____

13. When is a plastic periodontal probe used?

_____

_____

14. Describe the purpose and use of a probe with a curved working end.

_____

_____

_____

_____

15. What is the difference between a sulcus and a periodontal pocket?

_____

_____

_____

_____

16. What is measured during periodontal probing?

_____

_____

17. In addition to measuring the depth of a pocket/sulcus, what additional information can be identified with a probe?

_____

_____

18. List factors that influence the accuracy of the probing measurements.

_____

_____

_____

_____

_____

19. List five sources of error in periodontal probing.

_____

_____

_____

_____

20. List three factors that interfere with probing.

_____

_____

_____

_____

_____

21. The probe reading in part A of the following figure is _____. The probe reading in part B of the figure is _____.

A   B

22. Match the health status of the periodontium with the appropriate location of the probe tip.

Periodontal Status	Location of Probe Tip
_____ Gingivitis and early periodontitis	A. At the base of the sulcus or crevice, at the coronal end of the junctional epithelium
_____ Normal healthy tissue	B. Penetrates through the junctional epithelium to reach attached connective tissue fibers
_____ Advanced periodontitis	C. Within the junctional epithelium

23. What types of preliminary assessments should be done prior to the periodontal examination?

_____

_____

_____

_____

_____

_____

_____

24. When probing a sulcus, which tooth structure is touched by the probe?

_____

25. When probing a pocket, which tooth structures are touched by the probe?

_____

_____

26. Describe why it is important to keep the probe as parallel to the long axis of the tooth as possible.

_____

_____

_____

27. The probe is adapted to individual teeth and surfaces. In your own words, describe how to adapt the probe for each of the following structures.

- _Molars and premolars_

_____

_____

_____

_____

_____

_____

_____

_____

- _Anterior teeth_

_____

_____

_____

_____

_____

Proximal surfaces

_____

_____

_____

_____

_____

_____

_____

_____

_____

28. Identify the location of the six measurements recorded for each tooth in the periodontal probing record.

_____

_____

_____

_____

_____

_____

29. Describe what you would do if you encountered a significant calculus deposit during probing.

_____

_____

_____

_____

30. What is meant by the term "walking stroke"?

_____

_____

_____

_____

_____

_____

31. Describe CAL.

_____

_____

_____

_____

32. Explain the significance of CAL?

_____

_____

_____

33. List two fixed points that can be used during the calculation of CAL.

_____

_____

34. List two points that are used to measure pocket depth.

_____

_____

35. List the steps for determining CAL in the presence of visible gingival recession.

_____

_____

_____

_____

36. List the steps for determining CAL when the CEJ is covered by gingiva.

_____

_____

_____

_____

37. True or False (circle one). Provide a reason for your answer. The probing depth equals the clinical attachment level when the free gingival margin is level with the cementoenamel junction.

_____

_____

38. True or False (circle one). Provide a reason for your answer. When there is visible recession, the probing depth is greater than the clinical attachment loss.

_____

_____

39. List two reasons to conduct a mucogingival examination.

_____

_____

_____

40. Describe one method to make the facial mucogingival margin become visible.

_____

_____

_____

_____

41. Describe how to measure the width of the attached gingiva.

_____

_____

_____

_____

_____

42. Describe why it is important to use two single-ended metal instruments with wide blunt ends to measure mobility.

_____

_____

43. Match the level of mobility to its descriptor.

Miller Index of Tooth Mobility	Description
N	____ Slight mobility, greater than normal
1	
2	____ Vertical as well as horizontal movement
3	____ Physiologic mobility
	____ Greater than 1 mm displacement

44. What is fremitus?

_____

_____

45. Why are only maxillary teeth used to determine fremitus?

_____

_____

46. Briefly describe how to conduct the examination for fremitus.

_____

_____

_____

_____

_____

_____

_____

_____

_____

_____

47. Describe the clinical findings of each stage of furcation involvement.

Glickman Furcation Grade	Description
I	
II	
III	
IV	

48. Match each tooth with the appropriate anatomic features. There are two answers for each type of tooth.

Type of Tooth	Anatomic Features
Mandibular molars _____ and _____ Maxillary molars _____ and _____ Maxillary first premolars _____ and _____ Maxillary primary molars _____ and _____ Mandibular primary molars _____ and _____	A. Furcation area is accessible from the mesial and distal aspects, under the contact area B. Palatal root and two buccal roots (mesiobuccal and distobuccal); access for probing is from the mesial, buccal, and distal surfaces C. Bifurcation D. Widespread roots E. Furcation area is accessible from the facial and lingual surfaces F. Trifurcation

49. Match the tooth surface irregularities with the correct tactile sensation. Each answer is used more than once.

Tooth Surface Irregularity	Tactile Sensation
_____ Enamel pearl	A. Normal
_____ Smooth surface of enamel	B. Irregular: increases or elevations in tooth surface
_____ Carious lesion	C. Irregular: depressions, grooves
_____ Anatomic configurations, such as cingula, furcations	
_____ Abrasion	
_____ Root surface that has been planed	
_____ Calculus	
_____ Erosion	
_____ Irregular margins (overhang)	
_____ Pits such as those caused by enamel hypoplasia	
_____ Areas of cemental resorption on the root surface	
_____ Unusually pronounced cementoenamel junction	
_____ Deficient margins	
_____ Overcontoured restoration	
_____ Rough surface of a restoration	

50. Radiographic evidence of periodontal disease includes changes in:

_____

_____

_____

51. Describe how normal bone level appears in a dental radiograph.

_____

_____

52. What is vertical bone loss?

_____

_____

_____

53. Describe horizontal bone loss.

_____

_____

_____

54. How does the periodontal ligament appear in a dental radiograph?

_____

_____

COMPETENCY EXERCISES

Apply information from the chapter and use critical thinking skills to complete the competency exercises. Write responses on paper or create electronic documents to submit your answers.

1. Your employer, Dr. Harriet Golden, asks you put together instrument kits for the office and label them "basic assessment setup." Identify the instruments you have placed in the kit and discuss why you have included each one.

2. Whenever you are using air, you should take care to avoid some very specific situations that may hurt or startle the patient. List some of these situations and describe how you would avoid them.

3. When your instructor verifies your probing, many differences are found. You are having difficulty and need to look at the factors that affect probe determinations and probing procedures. Knowing the right question to ask yourself is a great way to solve a problem. Develop questions that will help you look at these factors and allow you to self-evaluate your own performance.

4. Identify the number on the handle of each explorer in your student kit. Describe the design of the working end, shank, and handle and construction of each part and specify its use.

5. Your patient Tony Wade presents with both mobility (III on teeth 22–27) and fremitus (+ on teeth 6–11). You note generalized bleeding and probe readings of 5–8 mm. The radiographs show horizontal bone loss in all posterior and anterior areas and vertical bone loss on the distal side of tooth 29. The crestal lamina dura is indistinct, irregular, and radiolucent throughout Tony's mouth. There are furcation involvements on teeth 30 and 31. The periodontal ligament spaces are thickened on teeth 28 and 29. Describe how the pocket depth, mobility, and fremitus findings were determined.

6. Label Tony's radiograph in the figure below with the following findings.

Findings
- *Horizontal bone loss*
- *Vertical bone loss*
- *Change in crestal lamina dura*
- *Furcation involvement*
- *Changes in the periodontal ligament*

EVERYDAY ETHICS

Before completing the learning exercises below, reread and reflect on the Everyday Ethics Scenario and Questions for Consideration in this chapter of the **textbook**. It may also be useful to review the Dental Hygiene Ethics discussion in Chapter 1, the Ethical Applications in the introduction pages for each section in the **textbook**, as well as the Codes of Ethics in **textbook** Appendices I–IV.

Individual Learning Activity

Imagine that you are the dental hygienist in this scenario. Answer each of the questions for consideration at the end of the scenario.

Collaborative Learning Activity

Work with a small group to develop a 2–5-minute role-play that introduces the everyday ethics scenario described in the chapter (a great idea is to video record your role-play activity). Then develop separate 2-minute role-play scenarios that provide at least two alternative approaches/solutions to resolving the situation. Ask classmates to view the solutions, ask questions, and discuss the ethical approach used in each. Ask for a vote on which solution classmates determine to be the "best."

Factors to Teach the Patient

This scenario is related to the following factors listed in this chapter of the **textbook**:

▷ The need for a careful, thorough examination if treatment is to be complete and effective.

▷ Information about the instruments and how their use makes the examination complete (e.g., the complete radiographic survey, probing 360° around each tooth, and exploring each subgingival tooth surface).

▷ Why bleeding can occur when probing. Healthy tissue does not bleed.

▷ The relation of probing depth measurements to normal sulci.

▷ The significance of mobility.

You have completed assessment procedures for Tony Wade (described in Competency Exercises 5 and 6). He is very confused about all the tests you have just performed and what all the information means. He wants you to take the time to explain all the data you have collected and the significance of the information you have identified.

Use the motivational interviewing approach (see **workbook** Appendix D) as a guide to create a conversation to explain to Tony the need for a careful examination, why bleeding can occur, the relationship of probing depth measurements to normal sulci, and the significance of the mobility. Be sure to refer to the figure you labeled in Competency Exercise 6 to illustrate some of your points. You may find it helpful to draw some pictures when discussing probing depths.

MeSH TERMS

Use a combination of MeSH terms and other key words to develop an effective and efficient PubMed literature search strategy.

Periodontium
Periodontal pocket
Periodontal ligament
Epithelial attachment
Gingiva
Gingival pocket

Gingival recession
Periodontal attachment loss
Alveolar bone loss
Tooth mobility

21

Indices and Scoring Methods

LEARNING OBJECTIVES

Upon successful completion of these exercises, you will be able to:

1. Identify and define the key terms and concepts related to dental indices and scoring methods.

2. Identify the purpose, criteria for measurement, scoring methods, range of scores, and reference or interpretation scales for a variety of dental indices.

3. Select and calculate dental indices for use in a specific patient or community situation.

KNOWLEDGE EXERCISES

Write your answers for each question in the space provided.

Dental Indices Infomaps

Infomaps are tables that place related information about different factors of one topic on a single page. This method of organizing not only allows you to learn information as you transfer key points from the textbook but also provides a study guide that lets you visually compare and contrast the different dental indices easily and effectively.

Transfer enough basic information about each index from the **textbook** to the appropriate Infomap so that you can use the collected data to complete the competency exercises for this chapter. The blank Infomaps 21-1 to 21-5 are found on the next few pages.

INFOMAP 21-1 | ORAL HYGIENE STATUS INDICES

INDEX	WHAT IS MEASURED?	TEETH AND/OR SURFACES SCORED	CRITERIA USED FOR MEASUREMENT	SCORING/CALCULATION OF INDEX	REFERENCE SCALES, RANGE OF SCORES, AND ADDITIONAL INFORMATION
Biofilm index					
Biofilm control record					
Biofilm-free score					
PHP					
OHI-S					

INFOMAP 21-2	GINGIVAL HEALTH INDICES				
INDEX	WHAT IS MEASURED?	TEETH AND/OR SURFACES SCORED	CRITERIA USED FOR MEASUREMENT	SCORING/CALCULATION OF INDEX	REFERENCE SCALES, RANGE OF SCORES, AND ADDITIONAL INFORMATION
SBI					
GBI					
EIBI					
GI					

INFOMAP 21-3	INDIVIDUAL AND COMMUNITY PERIODONTAL INDICES				
INDEX	WHAT IS MEASURED?	TEETH AND/OR SURFACES SCORED	CRITERIA USED FOR MEASUREMENT	SCORING/CALCULATION OF INDEX	REFERENCE SCALES, RANGE OF SCORES, AND ADDITIONAL INFORMATION
PSR					
CPI					

INFOMAP 21-4 — DENTAL CARIES INDICES

INDEX (AND AUTHOR)	WHAT IS MEASURED?	TEETH AND/OR SURFACES SCORED	CRITERIA USED FOR MEASUREMENT	SCORING/CALCULATION OF INDEX	REFERENCE SCALES, RANGE OF SCORES, AND ADDITIONAL INFORMATION
DMFT					
DMFS					
dft and dfs					
deft and defs					
dmft and dmfs					
ECC and S-ECC					
RCI					

INFOMAP 21-5	FLUOROSIS INDICES				
INDEX	WHAT IS MEASURED?	TEETH AND/OR SURFACES SCORED	CRITERIA USED FOR MEASUREMENT	SCORING/CALCULATION OF INDEX	ADDITIONAL INFORMATION
Dean's fluorosis index					
TSIF					

✓ COMPETENCY EXERCISES

Apply information from the chapter and use critical thinking skills to complete the competency exercises. Write responses on paper or create electronic documents to submit your answers.

Community Case Scenario #1: Answer the following questions based on this community case scenario.

You and your classmates conducted an oral health screening of 100 residents at the Mountain View Nursing Home using the ASTDD Basic Screening Survey for Older Adults as part of a statewide initiative to identify the oral health needs of this population. This statewide survey is being conducted because the Department of Community Health received a grant and is planning to set up a mobile clinic to provide dental services for nursing home residents in your city. There is not enough money to offer all possible services for this group of people, but the health department is hoping to provide enough care to meet most of the people's needs.

The screening revealed that 50 residents had both upper and lower dentures, no one presented with root fragments, 25 had untreated decay, and 25 demonstrated need for periodontal care. There were nine residents with suspicious lesions and 14 residents needing care within the next week.

Use the rough data in the scenario to answer the following questions.

1. How many residents participated in the basic screening survey?

_____

2. What percentage of the residents have untreated decay?

_____

3. What percentage of the residents require evaluation of suspicious lesions?

_____

4. What percentage of the residents have an urgent need for care?

_____

5. What percentage of the residents need periodontal care?

_____

Community Case Scenario #2: Answer the following questions based on this community case scenario.

You, several student colleagues, and some of the faculty members at your school are asked to be part of a statewide, community-based oral health surveillance project conducted by your local Department of Community Health.

The project requires that you collect data during the local Toothtown Activity Center Health Fair for young adults aged 17–25 years.

You are excited to be participating in calibration exercises, collecting data with other members of your school team, and then actually calculating and interpreting the results of your own data collection. What a great way to learn about the dental indices you have just been studying!

6. The Department of Community Health has decided to use the DMFT index to collect data about the caries experience of the group of individuals at the activity center. Discuss the advantages and disadvantages of using this index instead of the DMFS index for community screening.

7. After participating in the screening day at the Toothtown Activity Center, you feel quite confident about using the DMFT index and OHI-S to score individuals as well as the GI that your team decided to use. Now it is time to calculate the results and practice interpreting your findings. Using the information in Table 21-1, calculate the individual DMFs, the total group DMF, and the group average DMF.

8. Using the data in Table 21-1, calculate the percentage of DMF teeth in this group that currently have decay.

TABLE 21-1	CALCULATING DMF DATA			
INDIVIDUAL	D	M	F	INDIVIDUAL DMF
Abbe	12	0	14	
Bill	0	0	6	
Charlie	4	2	0	
David	1	0	6	
Edwin	3	0	0	
Frank	0	1	1	
Grace	4	0	6	
Harry	6	0	7	
Ida	18	2	0	
Joe	2	0	5	
Total				
Group average DMF				

9. Using the data in Table 21-1, calculate the percentage of DMF teeth that have been restored.

10. Using the data in Table 21-1, calculate the percentage of individuals in this group who have at least one decayed tooth.

11. Using the data in Table 21-1, calculate the percentage of individuals in this group who have treatment needs.

12. Use Tables 21-2 and 21-3 to calculate a GI score for Grace and an average GI score for all the individuals in the group.

13. What does Grace's GI score mean?

14. What is your interpretation of the average gingival health of the group?

15. Imagine that you have calculated GI scores for more than 150 individuals who were screened at the Activity Center Health Fair. You calculate that this group's average score is 2.78. How can you use this group average score as baseline data to evaluate the effect of oral hygiene presentations that you and your students will provide at a later time? In other words, explain how you might use this baseline average GI score to determine whether the people in this community were motivated to better oral health because of your education project.

16. Use Table 21-4 to calculate a DI score, a CI score, and an OHI-S score for Bill.

TABLE 21-2	CALCULATING GI DATA: AREA SCORES FOR GRACE			
Tooth	D	M	F	L
3 (16)	2	0	2	0
9 (21)	0	0	0	0
12 (24)	1	0	1	0
19 (36)	2	0	2	0
25 (41)	0	0	0	0
28 (44)	1	0	1	0
Total				
GI score				

TABLE 21-4	OHI-S DATA FOR BILL	
Tooth	DI	CI
3 (16)	3	0
8 (11)	3	0
14 (26)	3	2
19 (36)	3	0
24 (31)	3	0
30 (46)	2	0
Total		
Scores		
OHI-S score		

17. Use Table 21-5 to calculate a group OHI-S score. Make sure to include Bill's score.

TABLE 21-3	CALCULATING THE GROUP AVERAGE GI SCORE
Name	GI SCORE
Charlie	2.9
Harry	1.0
Ida	1.7
Joe	2.6
Grace	?_____
Total	
Group average GI	

TABLE 21-5	CALCULATING GROUP OHI-S DATA
INDIVIDUAL	OHI-S SCORE
Abbe	4.33
Bill	?_____
Charlie	1.20
David	1.03
Edwin	1.00
Group OHI-S score	

18. What does each individual person's OHI-S score indicate about his or her oral cleanliness? What does the average group score indicate?

DISCOVERY EXERCISE

Explore the Association of State and Territorial Dental Directors website (http://www.astdd.org) to locate information about the Basic Screening Surveys: An Approach to Monitoring Community Oral Health community data collection system. Many states in the United States use this system to gather oral health surveillance data. Download and study all of the components that are available on the website to help you learn about how this oral health surveillance system works. Consider purchasing the training videotape so you and your classmates can be trained to use the system in a future community screening.

MeSH TERMS

Use a combination of MeSH terms and other key words to develop an effective and efficient PubMed literature search strategy.

Data collection	Population surveillance
Dental health surveys	Public health surveillance
Dental plaque index	Incidence
DMF index	Prevalence
Oral hygiene index	World Health
Periodontal index	Organization

EVERYDAY ETHICS

Before completing the learning exercises below, reread and reflect on the Everyday Ethics Scenario and Questions for Consideration in this chapter of the **textbook**. It may also be useful to review the Dental Hygiene Ethics discussion in Chapter 1, the Ethical Applications in the introduction pages for each section in the **textbook**, as well as the Codes of Ethics in **textbook** Appendices I–IV.

Individual Learning Activity

Identify a situation you have experienced that presents a similar ethical dilemma. Write about you would do differently now than you did at the time the incident happened—support your discussion with concepts from the dental hygiene codes of ethics.

Collaborative Learning Activity

Answer each of the questions for consideration at the end of the scenario in the **textbook**. Compare what you wrote with answers developed by another classmate and discuss differences/similarities.

Factors to Teach the Patient

This scenario is related to the following factors listed in this chapter of the **textbook**:

▷ How an index is used and calculated and what the scores mean.

▷ Correlation of index scores with current oral health practices and procedures.

▷ Procedures to follow to improve index scores and bring the oral tissues to health.

As you are marking the areas of biofilm on the patient form, Mrs. Combs asks why dental hygienists always bother to do all that "extra work" just to provide oral hygiene instructions. Apparently no one had ever explained it to her before.

Using a motivational interviewing approach (see **workbook** Appendix D), develop points you will want to cover in an imaginary dialogue explaining these dental indices to your patient.

Use the conversation you create to role-play this situation with a fellow student. If you are the patient in the role-play, be sure to ask questions. If you are the dental hygienist, try to anticipate questions and answer them in your explanation.

CHAPTER 21 CROSSWORD PUZZLE

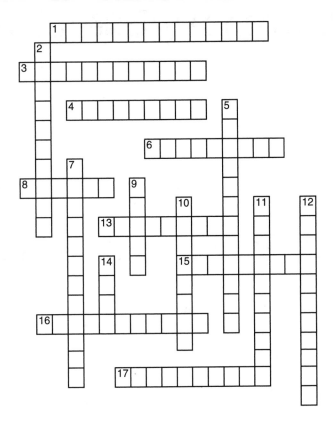

Puzzle Clues

Across

1. The process of gathering information.

3. Ongoing systematic collection, analysis, and interpretation of data for use in planning, implementing, and evaluating public health programs and practices.

4. Assessment of characteristics in a population that can disclose incidence or prevalence of specific diseases.

6. Process to determine accuracy and consistency between examiners.

8. Type of index that measures the presence or absence of a condition.

13. A factor measured and analyzed to describe health status.

15. The rate at which new cases of a specific disease occurs.

16. Ability of an index to measure consistently at different times and under a variety of conditions.

17. Number of cases of a specific disease or condition in existence in a given population at a certain time.

Down

2. Type of index that measures all the evidence of a condition, past and present.

5. Type of index that measures conditions that will not change.

7. Study of health and disease in populations.

9. Describes oral status by expressing clinical observations as numeric values.

10. Ability of an index to measure what it is intended to measure.

11. Index that measures conditions that can be changed.

12. Factors that influence health outcomes of an individual or in a community.

14. Pieces of information.

IV Summary Exercises

Assessment

Chapters 11–21

 COMPETENCY EXERCISES

Apply information from the chapter and use critical thinking skills to complete the competency exercises. Write responses on paper or create electronic documents to submit your answers.

Read Section IV Patient Assessment Summary on the next page to help you answer the following questions.

1. Identify follow-up questions to ask Mrs. Patel that will help you determine any additional information you need to complete this patient's dental hygiene care plan.

2. When you question her, Mrs. Patel states that she has been taking clindamycin, as prescribed by her physician, prior to each dental appointment for many years. Would you request a medical consultation with her physician prior to scheduling a scaling and root planing appointment for Mrs. Patel? Explain why or why not.

3. Use the assessment findings information you have for Mrs. Patel to complete the "At Risk For" sections of her Patient Assessment Summary.

4. Complete the "Periodontal Diagnosis" and "CAM-BRA" sections of the Assessment Summary form. What assessment information was available on the form that helped you to make those decisions? What additional information would be helpful as you completed those sections of the Assessment Form?

 DISCOVERY EXERCISES

1. Collect samples of the worksheets used for patient assessment record-keeping from several dental practices in your community. Compare these systems with those used in your school clinic. Discuss the advantages and disadvantages of each system with your student colleagues.

2. Many patients you provide dental hygiene care for will not speak English (or the language that most people in your country speak) as their first language. Those patients can often have a more difficult time accurately completing health history information. Explore the Internet to discover health history forms that are translated into other languages. A fine place to start is at using the Resource Center Link at the MetDental.com website, https://www.metdental.com/prov/execute/Content. This Web page includes a link leading you to a site where you can download and print health history forms in a variety of languages. Click on the resource center tab at the top of the page and then scroll down to find the link to Multilanguage Health History forms.

3. Look through the scientific literature to find periodontal disease studies that use some of the dental indices you learned about in Chapter 21 to collect data on periodontal disease status.

4. Explore the Internet to find oral health surveillance statistics for your community, state, or country. Analyze the statistics to describe the oral health status, and write a description of specific ways in which the oral health status of the population in your community might be improved by community-based dental hygiene interventions.

FOR YOUR PORTFOLIO

1. Include your personal written responses to the questions in the "Everyday Ethics" section from any of the chapters.

2. Complete patient assessment summaries for several patients who are scheduled with you in your clinic.

3. Demonstrate your interest and the development of your skills in providing culturally competent care by including any patient data collection or patient education materials that you discover for patients who are culturally different from yourself. Include a reflective journal entry describing ways that you can use these materials to enhance the quality of dental hygiene care you provide.

SECTION IV—PATIENT ASSESSMENT SUMMARY

Patient Name: *Mrs. Lorna Patel*	Age: *49*	Gender: F	☑ Initial Therapy
			☐ Maintenance
Provider Name: *D.H. Student*	Date: *Today*		☐ Re-evaluation

Chief Complaint:
Gum tissues bleed when brushing and flossing. Mouth is dry all the time.

Assessment Findings

Health History   **At Risk For:**

- History of high blood pressure managed by medication
- Cholesterol managed by medication
- Mitral valve prolapse
- Allergy to penicillin
- Zocar 20 mg/1 per day
- Caltrate 1 per day
- Enapril 10 mg/hydrochlorothiazide 15 mg/1 per day
- Multiple vitamin 1 per day
- Clindamycin 20.0 g taken 1 hour before appointment
- ASA Classification-II
- ADL level-0

Social and Dental History   **At Risk For:**

- 1.5 years since last recall
- Localized 4- to 5-mm probing depths
- Flosses daily
- Rinses with Listerine
- Mouth dry all the time
- Uses mints and candy for dry mouth
- Uses bottled water with no fluoride content

Dental Examination   **At Risk For:**

- Moderate dental biofilm along cervical margins and proximal surfaces
- Generalized supra- and subgingival calculus
- Light yellow stain
- Posterior gingiva red and bleeding on probing
- Generalized moderate attrition (evidence of bruxism)
- Numerous faulty MOD amalgam restorations
- Localized 4- to 5-mm maxillary and mandibular probing depths

Periodontal Diagnosis/Case Type and Status   **Caries Management Risk Assessment (CAMBRA) level:**

☐ Low   ☐ Moderate   ☐ High   ☐ Extreme

Dental Hygiene Diagnosis and Care Planning

Chapters 22 and 23

SECTION V LEARNING OBJECTIVES

Completing the exercises in this section of the workbook will prepare you to:

1. Use assessment data to write dental hygiene diagnostic statements.
2. Develop a formal dental hygiene care plan based on the dental hygiene diagnosis that sequences evidence-based dental hygiene interventions in order to address identified patient needs.
3. Identify and apply procedures for obtaining informed consent.
4. Document informed consent and the plan for patient care.

COMPETENCIES FOR THE DENTAL HYGIENIST (APPENDIX A)

Competencies supported by the learning in Section V

Core Competencies: C3, C4, C5, C7, C9, C10, C11, C12, C13

Health Promotion and Disease Prevention: HP1, HP2, HP3, HP4, HP5

Patient/Client Care: PC1, PC2, PC3, PC4, PC5, PC6, PC7, PC8, PC9, PC11, PC13

22

Dental Hygiene Diagnosis

KNOWLEDGE EXERCISES

Write your answers for each question in the space provided.

1. Supply the term or concept that matches each of the following descriptions:

   Measure of ability to perform self-care.

   _____

   A measure that integrates a combination of physical and cognitive ability.

   _____

   _____

   Statements that identify a problem.

   _____

   Prediction of outcomes that can be expressed as "good, fair, poor, or questionable."

   _____

   _____

   Systemic conditions, behavioral factors, or environmental factors that can lead to increased probability of oral disease.

   _____

2. Identify factors from the patient assessment that are analyzed and considered when planning dental hygiene care.

   _____

   _____

   _____

   _____

   _____

3. Identify and briefly describe the issues indicated by the mnemonic OSCAR:

   • O

   _____

   • S

   _____

   • C

   _____

   • A

   _____

   • R

   _____

4. Briefly define each of the five ASA classification levels.

_____

_____

_____

_____

_____

5. Define _dental hygiene diagnosis_ in your own words.

_____

_____

_____

6. List patient factors that determine overall prognosis after dental hygiene interventions.

_____

_____

_____

_____

_____

_____

_____

7. In your own words, explain anticipatory guidance.

_____

_____

_____

_____

_____

8. Your patient's clinical diagnosis, provided by the periodontist, is "chronic periodontitis." List the therapeutic goals of treatment for this patient.

_____

_____

_____

_____

_____

_____

_____

_____

_____

_____

_____

_____

_____

9. Explain the concept of oral health literacy.

_____

_____

_____

_____

✓ COMPETENCY EXERCISES

Apply information from the chapter and use critical thinking skills to complete the competency exercises. Write responses on paper or create electronic documents to submit your answers.

1. At which ASA classification levels would you be most likely to consider contacting the patient's physician prior to planning for dental hygiene care? Provide a rationale for your answer.

2. For each of patient scenarios described below:

Identify the OSCAR issue(s) that need to be evaluated.

Determine the ASA classification you will assign when assessing the patient during planning of dental hygiene care.

Write a justification for your selection.

Scenario A: Mrs. Kujath is 90 years old with very good physical and mental health. She has chronic arthritis, which is managed very well with daily pain medication, and only has minor problems with mobility, including sitting still for a long period of time. She doesn't really like the way her old denture looks, and she desires a new denture. She states that there is no problem about having the money to pay for the new denture.

Scenario B: Mr. Diamond has type I diabetes. His blood sugar levels indicate that his diabetes is not well controlled. Mr. Diamond has numerous posterior teeth that present with significant bone loss, generalized mobility, and class II or III furcations. Moreover, he is not particularly compliant with your recommendations for self-care for those furcation areas.

Scenario C: Mrs. Abdul must make a decision about treatment options for several teeth with severe periodontal involvement. Her health history indicates mild hypertension that is well controlled by medication. It has been many years since she has been to the dentist because of an extremely unpleasant dental experience she had as a child. She squirmed and protested when you measured her probing depths and, in general, had a very difficult time cooperating during the collection of assessment data. She says that she must talk with her son as he will be bringing her for her appointments and also be paying for whatever treatment is decided upon.

Scenario D: Ms. Anitha Jones has cerebral palsy. She arrives at the dental office in a wheelchair and is accompanied by an attendant. Because of extreme muscle spasticity caused by her condition, her arms and legs are in constant motion, sometimes lashing out unexpectedly, and she must have a variety of pads and restraints to maintain her position and safety in her wheelchair. You and her caregiver plan to transfer her from her wheelchair to the dental chair for treatment. Her health history indicates that she is not mentally disabled.

3. The best way to learn how to write dental hygiene diagnosis statements is to practice. After completing an initial assessment on a student colleague or patient, use the examples provided in Table 22-5 to help you develop dental hygiene diagnosis for each patient problem identified during the assessment.

4. After completing an initial assessment on a student colleague or patient, identify at least one area of low health literacy and write a dental hygiene diagnosis statement to address that area of need.

MeSH TERMS

Use a combination of MeSH terms and other key words to develop an effective and efficient PubMed literature search strategy.

Health literacy
Risk factors
Periodontal diseases
Diagnosis

Prognosis
Activities of daily living
Health education, dental

Factors to Teach the Patient

This scenario is related to the following factors listed in this chapter of the **textbook**:

▷ Why disease control measures are learned before and in conjunction with scaling?

▷ Facts of oral disease prevention and oral health promotion relevant to the patient's current level of healthcare knowledge and individual risk factors.

Your next patient, Jonathon Meyers, is a 26-year-old graduate student. He has not seen a dentist since he was a child. When his girlfriend told him about his bad breath, he decided to take advantage of the services offered at the dental clinic.

He presents with an aggressive periodontal condition in the lower anterior sextant of his mouth. Because he was not exposed to much dental education in his life, Jon has a low dental IQ and doesn't understand the cause and progression of dental disease. He smokes, demonstrates poor biofilm control, and states that he wants you to just "fix him up" with your treatments.

Using the motivational interviewing approach (see **workbook** Appendix D), write a statement explaining why disease control measures must happen before and in conjunction with scaling. Explain his role in attaining and maintaining oral health.

Use the conversation you create to role-play this situation with a fellow student. If you are the patient in the role-play, be sure to ask questions. If you are the dental hygienist, try to anticipate questions and answer them in your explanation.

EVERYDAY ETHICS

Before completing the learning exercises below, reread and reflect on the Everyday Ethics Scenario and Questions for Consideration in this chapter of the **textbook**. It may also be useful to review the Dental Hygiene Ethics discussion in Chapter 1, the Ethical Applications in the introduction pages for each section in the **textbook**, as well as the Codes of Ethics in **textbook** Appendices I–IV.

Individual Learning Activity

Imagine that you have observed what happened in the scenario, but are not one of the main characters involved in the situation. Write a reflective journal entry that:

- Describes how you might have reacted (as an observer—not as a participant),

- Expresses your personal feelings about what happened, or

- Identifies personal values that affect your reaction to the situation.

Discovery Activity

Ask a friend or relative who is not involved in health care to read the scenario and discuss it with you from the perspective of a "patient" who receives services within the healthcare system. Discuss what you learned from the concerns, insights, or difference in perspective that person expressed.

The Dental Hygiene Care Plan

KNOWLEDGE EXERCISES

Write your answers for each question in the space provided.

1. Define the following terms in your own words.
   - Dental hygiene intervention:

   - Informed consent:

   - Implied consent:

   - Informed refusal:

2. Identify and define the three parts of a dental hygiene care plan.

_____

3. List the 11 components of a written care plan.

_____

4. List three individual patient characteristics that can require significant adaptations in the written dental hygiene care plan.

_____

5. Which of the following is a factor that might affect the *sequence* you select for quadrant scaling and root planing in a dental hygiene care plan? (Circle the correct answer.)

   a. Availability of a power-driven scaler

   b. Patient complaint of pain associated with a periodontal abscess

   c. The amount of calculus in the lower anterior sextant

   d. Chronic systemic disease

6. What is the purpose for explaining the entire treatment plan to the patient?

_____

7. What are some important points to consider when explaining the dental hygiene care plan to the patient?

_____

8. Identify five areas of information you will discuss with the patient when you are obtaining informed consent.

_____

✓ COMPETENCY EXERCISES

Apply information from the chapter and use critical thinking skills to complete the competency exercises. Write responses on paper or create electronic documents to submit your answers.

1. Explain the role of the patient in developing a plan for care that prioritizes the patient's needs.

2. Explain the relationship between the master treatment plan and the dental hygiene care plan.

3. Why are medical, personal, and clinical findings linked to actual or potential risk factors in the assessment findings section of a written dental hygiene care plan?

4. Using your institution's guidelines for writing in patient records, document that the dental hygiene care plan was presented to the supervising dentist prior to explaining the plan to the patient.

5. Use the following information from the case of Jonathon Meyers to answer the questions below. Jon has not seen a dentist since he was a child. When his girlfriend told him about his bad breath, he decided to take advantage of the services offered at the dental clinic in your school.

   Jon presents with an aggressive periodontal condition in the lower anterior sextant of his mouth. He has a low dental IQ and doesn't understand the cause and progression of dental disease. He smokes, demonstrates poor biofilm control, and states that he wants you to just "fix him up" with your treatments.

   a. Write at least one dental hygiene diagnosis statement related to the information provided about the patient in this scenario.

   b. What interventions will you plan to target the problem(s) you identified?

   c. Write a goal for each problem you identified. Include a time frame for meeting the goal. How will you measure whether Jon met the goal?

EVERYDAY ETHICS

Before completing the learning exercises below, reread and reflect on the Everyday Ethics Scenario and Questions for Consideration in this chapter of the **textbook**. It may also be useful to review the Dental Hygiene Ethics discussion in Chapter 1, the Ethical Applications in the introduction pages for each section in the **textbook**, as well as the Codes of Ethics in **textbook** Appendices I–IV.

Individual Learning Activity

Imagine that you have observed what happened in the scenario, but are not one of the main characters involved in the situation. Write a reflective journal entry that:

- Describes how you might have reacted (as an observer—not as a participant),
- Expresses your personal feelings about what happened, or identifies personal values that affect your reaction to the situation.

Discovery Activity

Ask a friend or relative who is not involved in health care to read the scenario and discuss it with you from the perspective of a "patient" who receives services within the healthcare system. Discuss what you learned from the concerns, insights, or difference in perspective that person expressed.

Factors to Teach the Patient

This scenario is related to the following factors listed in this chapter of the **textbook**:

▷ Why patient input into the final care plan is important.

▷ The patient's rights and responsibilities regarding informed consent.

Using the motivational interviewing approach (see **workbook** Appendix D), write a statement explaining to Mrs. Kwan, the patient in the **textbook** everyday ethics scenario for this chapter, what informed consent means.

MeSH TERMS

Use a combination of MeSH terms and other key words to develop an effective and efficient PubMed literature search strategy.

Patient care planning
Comprehensive dental care
Informed consent

Treatment refusal
Patient-centered care
Health education, dental

V Summary Exercises

Dental Hygiene Diagnosis and Care Planning

Chapters 22 and 23

 COMPETENCY EXERCISES

Apply information from the chapter and use critical thinking skills to complete the competency exercises. Write responses on paper or create electronic documents to submit your answers.

SECTION V—PATIENT ASSESSMENT SUMMARY #1

Patient Name: *Mrs. Diane White*   Age: *27*   Gender: F   ☐ Initial Therapy
☑ Maintenance

Student (Clinician) Name: *D.H. Student*   Date: Today   ☐ Re-evaluation

Chief Complaint:

Gum tissues bleed when brushing and flossing.
First trimester of pregnancy with nausea.

Assessment Findings

Medical History

- First trimester of first pregnancy
- Husband smokes cigarettes in house and car
- ASA-II and ADL level-0

Social and Dental History

- One year since last recall
- Generalized 4-mm probing depths
- Infrequent flossing
- Several white spot lesions on cervical surfaces of posterior teeth
- Uses bottled water with no fluoride content
- Smell of fluoridated toothpaste makes her nauseated
- Uses frequent, high-carbohydrate snacking to control nausea

Dental Examination

- Moderate dental biofilm along cervical margins and proximal surfaces
- Posterior gingiva red and bleeding on probing
- No radiographic bone changes

Periodontal Diagnosis/Case Type and Status:

- Biofilm-induced gingivitis

At Risk For:

- Embryo susceptible to injuries and malformations
- Infant at risk for secondhand-smoke exposure

At Risk For:

- Increased incidence of dental caries risk of periodontal conditions

At Risk For:

- Increased incidence of dental caries
- Increased risk of periodontal conditions

Caries Management Risk Assessment (CAMBRA) level:
☐ Low   ☐ Moderate   ☐ High   ☐ Extreme

SECTION V—PATIENT ASSESSMENT SUMMARY #2

Patient Name: *Melody Crane*   Age: *15 months*   Gender: F   ☑ Initial Therapy
                                                                                                                                              ☐ Maintenance
Student (Clinician) Name: *D.H. Student*   Date: *Today*   ☐ Re-evaluation

Chief Complaint:
Gum tissues bleed when mother brushes Melody's teeth.
Melody fights with mother when she brushes her teeth.

Assessment Findings

Medical History
- Frequent ear infections—three since birth
- Liquid antibiotics—contain sweeteners

At Risk For:
- Early childhood caries

Social and Dental History
- Melody's initial dental visit
- Teeth present at 6 months
- Fluoridated water supply—but family drinks mostly bottled water
- Fluoride toothpaste used four times per week—unspecified amount of paste
- Bottle fed two times daily at naptime and bedtime
- At-will use of sippy cup for juice
- Five-year-old brother with restorations on all primary molars and some anteriors
- Parental lack of dental knowledge

At Risk For:
- Early childhood caries
- Fluorosis

Dental Examination
- Moderate dental biofilm along cervical margins of maxillary incisors
- White-spot lesions cervical of four maxillary incisors
- Red maxillary anterior gingiva

At Risk For:
- Early childhood caries
- Gingivitis

Periodontal Diagnosis/Case Type and Status
- Gingivitis

Caries Management Risk Assessment (CAMBRA) level:
☐ Low   ☐ Moderate   ☐ High   ☐ Extreme

Read Section V Patient Assessment Summaries to help you answer questions #1 and #2.

1. Use a copy of the dental hygiene care-plan template in **workbook** Appendix B, or use the care-plan format your school provides to write dental hygiene diagnosis statements for either of the patient summaries above.

2. Use the care-plan template or your school format to write a plan for clinical, education/counseling, and oral hygiene instruction/home care interventions for either Mrs. White or Melody Crane and her parents.

3. Use the careplan template in **workbook** Appendix B or the careplan form used in your clinic to write a formal care plan from assessment data collected during an initial appointment of a patient you are providing care for in your school clinic.

4. Write an outline of important points to address when presenting the care plan to the patient in order to obtain informed consent to proceed with the dental hygiene interventions you have planned.

5. Role-play to present the care plan to the patient.

6. Write a progress note documenting that you have presented the care plan and obtained informed consent.

DISCOVERY EXERCISES

1. Remember Jonathon Meyers, the graduate student from the exercises in Chapters 22 and 23? Imagine that you have now completed his initial therapy plan and are evaluating the results. He has reached most of the goals you set together in the plan, and his oral health status has much improved.

   You recommend a 3-month periodontal maintenance interval, but he wants to wait at least 6 months before coming to see you again. He cites recent toothpaste television commercials that recommend seeing a dentist every 6 months. You know that patients with a history of periodontal infection need to be seen more often.

   Conduct a brief review of recent literature to determine what scientific evidence supports a shorter periodontal maintenance interval. Write an outline of points you will cover when you explain to Jonathon why those research findings influence your recommendations for his continuing care plan.

2. Develop a PICO question related to determining the best fluoride regimen to recommend for a preschool-age child with extreme caries risk.

3. Select two or three current articles from your literature search that seem as if they would be useful for helping you decide which fluoride therapies you will recommend for this preschool-age patient. Either go to the library to find the paper journal or use online full-text sources to read the articles you have selected. Read the articles and evaluate the strength and usefulness of the information that is in them.

 FOR YOUR PORTFOLIO

1. Using the patient-specific dental hygiene care-plan template in **workbook** Appendix B or the care-plan format used in your dental hygiene program, complete comprehensive dental hygiene care plans for a variety of patients you have assessed in your school clinic. Demonstrate your ability to plan for a diverse selection of patients by selecting care plans prepared for patients with a variety of systemic conditions, risk factors, and levels of dental disease.

2. In your portfolio, include a care plan prepared at the beginning of your education and one for a similar patient prepared near the end of your education. Provide a written statement that reflects on and analyzes the ways in which a comparison of the two care plans demonstrates what you have learned about planning patient care.

 QUESTIONS PATIENTS ASK

What sources of information can you identify that will help you answer your patient's questions in this scenario?

"I saw something on the Internet recently about new research that proves that a certain new kind of treatment is more effective than the recommendations you have made in my dental hygiene care plan. Can you change my dental hygiene care plan?"

CHAPTER 23 WORD SEARCH PUZZLE

```
A L J Z L Y O R V E Z I Q J S I S O N G O R P Y
I K I G E V P W U Q F F P F M G Q W C Q Y Q L D
I O D E N T A L H Y G I E N E C A R E P L A N V
V N A I U Z C C J F V P E N I L B C E P U B O T
S Y F W Q R L D A I N O I T N E V R E T N I G S
S I B O Q G M V C H I E F C O M P L A I N T S M
L Y S S R A L K K Q N T W F E B J K C R U X N C
V C I O T M N Y H Y D M R D S E L T X D P B L Y
R A N J N Y E W T Q F W I F G S I T V X L O X D
I R L U R G G D D D K B L O P T A L A I D D R U
S E S B B A A T R U J S S U W P R S I C A G N E
K T G T H S C I H E Y E K O V R Y Y K A Z R Z H
F I J M Y S A M D Y F Q Y I K A I M R M G I V N
A L Y E R E L E R H Q U K V V C Q D Q I T B Z Y
C H V H S S X X F E U E S R S T Z S D I I N B H
T T D X T S X I E U E N L A S I F R R O D V X U
O L L G G M Q A K V F C Q N L C N O L E H D R F
R A I F J E M Y D R C E C O N E I S V P P I A Y
I E T Z C N A T A H Q K W B M R F H H X M Z L U
I H T A B T P Y F G J W R Y P E Y D L O P P E A
D D E N T A L H Y G I E N E D I A G N O S I S R
H I N F O R M E D C O N S E N T Z E X V B I W N
K E N I M O D I F I A B L E K H U L P I B F D A
O U J T X P V Z F N R Q T S J B Q W J O I P U X
```

Puzzle Clues

1. Measure of the ability to carry out the basic tasks needed for self-care.

2. A patient's stated primary concern or reason for seeking professional care (two words).

3. A measure of tasks that require a combination of physical and cognitive ability.

4. Detailed description of the oral health services to be carried out by the dental hygienist and based on the dental hygiene diagnosis (four words).

5. Critical analysis and evaluation of a particular condition or situation.

6. An individual's capacity to obtain, process, and understand basic health information and services needed to make appropriate health decisions (two words).

7. Intervention shown by research and experience to produce optimal results and is established as a standard (two words).

8. Patient's voluntary agreement to a treatment plan after details of the proposed treatment have been presented and comprehended by the patient (two words).

9. Patient's decision to refuse recommended treatment after all options, potential risks, and potential benefits have been thoroughly explained (two words).

10. Arrange a series of events to follow in a certain order or succession.

11. Identification of an oral health problem that a dental hygienist is qualified and licensed to treat (three words).

12. A statement of the problem.

13. Prediction of outcome.

14. Arrange in order of importance.

15. Specific treatment that happens or take place between other events.

16. Attribute or exposure that increases the probability of disease (two words).

17. Risk factors for disease that can be changed by intervention.

Implementation: Prevention

Chapters 24–35

SECTION VI LEARNING OBJECTIVES

Completing the exercises in this section of the workbook will prepare you to:

1. Educate patients regarding the prevention of oral disease.
2. Promote patient behaviors and practices that enhance oral health.
3. Select patient-specific dental hygiene interventions that will prevent oral disease and promote oral health.
4. Document prevention interventions and recommendations.

COMPETENCIES FOR THE DENTAL HYGIENIST (APPENDIX A)

Competencies supported by the learning in Section VI

Core Competencies: C3, C4, C5, C7, C9, C10, C11, C12, C13

Health Promotion and Disease Prevention: HP1, HP2, HP4, HP5

Patient/Client Care: PC10, PC11, PC12, PC13

24

Preventive Counseling and Behavior Change

LEARNING OBJECTIVES

Upon successful completion of these exercises, you will be able to:

1. Explain the steps in a preventive program to motivate patient behavior change, identify the need to conduct preventive counseling, and describe the proper setting.

2. Explain the elements, principles, and processes of motivational interviewing (MI).

3. Describe key factors, core skills, and strategies for implementing an MI approach to patient counseling.

4. Document the outcomes of a patient counseling session.

 KNOWLEDGE EXERCISES

Write your answers for each question in the space provided. Note: **Workbook** Appendix D provides an overview of motivational interviewing (MI) that may be helpful as you study the questions below.

1. Order the steps in a preventive program.

Order	Description
_____	Evaluate progressive changes
_____	Plan for intervention
_____	Plan short- and long-term continuing care
_____	Perform clinical preventive services
_____	Assess the patient's needs
_____	Implement the plan

2. List the factors that need to be considered during the assessment phase of a preventive program.

_____

_____

_____

_____

3. When is preventive counseling conducted?

_____

_____

_____

4. Describe the role of active listening in the MI approach to patient counseling and behavior change.

_____

_____

_____

_____

_____

_____

5. List the things a good listener *does not* do during patient counseling.

_____

_____

_____

_____

6. Why is it necessary to review the patient's behavior change goals during *each* patient appointment?

_____

_____

_____

_____

_____

7. What body language factors lead to a more successful preventive counseling session?

_____

_____

_____

8. Which two behavior change theories form the basis of MI?

_____

_____

9. What are the two essential characteristics of MI?

_____

_____

_____

10. When is brief motivational interviewing (BMI) effective?

_____

_____

_____

11. List the four interrelated elements of the spirit of MI.

P _____

A _____

C _____

E _____

12. List the four patient-centered conditions that demonstrate the clinician's attitude of acceptance.

_____

_____

_____

13. What are the four guiding principles of MI?

R _____

U _____

L _____

E _____

14. Explain why it is necessary for the dental hygienist to resist the "righting reflex" during patient counseling.

_____

_____

_____

_____

_____

_____

_____

15. What is the significance of understanding the patient's motivation?

_____

_____

_____

_____

16. In your own words, describe what is meant by "empower the patient."

_____

_____

_____

_____

_____

_____

_____

17. Identify the four processes of MI based on the brief definitions provided in the table below.

_____	Establish a helpful connection and working relationship
_____	Develop and maintain a specific direction in the conversation about change
_____	Elicit the patient's own motivations for change
_____	Develop the commitment to change and formulating a concrete plan of action

18. List three elements of MI implementation.

_____

_____

_____

19. List two elements of information exchange.

_____

_____

20. List two techniques of asking permission.

_____

_____

21. List two reasons why an exploration of the patient's prior knowledge is necessary.

_____

_____

_____

_____

22. Why is it important to let the patient set the agenda for the information and recommendations to be discussed?

_____

_____

_____

_____

23. List the core skills of MI, which are represented by the acronym OARS.

O _____
A _____
R _____
S _____

24. What is the purpose of asking open-ended questions during an MI session?

_____

_____

_____

25. In your own words, describe affirmation.

_____

_____

_____

_____

26. How does affirmation by the clinician contribute to a patient's health behavior change?

_____

_____

27. Fill in the blank: Good affirmations contain the word _____. Using statements that begin with the word _____ will focus the conversation more on the clinician than the patient.

28. In your own words, define the term "reflective listening."

_____

_____

_____

29. Describe the difference between the two types of reflection responses used in MI.

_____

_____

_____

_____

_____

30. In your own words, describe the difference between sustain talk and change talk.

_____

_____

_____

_____

_____

31. _____ is the point at which the patient is determining whether the benefits of change outweigh the risks of the current behavior.

32. When the clinician takes a neutral position, it allows the patient to:

_____

_____

33. What is the purpose of the Pro/Con matrix?

_____

_____

_____

_____

34. What is the purpose of the readiness ruler?

_____

_____

_____

_____

35. Fill in the blank boxes in Infomap 24-1 to organize concepts related to the four components of preparatory change talk.

36. List the signs that indicate the patient is ready to make changes in a current oral health behavior.

_____

_____

_____

_____

37. Match the type of planning scenario to the description.

Plan Type	Description
A. Clear plan	_____ The patient is developing the plan from scratch
B. Several clear options	_____ The patient knows what they want or need to do
C. Brainstorming	_____ The patient has determined there is more than one way to move toward the goal

38. What two factors most influence whether patient counseling is directed to the caregiver, to the child, or to both?

_____

_____

INFOMAP 24-1	COMPONENTS OF PREPARATORY CHANGE TALK	
COMPONENT	**EXAMPLES OF PATIENT STATEMENTS**	**EXAMPLES OF PHRASES TO STIMULATE CHANGE TALK**
D	I wish to, I want to, I would like to…	
A	I could, I might be able to	
R	Statements identifying a rationale for making a change	
N	I must, I need to, I should do…	

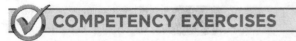

COMPETENCY EXERCISES

Apply information from the chapter and use critical thinking skills to complete the competency exercises. Note: **Workbook** Appendix D provides an overview of MI that may be helpful.

Each of the following patient conversations contains clinician responses that illustrate MI principles and tools. Complete the BMI Session exercises below by indicating the appropriate MI skill or tool on the lines provided for each of the clinician's statements.

BMI Session #1	ENGAGING THE PATIENT	
PERSON SPEAKING	**CONVERSATION STATEMENTS**	**CORE SKILLS AND TOOLS OF MI**
Clinician:	Now that we have updated your medical history and current medications, may I take some time to discuss your systemic health in more detail?	_____
Patient:	Sure ... that's fine.	
Clinician response:	You are insulin diabetic and on a few medications including a calcium channel blocker and statin cholesterol medication. What do you know about your diabetes and your medications and how they affect your oral health?	_____ _____
Patient:	Well ... I read somewhere that diabetics can have problems with their gums and medications can cause dry mouth. I think my gums are good; I brush and floss two times a day. I do drink a lot of water throughout the day because my mouth is dry.	
Clinician response:	So, you are aware of the link between diabetes and gum health. It is great you are taking the necessary daily home care steps to maintain your gum and bone health. Drinking water throughout the day is also good for your oral and systemic health.	_____ _____
	May I discuss the connection of your systemic conditions and medications that are relevant to your oral health?	_____
Patient:	Yes please ... I do my best to stay healthy. My diabetes is well controlled by the insulin pump I have and I never miss a dose of my blood pressure or cholesterol medications.	
Clinician response:	Your health is very important to you. You are really diligent about taking your medications. Would you like to know more about diabetes and periodontal disease or more about your medications first?	_____ _____

BMI Session #2	FOCUSING THE DISCUSSION/EVOKING REASONS	
PERSON SPEAKING	**CONVERSATION STATEMENTS**	**CORE SKILLS AND TOOLS OF MI**
Patient:	I really hate having my teeth cleaned, they always make me bleed, and my gums hurt for days afterward.	
Clinician response:	Having your teeth cleaned is painful and you don't like the bleeding.	_____
Patient:	I know I need to come, but I just don't like it.	
Clinician response:	You know it's important for your health and to keep your teeth, but it's really uncomfortable for you and you wonder if it's worth it.	_____
	What can we do to help make it more comfortable for you so you can come more regularly for your preventive care?	_____

BMI Session #3	EVOKING/ELICITING CHANGE TALK	
PERSON SPEAKING	**CONVERSATION STATEMENTS**	**CORE SKILLS AND TOOLS OF MI**
Patient:	I'm really upset I have all these new cavities this time.	
Clinician response:	You're not happy with what's going on in your mouth.	_____
Patient:	I never had cavities until I stopped smoking. It must all the candy and gum.	
Clinician response:	It is fabulous you have quit smoking! Your health is really important to you.	_____
	What do you already know about how snacking habits cause cavities?	_____
Patient:	Well, I know candy causes cavities, but I have to eat candy or chew gum so I don't smoke.	
Clinician response:	Can I share with you some alternatives that won't cause cavities?	_____
		_____
Patient:	Sure.	
Clinician response:	Gums and mints that are sugarless won't cause cavities. There are many on the market.	_____
	What do you think about that?	_____

BMI Session #4	EXPLORING AMBIVALENCE/DECISIONAL BALANCE	
PERSON SPEAKING	**CONVERSATION STATEMENTS**	**CORE SKILLS AND TOOLS OF MI**
Patient:	I know I shouldn't drink those energy drinks, but I need them to get me through the day.	
Clinician response:	On one hand, you really like the energy you get from them, but, on the other hand, you also realize they're causing your cavities.	_____
Patient:	Yeah, I can't imagine trying to get through the day without them.	
Clinician response:	So, can you tell me some of the good things and bad things about drinking energy drinks?	_____ Exploring decisional balance using the: _____
Patient:	Well, I drink them all day long and they give me energy and keep me going. Sometimes I don't have time for meals, and they help me get through the day. The problem is that now I have a bunch of cavities that's probably from all the sugar.	
Clinician response:	So, on one hand, you feel powerless over this energy drink, but yet you know it's ruining your teeth.	_____
Patient:	Yeah, I don't know what I'm going to do now.	
Clinician response:	What are some advantages and disadvantages of changing your energy drink habit?	_____
Patient:	Well, I sure will save a lot of money and time coming to the dentist!	
Clinician response:	(laughing) Well, that would make anybody happy, right? What else?	_____ _____

Now that you have had a bit of practice identifying the MI skills and tools in some clinician's responses, the next exercise will let you practice responding to a patient statement. As you think about what you will say, remember how important it is to "Resist Righting Reflex" in your response.

As you write your response in the space at the end of BMI Session #5 on the next page, make sure to include statements that:

• Indicate you are listening with compassion.

• Reflect empathetically on the patient's beliefs and values.

• Provide affirmation for the patient's current oral health behaviors.

• Help move the conversation forward toward a solution in a way that empowers the patient.

• Compare your response with those developed by your student colleagues.

BMI Session #5	RESIST RIGHTING REFLEX	
PERSON SPEAKING	**CONVERSATION STATEMENTS**	**CORE SKILLS AND TOOLS OF MI**
Patient:	I hate getting my teeth cleaned ... those metal instruments hurt! My teeth are so sensitive ... to ice cream and coffee too, but those instruments are the worst!	
Clinician response:	Your teeth are supersensitive and you would prefer if we didn't use the metal instruments that hurt so much. What do you know about sensitive teeth?	Simple reflection Empathy open-ended question (elicit)
Patient:	Nothing ... and I don't care "why" my teeth hurt all the time. I just want the sensitivity gone!	
Clinician response:	Okay, you don't want to know what causes sensitive teeth, but you would like a solution. May I suggest some products to reduce your sensitivity?	Simple reflection Asking permission
Patient:	Yes ... but I don't want to hear anything about fluoride! My last hygienist tried to get me to use fluoride toothpaste and rinses. I use all natural toothpaste because fluoride is poison!	
Your response:	_____ _____ _____	Reflection Affirmation Asking permission

EVERYDAY ETHICS

Before completing the learning exercises below, reread and reflect on the Everyday Ethics Scenario and Questions for Consideration in this chapter of the **textbook**. It may also be useful to review the Dental Hygiene Ethics discussion in Chapter 1, the Ethical Applications in the introduction pages for each section in the **textbook**, as well as the Codes of Ethics in **textbook** Appendices I–IV.

Individual Learning Activity

Identify a situation you have experienced that presents a similar ethical dilemma. Write about

you would do differently now than you did at the time the incident happened—support your discussion with concepts from the dental hygiene codes of ethics.

Collaborative Learning Activity

Answer each of the questions for consideration at the end of the scenario in the **textbook**. Compare what you wrote with answers developed by another classmate and discuss differences/similarities.

Factors to Teach the Patient

This scenario is related to the following factors listed in this chapter of the **textbook**:

▷ Elicit from the patient's short- and long-term goals pertaining to what the patient would like to achieve regarding disease status and overall self-care.

▷ Your patient Melina expresses her desire to implement a daily flossing routine. She understands that her bleeding gums are directly related to the fact that she does not floss and has demonstrated her ability to use the floss. During your discussion today, Melina is able to articulate reasons she *should* floss every day. She tells you she tries hard to remember to floss when she brushes, but states how difficult it is for her to fit the extra time for flossing into her daily routine.

Use a motivational interviewing approach (see **workbook** Appendix D) and role-play with a student colleague to develop a conversation that can help this patient set both short- and long-term goals for daily oral care.

MeSH TERMS

Use a combination of MeSH terms and other key words to develop an effective and efficient PubMed literature search strategy.

Health communication
Health education
Health education, dental
Health behavior

Motivational interviewing
Health knowledge, attitudes, practice

Protocols for Prevention and Control of Dental Caries

LEARNING OBJECTIVES

Upon successful completion of these exercises, you will be able to:

1. Identify and define the key terms and concepts related to dental caries.

2. Identify the stages of dental caries and describe the caries process.

3. Plan protocols for prevention, remineralization, and maintenance based on individualized assessment of risk factors for dental caries.

KNOWLEDGE EXERCISES

Write your answers for each question in the space provided.

1. In your own words, describe how the metabolic action of *Streptococcus mutans* and *Lactobacillus* bacteria contributes to the destruction of tooth structure and causes dental caries.

_____

_____

_____

_____

_____

_____

_____

2. A child can be at risk for dental caries as soon as tooth eruption begins. Why?

_____

_____

_____

_____

_____

_____

3. List the types of fermentable carbohydrates.

_____

_____

_____

_____

4. Identify the acids produced during the metabolic process of the bacteria in dental biofilm.

_____

_____

_____

_____

5. The _____ of carbohydrate ingestion in your patient's diet has a strong influence on the amount of acid produced and the extent of tooth destruction.

6. In what ways does the presence of adequate saliva protect your patient against dental decay?

_____

_____

_____

_____

_____

_____

_____

7. In your own words, describe how fluoride protects your patient against dental decay.

_____

_____

_____

_____

_____

_____

_____

_____

8. What is the normal salivary pH?

_____

9. How long does it take once fermentable carbohydrates enter the mouth for the salivary pH to drop from normal to the point at which demineralization occurs? What pH level facilitates demineralization?

_____

_____

_____

10. What is the significance of cavitation?

_____

_____

_____

_____

_____

_____

_____

11. What is the purpose of discussing individualized caries risk assessment with each patient?

_____

_____

_____

_____

_____

_____

12. List the five risk factor categories associated with the CAMBRA guidelines for caries management.

_____

_____

_____

_____

13. List the four CAMBRA risk levels.

_____

_____

_____

14. List the four intervention categories identified in the CAMBRA management protocol.

_____

_____

15. Why is risk assessment used in caries management?

_____

_____

_____

_____

16. How can you best gather data to assess your patient's individual caries risk factors?

_____

_____

_____

_____

_____

_____

_____

17. What topics should be considered when developing an individualized caries management strategy?

_____

_____

_____

_____

_____

_____

_____

_____

_____

_____

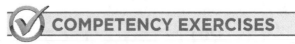 **COMPETENCY EXERCISES**

Apply information from the chapter and use critical thinking skills to complete the competency exercises. Write responses on paper or create electronic documents to submit your answers.

1. Seventeen-year-old Tren Nguyen immigrated to the United States with his family about 6 years ago. Since he arrived, Tren has embraced all things American and spends his free time playing computer games, snacking on fast food, and hanging out with friends. Tren's history of dental visits has been infrequent. He has been seen in your office only twice before—right after he arrived in the United States and then again about 3 years ago for a prophylaxis. No significant dental findings were charted at either of those visits. He has no history of previous dental restorations. He came to the clinic today because a dental checkup is required as part of his physical examination to play sports when he goes off to college next fall.

   When you examine Tren's mouth today, you find significant early and late white spot lesions on the facial surfaces of almost all of his teeth. It is interesting that there are no observable caries in the pits and fissures on the occlusal surfaces of any of his teeth and the surfaces are not deeply grooved. Make a list of the questions you will ask Tren as you gather caries risk assessment data before you write his dental hygiene care plan.

2. Now comes the fun part. You don't usually get to make up answers for all the questions that you ask your patients, but this time we can't go any further with these exercises unless we have some data. In the interest of your own learning, make up reasonable-sounding answers for each of the questions you asked Tren during your discussion of caries risk factors.

   Using the data you have collected from Tren's caries risk assessment, determine his CAMBRA level.

3. Write two dental hygiene diagnosis statements for Tren's care plan.

4. List the dental hygiene interventions you will plan to help Tren _arrest or control_ disease and _regenerate, restore, or maintain_ his oral health.

EVERYDAY ETHICS

Before completing the learning exercises below, reread and reflect on the Everyday Ethics Scenario and Questions for Consideration in this chapter of the **textbook**. It may also be useful to review the Dental Hygiene Ethics discussion in Chapter 1, the Ethical Applications in the introduction pages for each section in the **textbook**, as well as the Codes of Ethics in **textbook** Appendices I–IV.

Individual Learning Activity

Imagine that you have observed what happened in the scenario, but are not one of the main characters involved in the situation. Write a reflective journal entry that:

• Describes how you might have reacted (as an observer—not as a participant),

• Expresses your personal feelings about what happened, or

• Identifies personal values that affect your reaction to the situation.

Collaborative Learning Activity

Work with a small group to develop a 2–5-minute role-play that introduces the everyday ethics scenario described in the chapter (a great idea is to video record your role-play activity). Then develop separate 2-minute role-play scenarios that provide at least two alternative approaches/solutions to resolving the situation. Ask classmates to view the solutions, ask questions, and discuss the ethical approach used in each. Ask for a vote on which solution classmates determine to be the "best."

Factors to Teach the Patient

This scenario is related to the following factors listed in this chapter of the **textbook**:

▷ What causes dental caries and how they develop.

▷ That initial dental caries is not a cavity; what demineralization means.

▷ How remineralization can be accomplished using fluoride toothpaste and drinking fluoridated water daily.

▷ That the use of fluorides is necessary throughout life.

Use the motivational interviewing approach (see **workbook** Appendix D) as a guide to write a conversation explaining the components of Tren's care plan to him in such a way that you will motivate him to comply with your recommendations. (This patient was introduced in the Competency Exercises for this chapter.)

MeSH TERMS

Use a combination of MeSH terms and other key words to develop an effective and efficient PubMed literature search strategy.

Dental caries	Risk assessment
Dental caries susceptibility	Risk factors
Diet, cariogenic	Tooth demineralization
Cariogenic agents	Tooth remineralization

CHAPTER 25 CROSSWORD PUZZLE

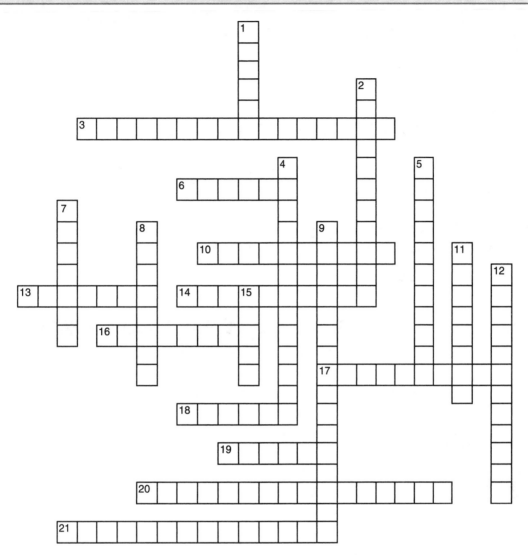

Puzzle Clues

Across

3. Management of dental caries through use of fluoride, calcium phosphate, or other agents.
6. A protocol for caries management.
10. Refers to bacteria that are capable of turning fermentable carbohydrates into acid.
13. Designates the highest level of risk for determining dental caries management protocols.
14. Breakthrough of the enamel surface.
16. Dental biofilm bacteria that thrive in an acidic environment.
17. Process that determines a patient's risk factors for disease.
18. Professional term for dental decay.
19. Buffers acids in the mouth and supplies minerals to replace the calcium and phosphate ions dissolved during demineralization.
20. Process in which minerals are removed from the tooth structure by acids.
21. Reduced salivary flow.

Down

1. Capable of neutralizing acid in a solution; one function of saliva.
2. This lesion gives evidence of subsurface demineralization (two words).
4. A species of bacteria that is more active in the later stages (progression) of decay.
5. Habits, behaviors, lifestyles, or conditions that increase the probability of a disease occurring (two words).
7. Ingredient in chewing gum that reduces levels of *Streptococcus mutans* and promotes remineralization.
8. Type of radiograph that can reveal caries on proximal surfaces of teeth.
9. Aided by sufficient saliva and by the action of topical fluorides.
11. Describes the caries process that has been halted.
12. A specific species of bacteria that predominates in the initial stages of the caries process.
15. A caries management system based on evidence and consensus (acronym).

26

Oral Infection Control: Toothbrushes and Toothbrushing

KNOWLEDGE EXERCISES

Write your answers for each question in the space provided.

1. Define *toothbrush abrasion*.

_____

_____

2. In your own words, describe an effective toothbrush handle.

_____

_____

_____

_____

3. Describe a tuft in the head of a toothbrush.

_____

_____

4. List two factors that affect the stiffness or firmness of toothbrush filaments.

_____

_____

_____

_____

5. List four factors that influence the type of toothbrush selected for an individual patient.

_____

_____

_____

_____

6. In your own words, describe the procedure for holding a toothbrush and positioning it in the mouth for effective removal of dental biofilm.

_____

_____

_____

_____

_____

7. Identify methods you can suggest to your patient for timing brushing in order to enhance effectiveness.

_____

_____

_____

_____

8. The Bass method of brushing is widely taught by dental hygienists to enhance effectiveness of their patients' oral cleaning. What problems are sometimes encountered as patients try to learn this technique?

_____

_____

_____

_____

9. Which two methods of toothbrushing are sometimes taught to young children when they have difficulty mastering a sulcular brushing technique?

_____

_____

10. Describe the procedure for the modified Stillman method of toothbrushing.

_____

_____

11. Which toothbrushing methods instruct the patient to direct the brush filaments at a 45° angle toward the gingival margin?

_____

_____

12. Which toothbrushing method instructs the patient to direct the brush filaments at a 45° angle toward the occlusal plane?

_____

13. What are the problems with biofilm removal when the patient uses the method described in question 12?

_____

_____

_____

14. List six factors in toothbrushing that are most likely to contribute to gingival recession or tooth abrasion.

_____

_____

_____

_____

15. List two methods for brushing occlusal surfaces.

_____

_____

16. What two anatomic features contribute to retention of dental biofilm on a patient's tongue?

_____

_____

17. Identify two methods for cleaning the tongue.

_____

_____

18. In your own words, define _neutropenia_.

_____

_____

19. What is the relationship of _neutropenia_ to oral health?

_____

_____

20. Identify at least three special circumstances in which the use of a powered toothbrush can enhance the removal of bacterial biofilm.

_____

_____

_____

_____

21. In your own words, describe the motion of an oscillating power toothbrush head. (_Hint:_ Use your hand to demonstrate the motion described in Table 26-2 in the **textbook**.)

_____

_____

_____

_____

_____

_____

✓ COMPETENCY EXERCISES

Apply information from the chapter and use critical thinking skills to complete the competency exercises. Write responses on paper or create electronic documents to submit your answers.

1. Nicholas Bean, a 12-year-old who is your first patient of the day, is going right from his prophylaxis appointment to the orthodontist's office, where they will be placing full-mouth bands and brackets on his teeth. You know that the best toothbrush to recommend for him to use is a bi-level orthodontic toothbrush, but you do not happen to have a sample to give him. You decide to tell his mother what it looks like so she can get one. Using terminology that describes the parts of a toothbrush from Figure 26-1 in the **textbook** and the pictures from Figure 26-2 in the **textbook**, develop a brief description of this type of toothbrush trim profile.

2. Mr. Gabriel Chin is one of your favorite patients, and he loves to share stories of his travels around the world. Today when he presents for his recall appointment, he shows you some toothbrushes that he recently brought back from a trip to visit relatives in his native country. The toothbrush, he states proudly, is the type his family has been using for many years and is made from the hairs of wild boars. You want to educate him without belittling his enthusiasm for his family's history. To help him understand about a better alternative, list three reasons why nylon or synthetic filaments are used today for toothbrushes instead of natural bristles.

3. Mr. Spiros Pappas is a long-standing patient who in the past has always presented with excellent oral health. During the medical history update, he shares that he is now undergoing chemotherapy treatment for cancer. As you conduct the intraoral soft tissue examination, you notice that his gingiva is quite inflamed with multiple areas of ulceration. Given his history, you suspect this is mucositis. He tells you that brushing has become very painful and asks what he can do to maintain his oral health. How would you reply?

4. Mrs. Janette Evans has been diagnosed with active periodontal disease. You will be working closely with her once a week for the next 2 months to control oral disease and obtain periodontal health because she will soon be going into the hospital for open-heart surgery. What important information should you give her about how to care for her toothbrush?

5. As you are providing oral hygiene instructions using the Bass method for Mrs. Evans, she asks you how much time she should spend brushing her teeth in order to thoroughly remove all of the biofilm, as you are recommending. Explain one of the methods she can use to monitor her toothbrushing.

6. When you are showing Mrs. Evans how to brush, you note that she needs some extra help with the distal surfaces of tooth 19, the most posterior tooth in that arch. Explain how she should position her toothbrush.

7. Explain how Mrs. Evans can effectively use her toothbrush to clean the mesial surface of tooth 7, which is extremely rotated and tilted in a labial direction.

8. Using your institution's guidelines for writing in patient records, document the oral hygiene instructions you provided for Mrs. Evans. Be sure to include enough detail so that you can use the comments at a subsequent visit to reinforce the information you provided.

9. When you see Mrs. Evans a week later, her biofilm scores are a bit lower but still not up to the levels you would like to see after your extensive oral hygiene instructions. When you do your intraoral examination, you notice a scuffed epithelial surface, several red pinpoint spots, and some generalized redness along the lingual gingival margin of teeth 13–15 and the facial margins of teeth 29–31. You determine that these acute lesions may be the result of toothbrushing activity during the previous week. Identify three possible precipitating factors and explain measures you or Mrs. Evans should take to eliminate the problems.

10. What are some reasons you might recommend a power toothbrush for Mrs. Evans instead of the manual toothbrushing technique you originally taught her?

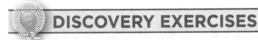

DISCOVERY EXERCISES

Collaborate with your classmates to gather samples of a variety of different power toothbrushes. (*Hint:* Contacting dental product companies is one way to do this, or you can use models that you, your classmates, or your faculty already own.)

1. For each brand or model of power toothbrush, determine the following information:
   - Motion
   - Brush head shape
   - Filaments
   - Handle size and shape
   - Overall weight
   - Power source
   - Speed
2. Discuss which model would be best for a variety of situations—for example, which one would you recommend for a child? For a caregiver to use when brushing someone else's teeth? Think of other situations and types of patients.
3. Conduct a PubMed search and review professional literature to evidence to support the recommendation of the type of power toothbrush you like best.

QUESTIONS PATIENTS ASK

What sources of information can you identify that will help you answer your patient's questions in this scenario?

"What toothbrush is right for me?" "Is a power toothbrush really worth buying? Will it help keep my teeth cleaner and my gums healthier?" "How do you know that the toothbrushing method you are teaching me is right for me?" You will hear these types of questions from your patients many, many times.

EVERYDAY ETHICS

Before completing the learning exercises below, reread and reflect on the Everyday Ethics Scenario and Questions for Consideration in this chapter of the **textbook**. It may also be useful to review the Dental Hygiene Ethics discussion in Chapter 1, the Ethical Applications in the introduction pages for each section in the **textbook**, as well as the Codes of Ethics in **textbook** Appendices I–IV.

Collaborative Learning Activity

Work with a small group to develop a 2–5-minute role-play that introduces the everyday ethics scenario described in the chapter (a great idea is to video record your role-play activity). Then develop separate 2-minute role-play scenarios that provide at least two alternative approaches/solutions to resolving the situation. Ask classmates to view the solutions, ask questions, and discuss the ethical approach used in each. Ask for a vote on which solution classmates determine to be the "best."

Discovery Activity

Ask a friend or relative who is not involved in health care to read the scenario and discuss it with you from the perspective of a "patient" who receives services within the healthcare system. Discuss what you learned from the concerns, insights, or difference in perspective that person expressed.

Factors to Teach the Patient

This scenario is related to the following factors listed in this chapter of the **textbook**:

▷ How dental biofilm forms and its effects on the teeth and gingiva.

▷ Why it is necessary to remove dental biofilm from the teeth daily, especially before going to sleep.

Thomas Raveli, 18 years old, is home for the holiday from his first term at college, and his mother has insisted that he keep his appointment with you for his regular 6-month cleaning. As you collect assessment data before providing dental hygiene care, you become very aware that his overall oral status is not the same as it has been at previous visits. You note generalized bleeding on probing and overall red and inflamed gingiva. Fortunately, there is no radiographic evidence of bone level changes.

Further questioning reveals that his overall home care routine has not been adequate and his eating patterns include frequent snacking because he doesn't particularly like the regular meals served in his dorm. He tells you about how hard it is to keep a regular schedule when he is so stressed by his college workload. He comments that it has been especially tough during the last several weeks when he was writing final exams. That's when he started noticing that his gums were bleeding every time he brushed his teeth! It hurt to brush, so he admits that he has been neglectful of his daily oral care.

Use the motivational interviewing approach (see **workbook** Appendix D) to write a statement explaining how using the proper brushing techniques can help prevent future problems for Thomas.

Use the conversation you create to role-play this situation with a fellow student. If you are the patient in the role-play, be sure to ask questions. If you are the dental hygienist, try to anticipate questions and provide evidence-based answers for them in your explanation.

MeSH TERMS

Use a combination of MeSH terms and other key words to develop an effective and efficient PubMed literature search strategy.

Dental devices, home care	Toothbrushing
Health education, dental	Gingival recession
Oral hygiene	Tooth abrasion

CHAPTER 26 WORD SEARCH PUZZLE

```
B X Q M G O F O M R X D D I Z F G P V U B O S Z
H D H A N C Q Z O U E Q K J M A M A R S C G D Q
U S P G S Q R A S G P O L A Z D O O K H A Y Q U
Y W U Q T X I T I N V S W R D D W U T T C H Y X
G P E W S O I L J S R E T R A H C K R I L N X H
U R B W L L Y F Q T M M R G C H Z M G M T S L J
U E S U L C U L A R E C N G C V U W Z S S T O O
A E C M X C K L J D H J R N Q Q U M A Y A Y P G
L B A L O D A U I I E V T B F F Z A D S U G W X
E N O M Z R J S R S U U P T J N O Y I E B J A Q
T X L A R A B E F E D W C V D W E N J H G Y V I
T F F T R N A X D X M I L Z E Z F N E S K Y I R
M I G Q D O S U Z L R Z A D D X H E K S M N D N
O V Z C Q E S E X C V D T Z U F Y I H S S A J L
E Z M W T L S I U R A W N D L T V T W F P W F J
D Z I Q B L L L V P U U O C M E J C S G J R W L
T M C R R V A C S W H P Z K C F R L Z C Q U X A
K E O U R R C D D G O R I B B U L Y P D R V O C
X M U D L V X T T G V M R L E O R A G W F U P I
Q U A K I E T I T U Y K O H R X K B E K G G B T
A K M V Q F Y D K C R T H P E M V I U J G L U R
Y X F L F M I D W K J Z P E X R U H G L J D W E
M K B Z M A Z E L E S O U G Y G V S X V F L A V
R S I U D Z N F D R A K J V J L A Q J E K X I G
```

Puzzle Clues

There are a variety of different toothbrushing methods you can teach your patients. Some are better than others for maximizing biofilm removal and minimizing damage to oral tissues. But all of them are included in this word search puzzle.

1. Bass
2. Charters
3. Circular
4. Fones
5. Horizontal
6. Leonard
7. Modified
8. Roll
9. Scrub
10. Smith's
11. Stillman
12. Sulcular
13. Vertical

Oral Infection Control: Interdental Care

 KNOWLEDGE EXERCISES

Write your answers for each question in the space provided.

1. Posterior teeth have _____ papillae with a col, and anterior teeth have _____ papilla that forms a small col under the contact area.

2. Identify tissue and anatomic characteristics of the col, the adjacent teeth, and the surrounding papillae that contribute to the increased risk of gingivitis in the interdental area.

_____

_____

_____

_____

_____

3. Describe the shapes of interdental brushes.

_____

_____

_____

_____

4. Describe a situation in which the interdental brush is a better choice than dental floss for complete biofilm removal or for application of chemotherapeutic agents on proximal surfaces of teeth.

_____

_____

_____

5. Identify the different types of floss that you and your patient can select based on individual preference and needs.

_____

_____

_____

6. Complete Infomap 27-1 to compare the benefits and limitations of waxed (or PTFE) and unwaxed floss, as noted in the **textbook**.

INFOMAP 27-1		
FLOSS TYPE	BENEFITS	LIMITATIONS
Waxed or expanded PTFE		
Unwaxed floss		

7. Identify the location, cause of, and methods for preventing floss cuts and clefts.

_____

_____

_____

_____

_____

_____

_____

_____

_____

8. List additional flossing aides you can recommend for a patient and identify indications for recommending each one.

_____

_____

_____

_____

_____

_____

_____

_____

_____

9. What kind of flossing motion can be applied with tufted floss, knitting yarn, or gauze strips that is not typically applied with regular floss?

_____

10. End-tuft brushes are usually recommended for a single area that is difficult to reach with a regular toothbrush. In what specific situations might you recommend the use of an end-tuft brush?

_____

_____

_____

_____

11. In your own words, describe a wooden interdental cleaner, state how it is used, and identify factors you must consider when recommending it for a patient.

_____

_____

_____

_____

_____

_____

_____

_____

_____

12. Describe an interdental tip and a toothpick in holder and explain how they are used.

- _Interdental tip_

_____

_____

_____

- _Toothpick in holder_

_____

_____

_____

_____

13. Describe oral irrigation.

_____

_____

_____

14. List the three delivery method categories for oral irrigation.

_____

_____

_____

15. List the advantages of patient-applied daily irrigation measures.

_____

_____

_____

_____

_____

16. List the patient assessment factors that provide information to help you assess your patient's individual needs before recommending a specific device for his or her interdental care.

_____

_____

_____

_____

_____

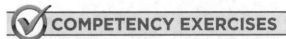

COMPETENCY EXERCISES

Apply information from the chapter and use critical thinking skills to complete the competency exercises. Write responses on paper or create electronic documents to submit your answers.

1. The best way to learn how to teach a patient about flossing is to practice doing it. Use all of the information you learned in the **textbook** chapter to teach a family member or friend (but not one of your student colleagues, because he or she has already read this chapter) about how and when to floss.

2. After careful assessment of his current oral hygiene measures, you find that your patient, Mr. Adamson, has very large hands and has a great deal of difficulty maneuvering dental floss in his posterior teeth. He also has an orthodontic band on tooth 3, which positions a temporary appliance being used to maintain an open space for the later placement of a permanent bridge. He has high levels of biofilm on all proximal areas and along the gingival margin of the orthodontic band. Write two dental hygiene diagnosis statements related to these issues.

3. Write a goal for the problems you identified in the dental hygiene diagnoses in question 2. Include a time frame for meeting the goal. How will you measure whether or not your patient met the goal?

4. You decide to recommend a floss holder for regular floss as well as the use of a "Perio-Aid" for Mr. Adamson. Obtain samples of these interdental devices, if you can, to help you with this exercise (they will also help with the Factors to Teach the Patient section). Write a progress note documenting your recommendations and the oral hygiene instructions that you provided for Mr. Adamson.

EVERYDAY ETHICS

Before completing the learning exercises below, reread and reflect on the Everyday Ethics Scenario and Questions for Consideration in this chapter of the **textbook**. It may also be useful to review the Dental Hygiene Ethics discussion in Chapter 1, the Ethical Applications in the introduction pages for each section in the **textbook**, as well as the Codes of Ethics in **textbook** Appendices I–IV.

Individual Learning Activity

Imagine that you are the dental hygienist in this scenario. Answer each of the questions for consideration at the end of the scenario.

Discovery Activity

Ask a friend or relative who is not involved in health care to read the scenario and discuss it with you from the perspective of a "patient" who receives services within the healthcare system. Discuss what you learned from the concerns, insights, or difference in perspective that person expressed.

Factors to Teach the Patient

This scenario is related to the following factors listed in this chapter of the **textbook**:

▷ By demonstration with disclosing agent, how the toothbrush doesn't clean the interdental area thoroughly.

▷ About dental biofilm and how it collects on the proximal tooth surfaces when left undisturbed.

▷ How vulnerable the interdental area is to gingival infection.

▷ How to use each recommended interdental aid to clean the proximal tooth surfaces.

Use motivational interviewing principles (see **workbook** Appendix D) to develop a conversation explaining to Mr. Adamson (introduced in question 2 of the Competency Exercises) how to assemble and use the interdental devices you are recommending.

MeSH TERMS

Use a combination of MeSH terms and other key words to develop an effective and efficient PubMed literature search strategy.

Oral hygiene
Dental devices, home care
Gingiva

28

Dentifrices and Mouthrinses

LEARNING OBJECTIVES

Upon successful completion of these exercises, you will be able to:

1. Identify and define the key terms and concepts related to dentifrices and mouthrinses.

2. Describe the components, action, and therapeutic or cosmetic benefits of a dentifrice.

3. Describe the purpose of, procedure for, and ingredients used in oral rinses.

4. Identify the considerations in selecting patient-specific dentifrices and oral rinses.

5. Define the purpose, requirements, and use of the revised ADA Seal Program.

 KNOWLEDGE EXERCISES

Write your answers for each question in the space provided.

1. What are the beneficial effects of the active ingredients in dentifrices?

2. Identify the three purposes of a dentifrice.

3. What is the purpose of the humectants in a dentifrice?

4. List at least three types of abrasives used as polishing agents in a dentifrice.

5. What are the purposes of sorbitol or glycerol as an ingredient in a dentifrice?

6. What is the purpose of essential oils (e.g., peppermint) used in dentifrices?

7. The amount of therapeutic agent in a dentifrice is about _____.

8. Which therapeutic ingredient in a dentifrice is related to prevention of dental caries?

9. Identify four therapeutic ingredients in a dentifrice that are related to reduction of supragingival calculus formation?

_____

_____

_____

_____

10. What is the most common ingredient used in dentifrices to aid in reducing sensitivity?

_____

11. List the six basic ingredients in commercial mouthrinses.

_____

_____

_____

_____

_____

_____

12. List at least four functions of chemotherapeutic agents found in mouthrinses and identify the purpose of each.

_____

_____

_____

_____

_____

_____

_____

_____

_____

_____

13. List at least three characteristics of an effective mouthrinse.

_____

_____

_____

14. Which therapeutic agent available in mouthrinses has the greatest substantivity?

_____

15. Which therapeutic agent available in mouthrinses acts by causing bacteriolysis?

_____

16. Which therapeutic agent available in mouthrinses acts by inhibiting bacterial enzymes?

_____

17. Which therapeutic agent available in mouthrinses is inactivated by a foaming agent frequently contained in commercial dentifrices? What is the agent?

_____

_____

18. Which two therapeutic agents available in mouthrinses are associated with the adverse effect of staining?

_____

_____

19. Describe the action and use of a mouthrinse containing peroxide.

_____

_____

_____

20. Explain why rinsing with a mouthwash that contains an effective therapeutic agent may not be effective for a patient with deep periodontal pockets.

_____

_____

21. List factors to consider when providing patient-specific recommendations for dentifrices.

_____

_____

_____

_____

_____

_____

22. What is the effect of using a mouthrinse with an oxidizing agent? List two oxidizing agents.

_____

_____

_____

_____

23. How are dentifrices classified by the United States FDA?

_____

_____

24. What is the website for the ADA Seal Program?

_____

_____

25. List the items that should be documented in the patient's chart concerning dentifrices and mouthrinses.

_____

_____

_____

_____

_____

_____

_____

_____

_____

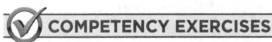 **COMPETENCY EXERCISES**

Apply information from the chapter and use critical thinking skills to complete the competency exercises. Write responses on paper or create electronic documents to submit your answers.

1. Using the information in the **textbook**, compare effectiveness, adverse effects, availability to the patient, and any other factors about therapeutic agents that might affect patient acceptance. (_Hint:_ Use a separate piece of paper to make a one-page infomap, or table, to aid in your comparison.) What additional information would you like to have about each of these agents that might help you inform your patients about using them?

2. Evan, a 7-year-old, has been prescribed a fluoride mouthrinse by Dr. Leiberman. Evan demonstrates a rinsing technique in which he fills his mouth with the liquid and rotates his head in all directions to distribute the rinse to all areas of his mouth.

You plan to teach him how to rinse using the steps outlined in Box 28-3 of the **textbook**. Write a dental hygiene diagnosis statement that identifies a problem related to Evan's current rinsing technique.

3. Write a goal for the problem identified in the dental hygiene diagnosis in question 2. How will you measure whether Evan met the goal? Include a time frame for meeting the goal.

4. Ms. Greene is a 45-year-old periodontal patient who develops a moderate amount of supragingival calculus. What type of dentifrice might you consider recommending to her?

5. Using your institution's guidelines for writing in patient records, document the recommendation of a toothpaste containing pyrophosphate during patient education.

 QUESTIONS PATIENTS ASK

What sources of information can you identify that will help you answer your patient's questions in this scenario?

After you answer her questions about the ADA Seal, Ms. Leffler is very impressed with your knowledge, and she clearly believes that _you_ are the expert to ask about dental products. Like many of your patients, she has questions about all kinds of oral-care products that she has heard or read about. "Does it really matter which toothpaste I use?" "There are so many different kinds with different ingredients that claim to do different things—which one is really the best?" "Are there any negative side effects that go along with any of those extra ingredients and chemicals?" "Which mouthrinse do you recommend?"

EVERYDAY ETHICS

Before completing the learning exercises below, reread and reflect on the Everyday Ethics Scenario and Questions for Consideration in this chapter of the **textbook**. It may also be useful to review the Dental Hygiene Ethics discussion in Chapter 1, the Ethical Applications in the introduction pages for each section in the **textbook**, as well as the Codes of Ethics in **textbook** Appendices I–IV.

Collaborative Learning Activities

Answer each of the questions for consideration at the end of the scenario in the **textbook**. Compare what you wrote with answers developed by another classmate and discuss differences/similarities.

Work with a small group to develop a 2–5-minute role-play that introduces the everyday ethics scenario described in the chapter (a great idea is to video record your role-play activity). Then develop separate 2-minute role-play scenarios that provide at least two alternative approaches/solutions to resolving the situation. Ask classmates to view the solutions, ask questions, and discuss the ethical approach used in each. Ask for a vote on which solution classmates determine to be the "best."

Factors to Teach the Patient

This scenario is related to the following factors listed in this chapter of the **textbook**:

▷ Significance of ADA product acceptance seal (especially because it is a voluntary program, and no seal on a product does not signify that it is unsafe or not effective).

Ms. Cerene Leffler usually prefers to use all-natural products. She has noticed that the dentifrice she likes does not display the ADA Seal on the package. She asks you during her dental hygiene appointment if that indicates that the toothpaste is not a good choice. Using patient-appropriate language, write a statement explaining to Ms. Leffler what the ADA Seal means.

MeSH TERMS

Use a combination of MeSH terms and other key words to develop an effective and efficient PubMed literature search strategy.

Dentifrices   Mouthwashes
Denture cleansers   Cariostatic agents
Toothpastes   Fluorides

CHAPTER 28 WORD SEARCH PUZZLE

```
D B E B P R C H V T Z E D I R O U L F H E H I A
J Y Q D A F J M M Z Q W N A D A S E A L U D Q A
P P L A I B O R C I M I T N A S U F T T Y V V S
P N A M U K K A L C W B Y F H R R L W J R P B Q
E Q F N Z J A M U H E I Y F Z O E B C E R I T V
V W O G O R N S I X I A B T O J H D N K F G H C
I N S Q D D E N U Z A O C S T V J I N X E S Z F
T N F H Q W Y M F O N O A I B B D N B I D N N Z
C N B V Z O H N I L N F K U D I G M R L B X B Y
A K V W X P I I E N F N T L X O L W Z R T B X P
C G D C D J S N A N E X A E I Q G L G H D Y K A
C M Z P Y S C D W S R R H T J D G E R X M T D R
W A S T R I N G E N T R A E S X G L N D Z I L E
I V K N V C M H V K O T A L M Q X A P I R V P H
S B E A M V R W H L B F O L I A G G R H C I I T
Q Z C T Y Q E Q H G G U N K W Z O X U Z Z T J O
W B I C Q H M C E K P T F N N W A P V P X N V M
V X R A Y M Y C K N A T E F U U A T I F Q A Y E
R V F F P B L Y Y I T T B M E F W G I V H T C H
S L I R N H O G F S D W Z S L R O A B O T S B C
V C T U O A P Z T R I C L O S A N J S Z N B G W
A C N S Z S O V C L O T I L Y X K D D H A U F E
I G E Y Q Y C Q Z D C Z S K U W U T B M H S D P
V Y D H U M E C T A N T G K L U T H L Y F M P V
```

Puzzle Clues

1. Type of chemotherapeutic agent that alleviates pain.
2. The term that means acid forming.
3. Substance that retains moisture and prevents hardening upon exposure to air.
4. Abbreviation for chlorhexidine.
5. A substance with a high molecular weight that results from chemically combining two or more monomers.
6. Restoration of mineral elements.
7. Treatment of disease by means of chemical substances or pharmaceutical agents.
8. A caries prevention agent found in dentifrices and mouthrinses.
9. A substance that causes contraction or shrinkage and arrests discharges.
10. Indicates that efficacy claims of a product have been tested by research studies and are valid (two words).
11. Ability of an agent to bind to surfaces and be released and retain potency over an extended period of time.
12. A chemotherapeutic substance usually used with a toothbrush.
13. Reduces oral acidity.
14. The effect of sodium lauryl sulfate in dentifrices.
15. A broad-spectrum antibacterial agent that has the ability to bind and remain in the oral cavity over a period of time.
16. A chemical with a bacteriostatic or bactericidal effect.
17. Refers to a type of ingredient added to a dentifrice to produce a specific preventive or treatment outcome.
18. A substance added to a dentifrice to prevent separation of the solid and liquid ingredients during storage.
19. This flavoring agent in dentifrices has been shown to provide anticaries benefits.
20. Type of fluoride that has been shown to help reduce oral biofilm.
21. This agent has been shown to have a beneficial effect on reducing the bacteria associated with VSC production.

The Patient with Orthodontic Appliances

 KNOWLEDGE EXERCISES

Write your answers for each question in the space provided.

1. In the _____ orthodontic system, a bracket is bonded to the surface of a tooth or group of teeth to hold an arch wire.

2. In a removable aligner system, an individualized series of _____ is used to progressively move the misaligned teeth.

3. What is the purpose of the mesh backing on the base of a bracket?

_____

_____

4. _____ hold the arch wire to the bracket.

5. The purpose of the arch wire is to:

_____

_____

6. List the advantages of using bonded brackets instead of circumferential bands.

_____

_____

_____

_____

_____

_____

_____

_____

7. List the disadvantages of bonded brackets.

_____

_____

_____

8. What materials are bonded brackets commonly made from?

_____

_____

_____

9. What is documented for each patient prior to placing bonded orthodontic brackets?

_____

_____

10. The procedure for applying the bonding agent is similar to the procedure for placing a dental _____.

11. The use of filler particles in bonding resin increases _____ _____ (multiple words); therefore, heavily filled resins are used for brackets placed on _____ teeth, which are subject to high forces of mastication.

12. Explain the significance of using a fluoride-releasing bonding system.

_____

_____

_____

13. A patient with orthodontic appliances is at risk for a higher incidence of which two oral diseases?

_____

_____

14. Describe how a regular toothbrush can be adapted on the facial surface of teeth with an orthodontic appliance?

_____

_____

_____

_____

_____

15. Explain how an orthodontic toothbrush, such as that pictured in Figure 29-4 in the **textbook**, is used.

_____

_____

_____

16. List the advantages of using an air polisher during dental hygiene treatment of the patient with orthodontic appliances.

_____

_____

_____

17. Explain the effect of the debonding process on tooth enamel.

_____

_____

_____

18. Use of a _____ can help reduce the effects of the debonding process on tooth enamel.

19. What is the purpose of frequent rinsing and drying during removal of the bonding resin?

_____

_____

20. List the final finish steps so that will leave help restore the pretreatment enamel surface finish following removal of the bonding resin.

_____

_____

_____

21. Along with careful periodontal examination, examination for demineralized areas, and removal of leftover composite resin, what other professional assessments and interventions are required after debonding orthodontic appliances?

_____

_____

_____

22. What is the purpose of an orthodontic retainer?

_____

_____

✓ COMPETENCY EXERCISES

Apply information from the chapter and use critical thinking skills to complete the competency exercises. Write responses on paper or create electronic documents to submit your answers.

1. Ms. Anna Moyer, a real-estate agent who really relies on her smile as she interacts with the public in her job, is very excited and yet extremely nervous on the day the brackets that have hidden her smile for so long are being removed. After the brackets and arch

wires are removed from Ms. Moyer's teeth, it is necessary to remove all residual adhesive. Discuss the steps you will take to ensure that all areas of each tooth are thoroughly free from adhesive.

2. Discuss the purpose of post-debonding preventive care that you, the dental hygienist, will provide for Ms. Moyer.

3. Two weeks after her fixed orthodontic appliances are removed, the orthodontist delivers a Hawley appliance to Ms. Moyer. You are responsible for educating and instructing her about the purpose and care of her retainer. What important points will you cover in your discussion?

4. Your next patient is Missy Breckenridge. She has had her orthodontic appliances for about 2 years now, and you notice that her gingiva is not as healthy as it was when you saw her 6 months ago. When you disclose her mouth, there is a large accumulation of dental biofilm between the brackets and her gingival margins. What topics will you be sure to include in your discussion with Missy as you provide oral hygiene instructions that address her need to ensure cleanliness on all surfaces.

Factors to Teach the Patient

This scenario is related to the following factors listed in this chapter of the **textbook**:

▷ The significance of biofilm around orthodontic appliances and teeth.

▷ How, when, and why to use fluoride rinses, toothpastes, and brush-on gels.

▷ The frequency for professional follow-up during and after orthodontic therapy.

Nicholas Bean is a 12-year-old patient. He is going directly from his prophylaxis appointment with you to the orthodontist's office, where they will be placing full-mouth bands/brackets and arch wires on his teeth. As they arrive for the appointment, Nicholas's mother comments that they won't be seeing you again until the braces come off. You want to begin to educate Nicholas and his mother right away about the importance of the use of fluorides, thorough daily oral hygiene measures, and especially why regular maintenance appointments are necessary during orthodontic treatment.

Using the information you learned from reading this chapter and the principles of motivational interviewing (see **workbook** Appendix D) as a guide, prepare an outline for a conversation with Nicholas' mother that provides anticipatory guidance about ways to maintain good oral health status while her son is undergoing orthodontic care.

MeSH TERMS

Use a combination of MeSH terms and other key words to develop an effective and efficient PubMed literature search strategy.

Orthodontic appliances
Orthodontic appliance design
Orthodontic brackets
Orthodontic extrusion
Orthodontic retainers
Orthodontic space closure

Orthodontic wires
Orthodontics, corrective
Orthodontics, interceptive
Orthodontics, preventive
Tooth movement
Tooth demineralization
Dental bonding
Dental debonding

EVERYDAY ETHICS

Before completing the learning exercises below, reread and reflect on the Everyday Ethics Scenario and Questions for Consideration in this chapter of the **textbook**. It may also be useful to review the Dental Hygiene Ethics discussion in Chapter 1, the Ethical Applications in the introduction pages for each section in the **textbook**, as well as the Codes of Ethics in **textbook** Appendices I–IV.

Individual Learning Activity

Identify a situation you have experienced that presents a similar ethical dilemma. Write about you

would do differently now than you did at the time the incident happened—support your discussion with concepts from the dental hygiene codes of ethics.

Discovery Activity

Ask a dental hygienist who has been practicing for a year or more to read the scenario. Provide them with a copy of the Code of Ethics as well. Share the responses you have made to answer each question and ask that person to discuss the situation with you. What insights did you have or what did you learn during this discussion?

30

Care of Dental Prosthesis

KNOWLEDGE EXERCISES

Write your answers for each question in the space provided.

1. What happens to bone after teeth are lost?

_____

_____

_____

_____

_____

2. Describe the difference between a torus and an exostosis.

_____

_____

_____

_____

_____

3. Identify reasons for wearing a fixed or removable prosthesis to replace the missing teeth.

_____

_____

_____

_____

_____

_____

_____

4. What happens if teeth are not replaced?

_____

_____

_____

_____

_____

5. List the components of a fixed partial denture prosthesis.

_____

_____

_____

6. List the criteria for an acceptable fixed partial denture prosthesis.

_____

_____

_____

_____

_____

7. What type of fixed partial denture is supported by one or more teeth at one end?

_____

_____

8. If your patient is unable to remove his or her own partial denture prosthesis, how do you help the patient remove it?

_____

_____

_____

_____

9. In your own words, describe an obturator.

_____

_____

_____

10. Label Figure 30-1 with the following components.

- *Denture border*
- *Impression surface*
- *Occlusal surface*
- *Polished surface*

11. List three reasons why a denture may be constructed to replace primary dentition for a child patient.

_____

_____

_____

12. What is the purpose of a provisional or interim dental prosthesis?

_____

_____

_____

_____

13. Why is it often necessary to reline or remake an immediate denture approximately 6 months after initial placement?

_____

_____

14. As a dental hygienist, you may provide counseling and education for your patient both before and after he or she receives a new denture. Explain the purpose of predelivery patient counseling.

_____

_____

_____

15. When a denture is placed immediately after extractions, you instruct your patient to leave the denture in place for _____ without removing it, to aid in control of bleeding and swelling.

16. Because adjustments can be expected when a new denture is placed over healed ridges, you instruct your patient to return within _____; you then make reappointments as needed.

17. What is the purpose of a postinsertion appointment with the dental hygienist after a new denture is placed? (*Hint:* The dentist will adjust the new denture, if needed, not the dental hygienist.)

_____

_____

18. List the potential effects of alveolar ridge remodeling after placement of a complete denture.

_____

_____

_____

_____

_____

19. Your patient may resort to _____ remedies to counter the effects of alveolar remodeling or poor denture fit, but you will counsel him or her to seek dental care if there are any problems, because other remedies are _____ if used improperly or over time.

20. List factors that contribute to the varying tissue reactions experienced by patients who wear dentures.

_____

_____

_____

_____

_____

_____

21. Xerostomia can adversely affect denture _____ and tissue _____.

22. List two negative oral effects related to the sensory changes that may be experienced by your patient who wears complete dentures.

_____

_____

23. For most of your patients who wear complete dentures, a _____ continuing care appointment frequency is adequate, unless they are experiencing problems.

24. Identify two kinds of liners that may be present on the impression surface of a complete denture prosthesis.

_____

_____

25. Identify two kinds of complete overdenture prostheses.

_____

26. What are the advantages of a complete overdenture prosthesis?

_____

_____

_____

_____

_____

_____

27. List factors that contribute to the success of an overdenture prosthesis.

_____

_____

_____

_____

28. What are the advantages of natural tooth and implant-retained overdentures?

_____

_____

_____

_____

_____

_____

_____

_____

_____

29. At dental hygiene appointments, it is important to thoroughly examine the oral tissues of a patient who wears complete dentures. In your own words, describe the tension test for examining the mouth of your edentulous patient.

_____

_____

_____

30. What characteristic of a removable partial denture prosthesis can negatively affect your patient's gingival health?

_____

_____

_____

_____

_____

_____

31. List the three most common causes of oral lesions under a dental prosthesis.

_____

_____

_____

32. What is the effect of xerostomia for your patient who wears dentures?

_____

_____

_____

_____

33. What is an epulis fissuratum?

_____

_____

_____

_____

34. Name the common fungal infection that can result in denture stomatitis.

_____

35. List three factors that can contribute to angular cheilitis in your patient who wears dentures.

_____

_____

_____

36. If you observe a localized ulcerated lesion related to an overextended denture border that persists longer than normal healing times, you should bring the situation to the attention of the dentist so that the lesion can be _____.

37. List the topics to include when you are educating your patient about ways to prevent damage to oral tissues related to wearing dentures.

_____

_____

_____

38. What dental hygiene interventions provide an added measure of protection for the oral health of a patient with a partial denture, single-arch complete denture with natural teeth remaining in the opposite arch, or overdenture supported by natural teeth?

_____

_____

_____

_____

_____

_____

39. What two procedures can be used to clean an oral prosthesis?

_____

_____

_____

_____

40. Describe the process you will use to remove your patient's complete denture if, for some reason, your patient is not able to remove it himself or herself.

- _Maxillary complete denture_

_____

_____

_____

_____

_____

_____

- _Mandibular complete denture_

_____

_____

_____

_____

_____

41. Identify two oral conditions that can be prevented with proper cleansing and care of dental prostheses and underlying tissues.

_____

_____

42. What is the purpose of instructing your patients to remove and properly store their dental prosthesis in liquid while sleeping at night?

_____

_____

43. What are the requirements for a denture cleanser you will recommend to your patient?

_____

_____

_____

_____

_____

44. Complete Infomap 30-1 to compare the various types of cleansers you can recommend for the care of full and partial dentures.

45. List three reasons to mark your patient's denture with identifying information.

_____

_____

_____

46. In your own words, briefly summarize the criteria for an adequate denture-marking system relative to the following issues.

- _The denture:_

_____

_____

- _The material used:_

_____

_____

- _The procedure used:_

_____

_____

47. List two areas in which identification information can be incorporated as a denture is fabricated.

_____

_____

Infomap 30-1			
TYPE	ACTIVE INGREDIENT	CLEANSER ACTION	DISADVANTAGES
Immersion type			
Alkaline hypochlorite (household bleach)			
Alkaline peroxide (commercial powder or tablet)			
Dilute acids (commercial ultrasonic solutions)			
Enzymes (in various cleansers)			
Abrasive type			
Pastes and powders (various commercial products)			
Household agents (salt, bicarbonate of soda, hand soap, scouring powders)			

48. Where an inclusion identification marker should be placed on an existing denture that was not previously labeled?

- *Maxillary denture:*

  _____

- *Mandibular denture:*

  _____

49. Identify two methods for marking identification information on the surface of a denture.

  _____

  _____

50. What information is included when marking the denture of a patient who is in a long-term care nursing home?

  _____

  _____

 COMPETENCY EXERCISES

Apply information from the chapter and use critical thinking skills to complete the competency exercises. Write responses on paper or create electronic documents to submit your answers.

1. Imagine that you have just joined the on-site dental team at a long-term care facility or nursing home. A short time after you begin your position, you discover that many of the residents wear full or partial dentures and those dentures are not being cleaned regularly by the nurses' aides who are responsible for providing daily personal care for the residents. Most of the dentures worn by the residents are complete-arch dentures made of acrylic resins. Many are old and stained, and some have calculus buildup on the surfaces of the denture. The dentures are seldom removed from the patients' mouths. When they are, they are often just placed on the bedside table or in the drawer until family members come for a visit and decide that the patient looks better with the denture back in place.

You plan to provide an in-service presentation for the caregivers about the importance of denture care and you also plan to provide hands-on training in denture-cleaning techniques for the caregiver staff.

- *List the information that you will include in your in-service presentation about denture care.*

- *Create a step-by-step checklist that the aides can use at the bedside to document daily cleaning of each resident's removable prosthesis as well as the resident's oral tissues.*

2. Explain why regular dental hygiene maintenance care is important for edentulous patients, whether they are wearing complete dentures.

3. Explain why caries-control methods are important to teach your patient who wears an overdenture.

 DISCOVERY EXERCISE

Investigate commercially available denture cleaners so you can make a recommendation to the long-term care center or nursing home staff. What is the active ingredient in each one? What is the relative cost of each type? Which type might be easiest for the caregivers to use in the nursing home setting? Which one (or ones) will you recommend in your in-service presentation? Provide a rationale for your choice(s).

 EVERYDAY ETHICS

Before completing the learning exercises below, reread and reflect on the Everyday Ethics Scenario and Questions for Consideration in this chapter of the **textbook**. It may also be useful to review the Dental Hygiene Ethics discussion in Chapter 1, the Ethical Applications in the introduction pages for each section in the **textbook**, as well as the Codes of Ethics in **textbook** Appendices I–IV.

Individual Learning Activities

Identify a situation you have experienced that presents a similar ethical dilemma. Write about what you would do differently now than you did at the time the incident happened—support your discussion with concepts from the dental hygiene codes of ethics.

Identify a situation in which you have resolved a similar ethical dilemma and share the story with a classmate. Discuss how that person might have acted differently to resolve the situation.

Discovery Activity

Ask a dental hygienist who has been practicing for a year or more to read the scenario. Provide them with a copy of the Code of Ethics as well. Share the responses you have made to answer each question and ask that person to discuss the situation with you. What insights did you have or what did you learn during this discussion?

Factors to Teach the Patient

This scenario is related to the following factors listed in this chapter of the **textbook**:

▷ How to make a self-examination of the oral tissues.

▷ Why all prostheses need cleaning more than once a day.

▷ The need to adapt toothbrushing, flossing, and use of other aids to the care of the abutment teeth.

▷ How tongue cleaning contributes to complete oral health.

▷ The significance of regular maintenance appointments to have the oral tissues checked and the prostheses professionally cleaned.

Evangeline Dada has just received a brand new six-unit anterior bridge, which spans her entire smile from abutment tooth #6 to abutment tooth #11. Before placement of the fixed prosthesis, she had a removable temporary appliance made of plastic. She had no trouble cleaning her teeth when she could remove the old appliance, and she has done a good job of keeping all her oral tissues healthy. She states she is completely at a loss as to how she must take care of this beautiful new smile of hers and asks you to spend some extra time providing oral-hygiene instructions for her today.

Use the principles of motivational interviewing described in **workbook** Appendix D as a guide to develop a conversation to educate Evangeline about her new bridge, the abutment teeth that support it, and maintaining the health of the oral tissues around and underneath this new fixed prosthesis.

Use the conversation you create to role-play this situation with a fellow student. If you are the patient in the role-play, be sure to ask questions. If you are the dental hygienist, try to anticipate questions and answer them in your explanation.

MeSH TERMS

Use a combination of MeSH terms and other key words to develop an effective and efficient PubMed literature search strategy.

Alveolar bone loss	Denture, partial, fixed
Dental prosthesis	Denture, partial, removable
Denture cleansers	Dentures
Denture design	Edentulous
Denture overlay	Stomatitis, denture
Denture, complete	

CHAPTER 30 CROSSWORD PUZZLE

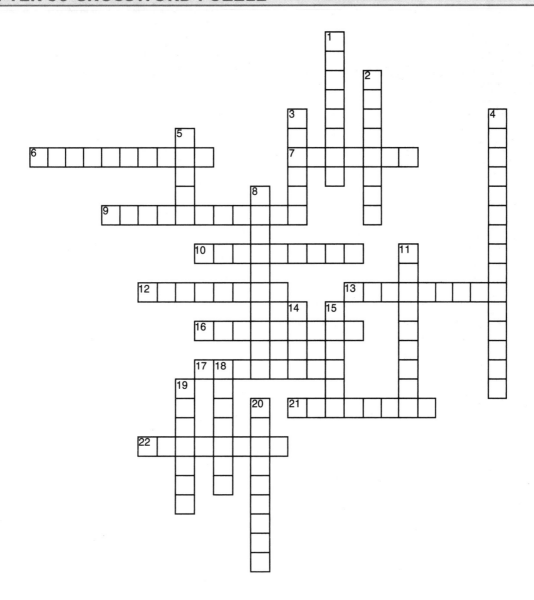

Puzzle Clues

Across

6. An artificial replacement for a body part.

7. Prosthesis worn for a limited time.

9. A type of removable dental prosthesis that is supported by both retained natural teeth or implants and the soft tissue of the alveolar ridge.

10. Directing a prosthesis to a desired oral location.

12. The external or outer surface of a dental prosthesis is a highly _____ surface, whereas the occlusal and impression surfaces are not.

13. A type of oral prosthesis that is cleaned and cared for outside of the oral cavity.

16. A dental prosthesis that closes a congenital or acquired opening in oral tissues.

17. A tooth or an implant used to support a fixed or removable dental prosthesis.

21. The surface of the dental prosthesis that makes contact with teeth in the opposing arch.

22. The clasp that holds a partial denture around abutment teeth.

Down

1. A caries preventative agent often placed on teeth that support an overdenture prosthesis.

2. A type of dental prosthesis that replaces the dentition and associated structures in an entire oral arch.

3. A term commonly used to refer to a fixed partial denture prosthesis.

4. Inflammation at the corners of the mouth (two words).

5. A type of partial denture prosthesis that is secured to natural teeth or dental implants and must be cleaned and cared for inside the oral cavity.

8. Continuous occlusal migration of a tooth.

11. Congenital absence of all teeth.

14. The part of a dental prosthesis that rests on the oral mucosa and to which teeth are attached.

15. Component of a fixed partial denture that replaces a missing natural tooth.

18. A substance that adheres to surfaces of a denture in the same way it can adhere to the surfaces of a natural dentition.

19. The type of dental prosthesis that replaces one or more teeth, but not all of the teeth in an arch.

20. A type of connector that attaches a removal prosthesis to a metal receptacle included within a restoration of an abutment tooth.

The Patient with Dental Implants

KNOWLEDGE EXERCISES

Write your answers for each question in the space provided.

1. Match the type of bone cell with its appropriate function.

Bone Cell	Function
___ Osteocyte	A. Repair and regeneration
___ Osteoblast	B. Remodeling and homeostasis
___ Osteoclast	C. Mediate activity

2. Explain how Wolff law is related to dental implants.

_____

_____

_____

3. Identify the bone density classification for each of the following descriptions.

Bone Density Classification	Description
_____	Immature, nonmineralized bone
_____	Dense cortical bone
_____	Thin cortical bone crest/fine trabecular bone
_____	Thick to porous cortical bone crest/coarse trabecular bone
_____	Fine trabecular bone

4. In your own words, define the following types of bone graft options.

Bone Graft Option	Definition
Xenograft	_____
Autograft	_____
Allograft	_____
Alloplast	_____

5. Describe osseointegration as you would for a patient.

_____

_____

6. What is the significance of fibrous encapsulation?

_____

_____

7. In your own words, describe the connection between the implant and the patient's oral soft tissue.

_____

_____

_____

_____

_____

_____

8. In your own words, briefly describe each of the three types of dental implants.
- _Subperiosteal:_

_____

_____

- _Transosseous (transosteal):_

_____

_____

_____

- _Endosseous (endosteal):_

_____

_____

_____

9. List the types of endosseous root form implants.

_____

_____

_____

_____

_____

10. Identify factors that can increase a patient's risk for poor outcomes if dental implants are placed.

_____

_____

_____

_____

_____

_____

_____

_____

_____

_____

_____

_____

_____

_____

11. Which conditions are absolute contraindications for dental implants?

_____

_____

_____

_____

_____

12. What are the components of a postrestorative evaluation?

_____

_____

_____

_____

_____

_____

13. Each time the patient with dental implants is scheduled for routine continuing care, you will examine the implant area carefully. List the basic criteria that indicate a healthy implant.

14. Briefly describe the basic technique for routine probing to check for tissue integrity and bleeding around the dental implant during a continuing care appointment.

15. Briefly describe methods of removing calculus from the surface of a dental implant.

16. Explain why it is important to instruct a patient with dental implants to select self-cleaning implements and agents carefully.

17. Identify two prominent contributing factors in the breakdown of the peri-implant environment.

18. What maintenance phase issues can contribute to implant failure?

19. In your own words, briefly describe each of the three classifications of peri-implant disease.
   • *Peri-implant mucositis:*

   • *Peri-implantitis without mobility:*

   • *Peri-implantitis with mobility:*

20. When signs of peri-implant disease are noted during an oral examination, at what point is the patient referred back to the oral surgeon for intervention?

✓ COMPETENCY EXERCISES

Apply information from the chapter and use critical thinking skills to complete the competency exercises. Write responses on paper or create electronic documents to submit your answers.

1. Describe the dental hygienist's role in collaborative treatment planning and preparing the patient for dental implant procedures.

2. Matthew Glenn, aged 45 years, is scheduled today for a periodontal maintenance appointment. You are very excited and anxious to check the area of his dental implant–supported bridge. The prosthesis he received 6 months ago is a three-unit replacement for teeth 3, 4, and 5, with each pontic supported by an individual dental implant. You provided oral hygiene instructions for him both before and after his implant procedure, but you haven't seen him since.

During your assessment today, you find out that he is not having any oral problems, and the implants have been comfortable and feel just fine. In fact, he is delighted with the implants. His daily oral care is generally very good, but you notice small areas of biofilm in the hard-to-reach areas of the prosthesis, such as the embrasure between teeth 4 and 5 and the distal surface of tooth 3. To your surprise, there is also significant calculus buildup on the facial and mesial surfaces of tooth number 2.

The gingival tissue around the implant looks generally healthy. Mr. Glenn also exhibits some very slight calculus buildup on the facial surfaces of the left-side maxillary molars and on the lingual surfaces of his lower anterior teeth. You find no other significant medical history, dental history, or dental examination findings for Mr. Glenn today.

Use a copy of the Individualized Patient Care Plan template (see **workbook** Appendix B) to develop a care plan for Mr. Glenn that emphasizes daily care techniques to ensure long-term success for his implants and prosthesis.

DISCOVERY EXERCISE

- Research websites for viewing a dental implant procedure.
- Research implant manufacturers and supply companies to discover the cost of the instruments.
- Research the current dental terminology codes from the American Dental Association to identify the correct insurance billing codes for implant maintenance procedures.
- Go to the American Association of Periodontology website to find more information about dental implants.

EVERYDAY ETHICS

Before completing the learning exercises below, reread and reflect on the Everyday Ethics Scenario and Questions for Consideration in this chapter of the **textbook**. It may also be useful to review the Dental Hygiene Ethics discussion in Chapter 1, the Ethical Applications in the introduction pages for each section in the **textbook**, as well as the Codes of Ethics in **textbook** Appendices I–IV.

Individual Learning Activity

Identify a situation you have experienced that presents a similar ethical dilemma. What did you learn from how the situation was (or was not) resolved at the time it happened?

Collaborative Learning Activity

Work with a small group to develop a 2–5-minute role-play that introduces the Everyday Ethics scenario described in the chapter (a great idea is to video record your role-play activity). Then develop separate 2-minute role-play scenarios that provide at least two alternative approaches/solutions to resolving the situation. Ask classmates to view the solutions, ask questions, and discuss the ethical approach used in each. Ask for a vote on which solution classmates determine to be the "best."

Factors to Teach the Patient

This scenario is related to the following factors listed in this chapter of the **textbook**:

How to care for implants: special needs related to titanium surfaces.

▷ How the health of the periodontal tissues and the duration of the implants and prostheses depend on meticulous daily self-care by the patient and regular professional maintenance.

▷ The role of biofilm in periodontitis and peri-implantitis; vulnerability of the implant to infection from periodontal pathogens that may be present on adjacent natural teeth.

▷ How cleaning a mouth with complex restorations takes longer.

Use the individualized patient care plan you developed for Mr. Glenn (introduced in Competency Exercise question 2) and the principles of motivational interviewing (see **workbook** Appendix D) as a guide to prepare a conversation to provide oral hygiene instructions for Mr. Glenn during his dental hygiene appointment today.

MeSH TERMS

Use a combination of MeSH terms and other key words to develop an effective and efficient PubMed literature search strategy.

Dental implantation	Osseointegration
Dental implants, single-tooth	Dental implantation, subperiosteal
Dental implantation, endosseous	Peri-implantitis
	Dental implants

32

The Patient with Nicotine Use Disorders

LEARNING OBJECTIVES

Upon successful completion of these exercises, you will be able to:

1. Identify and define the key terms and concepts related to the use of tobacco.

2. Explain the systemic and oral effects of tobacco use.

3. Describe the effects of nicotine addiction.

4. Describe strategies for tobacco cessation.

5. Plan dental hygiene care and tobacco cessation interventions for patients who use tobacco.

6. Identify the role of the community-based dental hygienist in community-based tobacco-free initiatives.

 ### KNOWLEDGE EXERCISES

Write your answers for each question in the space provided.

1. Tobacco contains many components that are _____ to humans. Tobacco use is the single most _____ cause of disease and premature death in the world.

2. The drug in tobacco products that causes addiction is _____.

3. **True or False** (circle one and provide a rationale for your answer). Tobacco use with a water-cooled hookah device is a safe alternative to traditional smoking.

   _____

   _____

4. **True or False** (circle one and provide a rationale for your answer). The electronic nicotine delivery device is *not* an approved method of smoking cessation.

   _____

   _____

5. List factors that affect the amount of nicotine absorbed into the bloodstream when smoking tobacco.

   _____

   _____

   _____

   _____

   _____

6. Nicotine from smokeless tobacco can be absorbed through which tissues?

   _____

   _____

7. After the onset of smoking a cigarette, peak concentration of nicotine in the blood plasma occurs within approximately _____ and rapidly _____ over the next 20–30 minutes.

8. With the use of moist snuff, plasma concentration of nicotine in blood plasma reaches a peak at about _____ and then slowly declines.

9. How is nicotine eliminated from the body?

_____

_____

10. Match each of the following descriptive statements with the appropriate component of tobacco. Each term may be used more than once.

Tobacco-Related Terms	Descriptive Statements
A. Cotinine	____ By-product of nicotine is found in body fluids
B. Nicotine	____ The chief psychoactive ingredient in tobacco
C. Nitrosamines	____ The chief addictive agent in tobacco
D. Pyrolysis	____ Refers to a group of cancer-causing chemicals found in tobacco
	____ The process of breaking down chemicals contained in tobacco by heat created at the end of a burning cigarette
	____ Substances measured to determine recent use of nicotine-containing products
	____ Substance found in the various aids used for smoking cessation
	____ Intensifies the release of dopamine by the brain
	____ Although addictive, this chemical is _not_ the most physically harmful substance found in tobacco
	____ Released with other substances when the tobacco is ignited

11. In your own words, briefly summarize the systemic effects of tobacco use.

_____

_____

_____

_____

_____

12. List as many negative health effects of tobacco use and/or exposure to secondhand ETS as you can.

_____

_____

_____

_____

_____

_____

_____

_____

_____

13. Identify as many potential oral health consequences of tobacco use as you can.

_____

_____

_____

_____

_____

_____

_____

_____

_____

14. Match each of the following descriptive statements with the appropriate tobacco-related term.

Tobacco-Related Terms	Descriptive Statements
A. Tolerance	____ The use of any drug in a way that causes harm to the person or other persons who are affected by the user's behavior
B. Dependence	
C. Abuse	
D. Addiction	
E. ETS	____ Refers to the user's need for increased tobacco use over time to create the desired feeling of well-being
F. TSNAs	
	____ Loss of control over the amount and frequency of use of tobacco and withdrawal symptoms occur when use of tobacco is discontinued

Tobacco-Related Terms	Descriptive Statements
	____ Formed by tobacco smoke reaction with nitrous acid on indoor surfaces
	____ Chronic, progressive, relapsing disease characterized by compulsive use of a substance
	____ Refers to passive exposure to second- or thirdhand tobacco smoke

15. Describe the *reinforcing effect* of tobacco.

_____

_____

_____

_____

_____

_____

_____

_____

16. Why are children of parents or caregivers who use tobacco also at high risk for disease?

_____

_____

_____

_____

_____

_____

_____

17. In your own words, explain each of the following terms as they relate to your role during dental hygiene care for your patient who uses tobacco products.

- *Detect:*

_____

_____

_____

- *Explain:*

_____

_____

- *Motivate:*

_____

_____

- *Refer:*

_____

_____

_____

- *Document:*

_____

_____

_____

18. Explain two strategies you can use to support a patient who is ready to quit using tobacco.

_____

_____

19. The five As provide the basis for a simple but effective tobacco dependence–intervention approach. Number the five As in the appropriate order (from 1 to 5) and then *briefly* outline the basic premise of each one.

- _____ *Advise:*

_____

_____

- _____ *Arrange:*

_____

_____

_____

- _____ *Ask:*

_____

- _____ *Assess:*

_____

- _____ *Assist:*

_____

20. List the methods available for delivering nicotine-replacement therapy if your patient is considering pharmacotherapy as a treatment for nicotine addiction.

21. Identify non-nicotine pharmacotherapies approved by the FDA for tobacco cessation.

22. In your own words, state the objectives and rationale for using pharmacotherapies to help your patient stop using tobacco.

23. What factors are considered when recommending pharmacotherapies to help your patients stop using tobacco?

24. What are the contraindications for use of pharmacotherapy-assisted tobacco cessation?

25. What are the most common *oral* side effects of the pharmacotherapies used for treatment of nicotine addiction?

✓ COMPETENCY EXERCISES

Apply information from the chapter and use critical thinking skills to complete the competency exercises. Write responses on paper or create electronic documents to submit your answers.

1. Use the Tobacco Use Assessment Form (Figure 32-3 in the **textbook**) to assess the tobacco-using habits of a friend or relative. Use the methods outlined in the Tobacco Cessation Flowchart (Figure 34-4 in the **textbook**) and a motivational interviewing approach (see **workbook** Appendix D) to explore the readiness of this individual to quit.

2. The Section V Summary exercises section of this workbook contains a Patient Assessment Summary for Mrs. Diane White, who is in her first trimester of pregnancy. Although Mrs. White does not smoke, her husband does. Describe the tobacco use and cessation information you would like to be able to provide as you talk to Mrs. White during her dental hygiene and reevaluation appointments. Describe how you will use motivational interviewing principles (see **workbook** Appendix D) as you educate Mrs. White on the detrimental health effects of her husband's tobacco habit.

3. Using your institution's guidelines for writing in patient records, document that you have provided education and counseling related to the health effects of tobacco use during Mrs. White's appointment.

4. As a dental hygienist, your role in addressing the oral and systemic health damage of tobacco use is wider than simply providing assessment, information, motivation, and guidance to individual patients in your

clinical practice. Discuss your role in tobacco education and cessation from a personal and community-based or advocacy perspective.

DISCOVERY EXERCISE

Collect a variety of patient education materials—such as brochures, posters, or videotapes—that address the health and/or oral health effects of tobacco use. Encourage each of your student colleagues to collect as many materials as possible from a variety of different sources. Get together in small groups to discuss the materials.

- Determine the scientific accuracy of the information included in the patient-education materials.
- Determine which type of patient each of the materials is best suited for.
- Determine how each of the materials might best be used as part of tobacco-cessation initiatives in your clinic.

EVERYDAY ETHICS

Before completing the learning exercises below, reread and reflect on the Everyday Ethics Scenario and Questions for Consideration in this chapter of the **textbook**. It may also be useful to review the Dental Hygiene Ethics discussion in Chapter 1, the Ethical Applications in the introduction pages for each section in the **textbook**, as well as the Codes of Ethics in **textbook** Appendices I–IV.

Collaborative Learning Activity

Answer each of the questions for consideration at the end of the scenario in the **textbook**. Compare what you wrote with answers developed by another classmate and discuss differences/similarities.

Discovery Activity

Summarize this scenario for faculty member at your school and ask them to consider the questions that are included. Is their perspective different than yours or similar? Explain.

Factors to Teach the Patient

This scenario is related to the following factors listed in this chapter of the **textbook**:

▷ Nonsmokers who breathe ETS can incur the same serious health problems as smokers. Children are especially susceptible.

Mrs. White's husband (see Competency Question #2 above) arrives to pick up his wife following her dental hygiene appointment. He wants to discuss their insurance coverage with the office manager, but she is on the telephone, so he must wait for a few minutes to speak with her. He sits down in a chair and immediately takes out a pack of cigarettes and some matches. He asks you for an ashtray.

Use the motivational interviewing principles (see **workbook** Appendix D) as a guide to prepare an outline for explaining the tobacco-free policy in your office to Mr. White. Mr. White is not your patient—how far can you go in approaching him about the dangers of his tobacco use for his unborn child or providing recommendations for smoking cessation measures?

Use the conversation you create to role-play this situation with a fellow student. If you are the patient in the role-play, be sure to ask questions. If you are the dental hygienist, try to anticipate questions and answer them in your explanation.

MeSH TERMS

Use a combination of MeSH terms and other key words to develop an effective and efficient PubMed literature search strategy.

Smoking	Tobacco use
Carcinogens	Gingival neoplasms
Tobacco	Tobacco use cessation
Head and neck neoplasms	Palatal neoplasms
Tobacco products	Tobacco use cessation
Mouth neoplasms	products
Tobacco smoke pollution	Laryngeal neoplasms
Lip neoplasms	Tobacco use disorder
Tobacco, smokeless	Leukoplakia, oral
Tongue neoplasms	

33

Diet and Dietary Analysis

 KNOWLEDGE EXERCISES

Write your answers for each question in the space provided.

1. List the major food categories included in the MyPlate icon (Figure 33-1 in the **textbook**).

   _____

   _____

   _____

   _____

2. Identify two additional food categories listed in Table 33-2, Healthy U.S. Style Patterns, that contribute to an individual's caloric intake.

   _____

   _____

3. The food intake pattern sheet contains a table that outlines the daily amount of food that is appropriate based on 12 different _____ (two words).

4. Identify three characteristics used to determine the appropriate calorie intake level for an individual person's diet.

   _____

   _____

   _____

5. Look at Table 33-1 in the **textbook** to find the appropriate calorie level for yourself. _____

   _____

6. What amount of food from the dark-green vegetable subgroup is suggested for your diet?

   _____

   _____

7. Table 33-3 in the **textbook** provides a comprehensive list of nutrients with their functions, associated disease states, and food sources. Your instructor will let you know the level of detail you are expected to recall from the information in that table. It is most important for you to be able to link deficiencies in nutritional intake with oral manifestations you may observe while providing dental hygiene care for your patients. Table 33-4 provides some oral manifestations that are associated with nutritional deficiencies.

   Infomap 33-1 (on the next page) reorganizes information from the **textbook** to help you associate nutrient deficiencies with specific intraoral findings. Use information throughout Chapter 33 of the **textbook** to help you complete the infomap with (a) the oral findings you might observe if your patient is deficient in each listed nutrient and (b) food sources for that nutrient you can recommend to your patient.

INFOMAP 33-1

NUTRIENT	ORAL MANIFESTATIONS OF DEFICIENCY	FOOD SOURCES
Vitamin A		
Thiamin (vitamin B$_1$)		
Niacin (vitamin B$_3$)		
Riboflavin (vitamin B$_2$)		
Pyridoxine (vitamin B$_6$)		
Cobalamin (vitamin B$_{12}$)		
Ascorbic acid (vitamin C)		
Vitamin D		
Calcium		
Fluoride		
Folate		
Iron		
Magnesium		
Phosphorus		
Zinc		
Protein		

8. Which vitamins and minerals are associated with healthy skin and mucous membrane?

_____

_____

_____

_____

_____

9. Which nutrients are important for healthy wound healing and tissue repair?

_____

_____

_____

10. Which nutrients are essential for development of healthy tooth structure?

_____

_____

_____

_____

_____

11. Dental caries is the result of intake of _____ foods and is not due to nutrient deficiency.

12. Identify four factors that interact to result in dental caries.

_____

_____

_____

_____

13. Any incident of sucrose intake lowers the pH in the dental biofilm. But what two major factors interact to enhance cariogenic exposure and increase your patient's risk for developing dental caries?

_____

_____

_____

14. In your own words, discuss the purposes of a dietary assessment.

_____

_____

_____

_____

_____

15. Summarize the information you will provide for your patient when you are explaining your dietary assessment intervention prior to asking the patient to complete a food diary.

_____

_____

_____

_____

_____

_____

16. Identify some common dietary omissions that you will want to be sure to review with your patient as you explain the dietary intake form.

_____

_____

_____

17. In your own words, explain how to calculate a patient's caries risk using the Sweet Score. (*Hint:* Use the information in Table 33-7 in the **textbook** to guide your answer.)

_____

_____

_____

_____

_____

_____

_____

_____

18. If, after calculating the Sweet Score, you determine that your patient is at moderate or high risk for dental caries, what recommendations will you be sure

to provide during your oral health education session with that patient?

_____

_____

_____

_____

_____

_____

_____

19. Identify _patient_ factors that can affect your success in providing nutritional counseling for your patients.

_____

_____

_____

_____

_____

20. Identify _communication_ factors that can affect your success in providing nutritional counseling for your patients.

_____

_____

_____

_____

_____

21. For a patient who is especially caries-susceptible, what ingredient in chewing gum will help promote remineralization if chewed immediately after each meal?

_____

22. In your own words, describe the term "nutrition" in terms your patient could understand.

_____

_____

_____

_____

_____

COMPETENCY EXERCISES

Apply information from the chapter and use critical thinking skills to complete the competency exercises. Write responses on paper or create electronic documents to submit your answers.

1. Make a food diary table similar to Table 33-5 in the **textbook** and create a food diary for everything you ate yesterday. (No cheating, now; no one will ever see this but you.) What nutrients are missing from your diet?

2. Make a copy of the scoring the sweets form (Table 33-7 in the **textbook**). Use the information in your 24-hour food diary to calculate your personal risk for dental caries. What recommendations will you give yourself to reduce your caries risk?

3. Ask a student colleague, friend, or member of your family to complete a 3- or 5-day food diary. Make a copy of the dietary analysis recording form (Table 33-6 in the **textbook**) to complete a dietary analysis for that person.

4. Identify topics you would include in a patient education program based on the dietary analysis you completed for question 3.

5. Use the MyPlate nutritional guidelines to create _your_ ideal caries-control diet that contains foods you like to eat. Create menus for several days and make sure that your diet provides adequate nutrition for a person who is just like you. Compare your menus with the menus created by your student colleagues.

Discuss how your colleagues' food preferences, cultural considerations, or personal eating practices compare with yours. What does this exercise help you realize about possible barriers when you are providing diet counseling for your diverse, individual patients?

6. Because individualized dental hygiene care plans are based on individualized patient needs determined by assessment data, not every dental hygiene care plan you write will include dietary assessment or dietary counseling. Discuss patient assessment findings that would indicate the need to include a 24-hour or 3- to 7-day dietary assessment as part of your patient's dental hygiene care plan.

EVERYDAY ETHICS

Before completing the learning exercises below, reread and reflect on the Everyday Ethics Scenario and Questions for Consideration in this chapter of the **textbook**. It may also be useful to review the Dental Hygiene Ethics discussion in Chapter 1, the Ethical Applications in the introduction pages for each section in the **textbook**, as well as the Codes of Ethics in **textbook** Appendices I–IV.

Individual Learning Activity

Imagine that you are the dental hygienist in this scenario. Answer each of the questions for consideration at the end of the scenario.

Discovery Activity

Ask a dental hygienist who has been practicing for a year or more to read the scenario. Provide them with a copy of the Code of Ethics as well. Share the responses you have made to answer each question and ask that person to discuss the situation with you. What insights did you have or what did you learn during this discussion?

Factors to Teach the Patient

This scenario is related to the following factors listed in this chapter of the **textbook**:

▷ Reasons to avoid frequent daily use of medications with sucrose.

▷ Reasons for rinsing with water after a medication contained in a syrupy sucrose mixture.

▷ How dental caries on the tooth surface starts and progresses.

▷ How the interaction of cariogenic foods, tooth surface, saliva, and microorganisms act together in the dental caries process.

▷ How repeated, frequent acid production and the pH in the dental biofilm adversely affect the teeth.

Your next patient, Nathan, is a 7-year-old boy with a lot of serious medical health issues. Because he often has a queasy stomach, his mother fixes him many small meals each day and states that mostly all he will eat are high carbohydrate foods.

In addition, Nathan is frequently placed on a (sucrose-enhanced) antibiotic liquid preparation prescribed by his physician. His mother states he absolutely refuses to take any medication in a pill form, so the antibiotic syrup is the only answer.

Use the principles of motivational interviewing (see **workbook** Appendix D) as a guide to prepare an outline for a conversation with Nathan's mother explaining his risk for caries and the importance of changing the boy's daily dietary habits. Make sure to adapt your recommendations for the barriers to behavior change that have been identified in the scenario.

Use the conversation you create to role-play this situation with a fellow student. If you are Nathan's mother in the role-play, be sure to ask questions and try to identify additional real-life barriers to behavior change. If you are the dental hygienist, try to anticipate questions and answer them in your explanation.

MeSH TERMS

Use a combination of MeSH terms and other key words to develop an effective and efficient PubMed literature search strategy.

Diet	Nutritional status
Nutritional requirements	Diet, cariogenic
Food habits	Nutrition assessment
Dietary carbohydrates	Cariogenic agents
Diet surveys	Nutrition disorders
Dietary sucrose	

CHAPTER 33 CROSSWORD PUZZLE

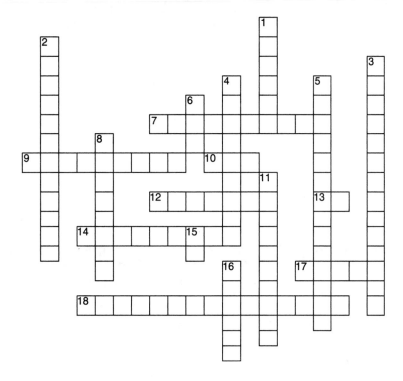

Puzzle Clues

Across

7. Foods that lower the pH of oral biofilm and increase risk for dental caries.

9. A factor in exposure to cariogenic food that is very significant for increasing risk for dental caries.

10. Average amounts of nutrients that should be consumed daily by healthy individuals (acronym).

12. Developed by the USDA to illustrate the food groups important for a balanced diet.

13. Maximum intake of a specific nutrient that is unlikely to create adverse health risks for an individual (acronym).

14. Lifestyle that includes only light physical activity on a day-to-day basis.

17. Diet consisting only of plant foods.

18. Refers to comparing the nutrient content of a food with the amount of energy it provides (two words).

Down

1. Lifestyle that includes an increased amount of physical activity.

2. Poor nourishment resulting from improper food intake.

3. Foods that do not lower the pH of biofilm or that encourage remineralization.

4. Listing of various foods and measurements of amounts eaten during a specific time period (two words).

5. Carbohydrate, protein, and fat are examples.

6. Comprehensive term that encompasses all categories of dietary reference guidelines (acronym).

8. Chemical substance in foods that is needed by the body for building and repair.

11. Term that refers to nutritional inadequacy of specific nutrients in body tissues.

15. Recommendations for adequate intake of essential nutrients (acronym).

16. United States Department of Health and Human Services (acronym).

34

Fluorides

 KNOWLEDGE EXERCISES

Write your answers for each question in the space provided.

1. Fluoride is made available to the tooth surface in two ways. Which method has the primary beneficial effect throughout life?

_____

_____

2. **True or False (circle one).** Fluoride can be lost slowly from the teeth over time due to resorption or remodeling.

3. Describe how dietary fluoride is absorbed by and distributed to body tissues.

_____

_____

_____

4. Dietary fluoride is excreted mostly through the _____.

5. Approximately 99% of fluoride in the body is located in _____ tissues, such as _____ and _____.

6. During the formation of enamel, fluoride is deposited starting at the _____.

7. Fluoride concentration is greatest in the area of dentin nearest the _____. (*Hint*: See Figure 34-1 in the **textbook**.)

8. Too much fluoride ingested during tooth development can result in _____.

9. Before the tooth erupts but after the crown is completely mineralized, systemic fluoride is deposited on the _____.

10. Fluoride, from drinking water or from topical fluoride treatments, continues to be deposited on the surface of the tooth after the tooth has _____.

11. Topical fluoride uptake on the tooth surface is most rapid during _____.

12. Topical fluoride concentration in the enamel is highest at the _____ of the enamel.

13. Fluoride level in cementum is high and increases _____.

14. In your own words, describe demineralization.

_____

_____

_____

15. Where does demineralization occur?

_____

_____

_____

_____

16. In early stages of demineralization, which area of the enamel has the greatest fluoride concentration?

_____

_____

_____

_____

17. In your own words, describe remineralization.

_____

_____

_____

_____

18. What is the role of fluoride in the demineralization–remineralization process?

_____

_____

19. What is the effect of fluoride on bacteria?

_____

_____

20. What is dental fluorosis?

_____

_____

_____

_____

_____

21. Who identified fluorine as the element related to the observed changes in tooth enamel and risk for dental caries?

_____

22. Who was Dr. H. Trendley Dean?

_____

_____

_____

_____

23. What is the optimal level of fluoride concentration in community drinking water currently advised by the U.S. Department of Health and Human services for caries prevention?

_____

24. Adding fluoride to the school water supply in communities that do not have access to a fluoridated community water system is one way to benefit children in rural areas. Why is the concentration of fluoride increased from the optimum level when fluoride is added to only the school water supply?

_____

_____

_____

_____

25. When fluoride is removed from the water in a community, one of two possible effects is noted. What are the two possible effects?

_____

_____

_____

_____

26. What compounds are used to fluoridate community water supplies?

_____

_____

_____

_____

27. List factors to investigate when you are trying to determine whether a child needs dietary fluoride supplements.

_____

_____

_____

_____

28. What level of fluoride is typically found in ready-to-feed and reconstituted infant formulas?

_____

_____

_____

29. In what forms can supplementary fluoride be given?

_____

_____

_____

30. If the fluoride water concentration in the community is 0.45 ppm and there is no additional fluoride in the water supply at school, what is the dose of supplemental fluoride that is recommended for a 5-year-old child and her 12-year-old brother?

_____

_____

31. The ideal fluoride regimen for most patients is high frequency, low concentration. That is why fluoridated water is so effective in preventing dental decay for most people. What factors indicate the need for you to include a professionally applied fluoride treatment in your patient's care plan?

_____

_____

_____

_____

_____

_____

32. What are the objectives for a professionally applied topical fluoride?

_____

_____

_____

33. What is the concentration of fluoride ions in a 1.23% acidulated phosphate gel, which you apply to your patient's teeth using a tray?

_____

Which professional fluoride preparation contains the highest concentration of fluoride ions?

_____

34. In your own words, describe the term *cariostatic effect*.

_____

35. Name the cariostatic agent in silver diamine fluoride.

_____

36. What professionally applied solution is recommended for infants and small children who are at high risk for dental caries?

_____

37. Which types of fluoride applications are considered effective to reduce dentinal hypersensitivity?

_____

38. If your patient presents with a four-unit porcelain anterior bridge, which fluoride preparation is *not* appropriate for you to recommend and why?

_____

_____

39. List the indications for silver diamine fluoride.

_____

_____

_____

_____

40. List three advantages of silver diamine fluoride.

_____

41. How are the patient's teeth prepared before painting on a fluoride solution, applying a fluoride varnish, or placing the trays during a professional fluoride application?

_____

_____

_____

42. Briefly list the steps for applying a fluoride varnish.

_____

_____

_____

_____

_____

_____

_____

43. Briefly describe techniques for using self-applied fluorides. _____

_____

44. Match each of the following descriptions with the appropriate self-applied fluoride *mouthrinse* preparation. Each type of mouthrinse is described more than once in the description column.

Description	Mouthrinse Type
____ Once per week use	A. Low potency/ high frequency
____ Recommended for daily use	
____ Available only as a sodium fluoride preparation	B. High potency/ low frequency
____ Available as a sodium fluoride or acidulated phosphate fluoride preparation	
____ Can be purchased as an over-the-counter preparation	
____ Is available in a 0.05% solution	
____ Is sometimes used in school-based fluoride rinse programs	
____ Has been shown to reduce the incidence of dental caries by 30%–40% with reports of a 42.5% reduction in caries in primary teeth	

45. Use Infomap 34-1 to help you compare type of fluoride ion and concentrations available in each type of preparation available for recommendation to patients who are at risk for dental caries.

INFOMAP 34-1		
PREPARATION TYPE	**APF**	**NaF (OR SODIUM MONOFLUOROPHOSPHATE)**
Professional topical fluoride foam or gel preparations		
Self-applied fluoride gel preparations		
Self-applied fluoride rinse preparations		
Fluoride dentifrice preparations		
Fluoride varnish preparations		
Optimally fluoridated water		

46. In your own words, briefly list important safety measures to discuss with your patient when educating about the use of home fluorides.

_____

_____

_____

_____

_____

_____

_____

47. Briefly describe the signs and symptoms of a toxic dose of fluoride.

_____

_____

_____

_____

_____

_____

_____

48. If your patient feels nauseated and has stomach pain after receiving a professional fluoride treatment in your clinic, what is the first thing you should do?

_____

49. What tooth-related, observable symptom is linked to a larger-than-safe dose of systemic fluoride ingested over a long period of time?

_____

50. Supply the acronym or chemical formula that can be used to document each type of fluoride preparation in a patient progress note—just one more time to help you remember!

- *Acidulated phosphate fluoride*

_____

- *Sodium fluoride*

_____

- *Silver diamine fluoride*

_____

- *Stannous fluoride*

_____

51. Consideration of any fluoride treatment requires you to communicate effectively with the patient/parent/legal guardian/advocate and consider use of a written informed consent form. List five specific reasons why this is particularly important when discussing SDF placement.

_____

_____

_____

_____

_____

✓ COMPETENCY EXERCISES

Apply information from the chapter and use critical thinking skills to complete the competency exercises. Write responses on paper or create electronic documents to submit your answers.

1. Refer to the patient assessment summary for Melody Crane (aged 15 months). Use the information in the summary to develop dental hygiene diagnosis statements and a plan for interventions related to her risk for early childhood caries.

2. A dental hygienist experienced an unfortunate incident a few days ago while preparing a fluoride treatment for a 6-year-old child who weighs 45 pounds. She filled a set of trays with the maximum allowable amount of 2.0% neutral sodium fluoride gel for children (*Hint:* consult the legend for Figure 34-5 in the **textbook**) and left the trays sitting on the counter while she exited the room briefly to get permission for the fluoride treatment from the child's mother. She returned moments later to find that the child had picked up the trays and licked every bit of the fluoride gel out of both the upper and the lower tray. **Calculate the dose of fluoride that the child received in this incident**. Does this amount exceed the safely tolerated dose or the certainly lethal dose? *Hint:* Consult **textbook** Box 34-4B (CLDs and STDs for Selected Ages) and Figure 34-6 (how to calculate amounts of fluoride).

3. What type of toxic reaction might the child described in the previous scenario experience after ingesting this dosage of fluoride?

4. Give an example of a situation that could lead to chronic fluoride toxicity and discuss what you would include in an education presentation for your patient (or patient's parent) to prevent this from happening.

CHAPTER 34—PATIENT ASSESSMENT SUMMARY

Patient Name: *Melody Crane*	Age: *15 Months*	Gender: F	☑ Initial Therapy
			☐ Maintenance
Provider Name: *D.H. Student*	Date: *Today*		☐ Reevaluation

Chief Complaint:

Toothache and swollen area in lower left jaw. Ulcerated lesion on upper left lip.

Assessment Findings

Health History

- *Frequent ear infections—three since birth*
- *Frequent use of liquid antibiotics—contain sweeteners*
- *ASA Classification—II*
- *ADL level—3*

At Risk For:

- *Early childhood caries*

Social and Dental History

- *Initial dental visit—first teeth present at 6 months*
- *Family drinks mostly bottled or filtered water*
- *Fluoride toothpaste used four times per week—unspecified amount of paste*
- *Bottle used two times daily at naptime and bedtime, at-will use of "sippy-cup" for juice*
- *Five-year-old brother with restorations on all primary molars and some anterior teeth*

At Risk For:

- *Early childhood caries*

CHAPTER 34—PATIENT ASSESSMENT SUMMARY (*continued*)

Dental Examination

- *Moderate dental biofilm along cervical margins of maxillary incisors*
- *White-spot lesions at cervical of four maxillary incisors*
- *Red maxillary anterior gingiva*

At Risk For:

Periodontal Diagnosis/Case Type and Status

Gingivitis

Caries Management Risk Assessment (CAMBRA) Level:

☐ Low ☐ Moderate ☐ High ☑ Extreme

Dental Hygiene Diagnosis

Problem

Related to (Risk Factors and Etiology)

Planned Interventions

(to arrest or control disease and regenerate, restore or maintain health)

Clinical

Education/Counseling   Oral Hygiene Instruction/Home Care

EVERYDAY ETHICS

Before completing the learning exercises below, reread and reflect on the Everyday Ethics Scenario and Questions for Consideration in this chapter of the **textbook**. It may also be useful to review the Dental Hygiene Ethics discussion in Chapter 1, the Ethical Applications in the introduction pages for each section in the **textbook**, as well as the Codes of Ethics in **textbook** Appendices I–IV.

Individual Learning Activity

Imagine the scenario from the patient's perspective. How might the patient's response to the questions following the scenario be different from those of the dental hygienist involved?

Collaborative Learning Activity

Work with another student colleague to role-play the scenario. The goal of this exercise is for you and your colleague to work through the alternative actions in order to come to consensus on a solution or response that is acceptable to both of you.

Factors to Teach the Patient

This scenario is related to the following factors listed in this chapter of the **textbook**:

▷ Personal use of fluorides.
▷ Need for parental supervision.
▷ Determining need for fluoride supplements.
▷ Fluorides being a part of the total preventive program.
▷ Fluoridation.
▷ Bottled drinking water.

In Competency Exercise question #1, you developed a plan for a patient-specific fluoride intervention for Melody Crane. Use the plan you developed and the example conversations in **workbook** Appendix D as a guide to prepare a conversation that you might use to educate Melody's mother about the fluoride intervention you have planned and about her role in preventing further caries activity for her children.

CHAPTER 34 WORD SEARCH PUZZLE

```
S R U D E M I N E R A L I Z A T I O N D
Q W M F Z D E F L U O R I D A T I O N J
W H Y L V Y P E F L U O R A P A T I T E
H Y T O X C I C I T Y J H D Q R U C M Y
R D J K F L U O R O S I S G N T K A E L
K R G S E D Q L U T K F E W Z K C Q Y K
U O N I P U S W S C L M G F U Q L T N R
I X K B J Z H Q S V M F Z L S B V K I I
Z Y B J J M C K A Y R P F L U O R I D E
V A T M B C A R I O S T A T I C X B H F
A P D T M V W H I T E S P O T H K V P K
R A H A L O E F F E C T Q V K D H A Y I
N T R E M I N E R A L I Z A T I O N M D
I I L C S U B S U R F A C E L E S I O N
S T H Y P O C A L C I F I E D E T U D E
H E N B C V F O J V Z W C F I T H C W Y
G A A J L Z D B V D P U N B I V M X F W
R O W K E F F I C A C Y D Z V X L S I N
N F I T H I X O T R O P I C J U U S W B
V G G M F C P P M F G Q J X T I Q Y H F
```

Puzzle Clues

1. Refers to a fluoride preparation with a pH of 3.5 that may etch porcelain (acronym).

2. The researcher who associated Colorado brown stain with drinking water.

3. The result, in a non-fluoridated community, of consuming fluoride that has been incorporated into food or beverages during processing (two words).

4. Over the counter (acronym).

5. A small area on the tooth that may be the first clinically detectable caries lesion or an area of demineralization (two words).

6. An area of demineralization below the enamel surface that can become remineralized with fluoride application (two words).

7. $Ca_{10} (PO_4)_6O_2$.

8. Inhibiting dental caries.

9. The removal of fluoride from a water supply that has a naturally occurring higher-than-optimum fluoride level.

10. Breakdown of the tooth structure with a loss of calcium and phosphorus.

11. Term referring to the ability of clinically tested products to produce a significant health benefit.

12. A less-soluble apatite that is more resistant to acids.

13. A systemic nutrient that enhances tooth remineralization.

14. Small white spots to severe brown staining and pitting of the enamel caused by pre-eruptive ingestion of excessive amounts of fluoride.

15. Most fluoride is excreted from the body through this organ.

16. Refers to enamel with deficient calcification.

17. Parts per million (abbreviation).

18. Fluoride enhances this process, which returns minerals to the tooth.

19. A type of gel that becomes fluid under stress to permit flow.

20. This can occur as a result of a rapid intake of high concentration fluoride over a short period of time.

21. A form of professional topical fluoride application that is easily applied to root surfaces and sets up in the presence of saliva.

Sealants

 KNOWLEDGE EXERCISES

Write your answers for each question in the space provided.

1. In your own words, describe the purpose of placing a dental sealant.

2. How does the placement of an acid etchant prepare the tooth for a dental sealant?

3. List the criteria for an ideal dental sealant.

4. The many types of dental sealants have, to some extent, combined or overlapping characteristics. For example, autopolymerized dental sealants can be either clear or opaque in color. Briefly describe the classifications and types of dental sealants.

5. What criteria determine that sealant placement is indicated for a specific patient or tooth?

6. Study Table 35-1 in the **textbook** and review the Section "Clinical Procedures" in Chapter 35 of the **textbook** to learn the basic procedures for application of dental sealants. List some general rules for sealant application.

_____

_____

_____

7. Number from 1 to 10 to place the action steps for application of dental sealants in the correct order.

Order	Description of Action Step
___	Check occlusion
___	Isolate tooth (or teeth in a quadrant)
___	Rinse and dry tooth
___ and ___	Evaluate (this step occurs twice)
___	Cure or wait for self-polymerization
___	Prepare tooth
___	Place sealant material
___	Dry area and place etchant
___	Prepare patient

8. What is the purpose of debriding and cleaning the tooth surface before etching for sealant placement?

_____

_____

_____

_____

9. What materials can be used to isolate the area receiving a dental sealant?

_____

_____

_____

_____

10. After the tooth surface is etched, rinsed, and completely dried, what should you observe?

_____

11. What anatomic feature may prevent the dental sealant material from penetrating to the bottom of the occlusal fissure?

_____

_____

_____

12. Identify the factors that affect sealant retention.

_____

13. What is documented in the patient record following the placement of a dental sealant?

_____

_____

_____

_____

 COMPETENCY EXERCISES

Apply information from the chapter and use critical thinking skills to complete the competency exercises. Write responses on paper or create electronic documents to submit your answers.

1. You are collecting assessment data during an initial dental hygiene appointment for Dimitri Albergo, who is 12 years old. Dr. Donovan expects you to evaluate the need for dental sealants, record your findings on an assessment form, and then discuss your specific recommendations when he comes in to examine the patient. Together, you will make decisions for including sealants in Dimitri's dental hygiene care plan. What oral findings indicate a potential need for the placement of dental sealants?

2. Discuss why Dimitri's second molars are the most important teeth to evaluate for sealant placement.

3. During your oral examination of Dimitri, you find a pit-and-fissure area on tooth 30 that is questionable for the placement of a dental sealant. What next step will you take to determine whether that specific tooth surface is appropriate for sealant placement?

4. When you evaluate Dimitri's bitewing radiographs, no occlusal or proximal surface dental caries are present on tooth 14. What is the next step in deciding whether to select that tooth for placement of a dental sealant?

🖥 **MeSH TERMS**

Use a combination of MeSH terms and other key words to develop an effective and efficient PubMed literature search strategy.

Pit-and-fissure sealants	Resins, synthetic
Light curing of dental adhesives	Curing lights, dental
Acid etching, dental	Self-curing of dental resins

EVERYDAY ETHICS

Before completing the learning exercises below, reread and reflect on the Everyday Ethics Scenario and Questions for Consideration in this chapter of the **textbook**. It may also be useful to review the Dental Hygiene Ethics discussion in Chapter 1, the Ethical Applications in the introduction pages for each section in the textbook, as well as the Codes of Ethics in **textbook** Appendices I–IV.

Individual Learning Activity

Imagine that you are the dental hygienist in this scenario. Answer each of the questions for consideration at the end of the scenario.

Collaborative Learning Activity

Answer each of the questions for consideration at the end of the scenario in the **textbook**. Compare what you wrote with answers developed by another classmate and discuss differences/similarities.

Factors to Teach the Patient

This scenario is related to the following factors listed in this chapter of the **textbook**:

▷ Sealants as part of a preventive program but not as a substitute for other preventive measures (e.g., limiting dietary sucrose, using fluorides, and controlling dental biofilm).

▷ What a sealant is and why such a meticulous application procedure is required.

▷ What can be expected from a sealant, including how long it lasts and how it prevents dental caries.

The dental hygiene care plan you develop for Dimitri (introduced in Competency Exercise question 1) recommends dental sealants for all four of his second permanent molars, plus teeth 14 and 3. Dimitri's mother has heard of dental sealants but does not understand why she should spend so much money to "fix" a tooth that has nothing wrong with it. In order to obtain consent from Dimitri's mother to apply the dental sealants, you must educate her.

Use the motivational interviewing principles (see **workbook** Appendix D) as a guide to develop a conversation to explain dental sealants to Mrs. Albergo.

CHAPTER 35 CROSSWORD PUZZLE

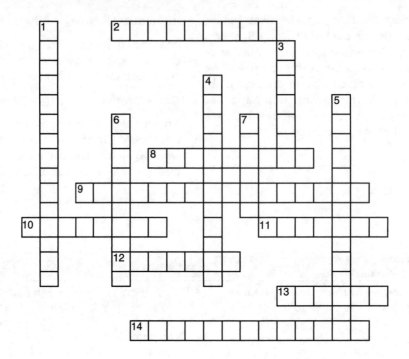

Puzzle Clues

Across

2. Early or beginning dental caries.

8. Resistance to flow or alteration of shape a result of molecular cohesion.

9. Polymerization with the use of an external light source.

10. Absorbent pad placed in the cheek over the opening of Stensen duct to aid in maintaining a dry field while placing sealants.

11. Physical adherence of one substance to another.

12. Phosphoric acid, which prepares the surface of the tooth to provide mechanical retention for the sealant.

13. Polymerization of resin-based sealant and composites.

14. Contains additional materials that make the sealant more resistant to abrasion.

Down

1. Self-curing dental sealant.

3. Organic polymer that bonds to an enamel surface by mechanical retention.

4. Paper that marks points of contact (occlusion) between the maxillary and mandibular teeth.

5. Reaction in which a high-molecular-weight product is produced by successive additions of a simpler compound.

6. Tiny openings.

7. Plastic material used for dental sealants (acronym).

Implementation: Prevention

Chapters 24–35

 COMPETENCY EXERCISES

Apply information from the chapters and use critical thinking skills to complete the competency exercises. Write responses on paper or create electronic documents to submit your answers.

SECTION VI—PATIENT ASSESSMENT SUMMARY			
Patient Name: *Harold Wilmot*	Age: *44*	Gender: M	☑ Initial Therapy
			☐ Maintenance
Provider Name: *D.H. Student*	Date: *Today*		☐ Re-evaluation
Chief Complaint:			
Recently moved into this community—"I need my teeth cleaned."			

Assessment Findings	
Health History	**At Risk For:**
• Asthma; uses steroid inhaler • Hypertension (148/82): controlled with beta-blocker medication • Tobacco use: $\frac{1}{2}$ to 1 pack per day for about 25 years • ASA classification-II • ADL level-0	
Social and Dental History	**At Risk For:**
• Has had regular dental visits (1 per year); last visit 1 year ago • Has received tobacco cessation education and regular oral hygiene instructions at previous dental visits • Has tried twice to quit smoking, but relapsed because of withdrawal symptoms	

Dental Examination

- Complete upper denture; lower partial denture (replaces 23–26, 19, and 30)
- Generalized recession 1–3 mm on remaining teeth; radiographic evidence of generalized slight horizontal bone loss
- Probing depths = 5 mm on 31 distal and on mesial and distal surfaces of all premolars; generalized slight bleeding on probing
- History of coronal and root caries; all current restorations intact; no new cavitated carious lesions
- Moderate calculus on mandibular anterior prostheses; proximal biofilm noted in premolars
- 3 mm × 3 mm area of leukoplakia on alveolar ridge distal to tooth #18

At Risk For:

Periodontal Diagnosis/Case Type and Status

Caries Management Risk Assessment (CAMBRA) Level:
☐ Low   ☐ Moderate   ☐ High   ☐ Extreme

DENTAL HYGIENE DIAGNOSIS statements related to PREVENTION interventions

Problem	Related to (Risk Factors and Etiology)

PLANNED INTEVENTIONS related to PREVENTION

(to arrest or control disease and regenerate, restore or maintain health)

Education/Counseling	Oral Hygiene Instruction/Home Care

Review Section VI Patient Assessment Summary for Mr. Harold Wilmot to help you answer questions #1–3. The template included with his assessment summary will provide spaces for you to record your answers for these questions.

1. Complete the blank "At Risk For," "Periodontal Diagnosis," and "CAMBRA" sections of the assessment form as best as you can with the information in the patient assessment.

2. Write at least three dental hygiene diagnosis statements for Mr. Wilmot's dental hygiene care plan.

3. List the prevention interventions you will plan to help Mr. Wilmot arrest or control disease and regenerate, restore, or maintain oral health.

4. Maria Hernandez is a 19-year-old single mother who has just received health insurance, including dental insurance. This is only her second visit ever to a dentist. The first was when she had a tooth extracted, because of dental caries, at age 14. She presents with swollen gingiva, multiple areas of severe dental caries, and extensive biofilm along the gingival margins of all her teeth. She is 5 months pregnant with her second child and has no other health issues.

Maria is nearly fluent in English, although Spanish is her first language; she lives with her mother and younger siblings. Maria's first child, who is 4 years old, has been receiving care in the clinic and has, within the last 6 months, had extensive dental work, including crowns and extractions because of dental caries.

What aspects of prevention will you focus on during a series of perhaps four dental hygiene appointments with Maria?

5. Today you examine Victor Azure, an 11-year-old child who lives on the nearby Navajo reservation with his mother, father, and two older brothers, who attend high school. The results of Victor's dental examination reveal multiple restorations in primary molars and dental sealants on first molars provided by the dental practice located on the reservation. He has currently no active caries, but you observe a few demineralized areas on the maxillary incisors. You also

observe swollen gingiva and extensive biofilm along the gingival margins of all of Victor's teeth.

Victor states that he brushes nearly every day with fluoridated toothpaste but really hates to do it because it is boring. Victor sometimes uses a home fluoride rinse, but more often uses a strong-tasting mouthwash that his father likes. Victor states that his father uses the mouthwash because he has bad breath and some of his teeth wiggle. Victor knows some of his remaining primary teeth are getting loose and hopes that the mouthwash will keep him from losing them.

The interview with Victor's mother, Skye, regarding his dental history indicates that Victor was exposed to fluoridated water for only the first 3 years of his life, before the family came back home from Chicago to live on the reservation, which does not have fluoridated water. Victor did not ever visit a dentist until last year, when all the restorative work was done, and his mother states that she plans to try to maintain the regular schedule of visits to the dentist that was recommended when Victor was there 6 months ago.

Skye states that the dentist told her that Victor's high rate of decay is linked to his diet, which is high in frequent carbohydrate intake, including large amounts of carbonated beverages, which he drinks all day long. But she also states that she isn't worried about the high rate of decay in the primary teeth because those are going to fall out soon anyway. She states proudly that she allowed the placement of the sealants to protect his adult teeth from decay.

When you go over Victor's medical history with his mother, you find that except for the fact he is extremely overweight, there are no current health problems. There is, however, a family history of diabetes.

Identify the factors in this case scenario you will address in your plan for preventive dental hygiene care for Victor.

6. Your patient, Mrs. Edmons, makes a frantic telephone call to the clinic this morning. Her normal, healthy, very curious 2-year-old son, Nick, has sucked out and eaten most of a small tube of fruit-flavored toothpaste. She estimates he has consumed about 3 oz. of toothpaste. You ask her to identify the kind and amount of fluoride in the toothpaste. She states the back of the tube indicates 0.15% sodium fluoride. The first step will be to determine the amount of toothpaste Nick has eaten in milliliters (see Figure 34-6 in Chapter 34). What will you tell Mrs. Edmons?

7. Get together with a group of your student colleagues and gather examples/samples of a variety of adjunctive dental hygiene aids, such as flossing aids or holders, oral irrigators, and different types of interdental cleaners. Each one of you will then be responsible for learning how to use one oral hygiene aid, demonstrating it to all the others in the group and providing feedback to each individual as he or she practices the technique for using the aid.

8. Explore the patient records available in your school clinic to find patients for whom the assessment data indicate a need for preventive interventions. A patient that you have personally collected the assessment data for is probably the best choice, but any patient record will do for this exercise. Use the assessment data to develop a patient-specific dental hygiene care plan for that patient that addresses all the relevant aspects of oral-disease prevention and oral-health promotion discussed in this section of the textbook.

DISCOVERY EXERCISES

1. Identify teaching materials currently available in your school to use for patient education in your clinic. Investigate sources for new or additional materials and request samples. When you receive them, analyze them for accuracy, readability, and appeal. Decide which ones are most appropriate and valuable for providing information for the patients you will see in your school clinic.

2. Create a product-comparison infomap. This discovery exercise will help you compare chemotherapeutic agents used in dentistry and is best done by working together in small groups of three to six students.

Step 1: Gather together a variety of mouthrinses, dentifrices, or other dental products that contain chemotherapeutic ingredients recommended by dental hygienists for prevention of dental disease. Have each group member be responsible for finding particular products. You can gather over-the-counter products as well as those that are commonly dispensed only by prescription. You will need to make sure that you have the available packaging information for each product.

Step 2: Assemble small plastic cups, long cotton swabs, and some paper towels so that you can do a taste test.

Step 3: Develop an infomap to help you compare these products. There are examples of infomaps throughout this workbook to give you ideas as you develop this one. Your infomap should allow you to compare similar products in such areas as active chemotherapeutic ingredients, alcohol content, ADA Seal of Approval, cost, taste, efficacy of the product based on current research findings, and any other topic areas you think are important for your comparison.

The infomap you create can be used to help you compare products when you are making recommendations to your patients. After your student group develops the basic framework for the infomap, you can continue to add products as you become aware of them in order to keep a currently updated review of products for recommending to your patients.

3. Use the information in the **textbook** to create an infomap that compares various kinds of manual toothbrushes you can recommend for your patients. How about an infomap comparing the various brands and types of dental floss? What other prevention products could you compare in an Infomap format?

4. Being able to apply evidence-based prevention protocols as we make recommendations for patients requires practice in accessing, analyzing, and applying information from the dental and oral-health literature. Select a prevention topic and perform a PubMed search to obtain a list of current scientific research articles related to that topic. Obtain the full-text articles either online or at the library. Write a short review of the literature to summarize what you learned from reading the articles. Be sure to include recommendations for patient care based on your analysis of the literature.

5. Work with your student colleagues to create an annotated list of websites that provide information on topics related to the prevention of oral disease. Each student should select a topic, and then perform an Internet search using the search engine of his or her choice. Make sure the websites you select provide valid, scientific, and reliable information. Write a brief summary of the information you learned from the website, and be sure to include the correct Internet address (URL) at the top of the page. Provide electronic copies of your brief description of the website to your instructor or to a student colleague who is willing to compile the information into one document that can be shared by all students.

6. Investigate prevention in the news. Collect articles from the current popular literature—such as newspapers, magazines, and television or radio announcements—that provide information on prevention of oral diseases. Also look for dental product advertisements that appear in the popular press. This is the information that your patients see and will probably ask you about when you are providing patient education.

   • Is the information that you find presented in the popular media valid and scientifically accurate?

   • How can this information affect the way in which the dental profession is perceived?

   • Does the media information you find agree with the recommendations you make for dental preventive care?

FOR YOUR PORTFOLIO

1. Read the definitions of behavior change, communication style, preventive counseling, and motivational interviewing provided in Chapter 24. Combine these definitions to write a personal "Dental Health Educator" philosophy statement.

2. Include a copy of the original product comparison infomap your student group created in the discovery exercise above. As you update the infomap with new product information, also include your most currently updated infomap in your portfolio. Having both the original and the updated infomaps will help demonstrate your commitment to continued learning.

3. Provide written examples to describe dental hygiene education and counseling interventions you have provided for specific patients. Select examples that illustrate your ability to communicate, motivate, and educate particular patients so that positive health outcomes result. Structure your examples so that each includes a discussion of the following:

   • Significant assessment findings

   • Use of the principles of motivational interviewing during patient discussions

   • Prevention topics and methods presented

   • Oral-health techniques demonstrated

   • Method of patient practice used

   • Methods for evaluating success of the patient's compliance, motivation levels, and learning styles (Discuss any factors that affected your ability to communicate with the patient and factors that affected compliance with your recommendations.)

4. Include copies of patient-specific care plans you have developed to illustrate your ability to plan individualized prevention for specific patient cases. Include some early attempts at developing care plans and also some care plans you developed near the end of your student career. Provide a short written analysis of how the early examples compare with the later examples of care planning to demonstrate your growth toward competency in care planning for prevention.

5. Include the literature review you wrote in the discovery exercise above. Later you can update your search to see if there is new information available that might change any recommendations you made in your first review.

6. Collect as many examples of prevention in the news as you can during the time you are a student and jot down notes analyzing each example. Later on you can use your notes to write an analysis of all the examples you collected. Take time to identify trends in how preventive dentistry is presented in the popular media. How does the popular view of dentistry affect the way your patients perceive and are motivated by your prevention interventions and recommendations?

Implementation: Treatment

SECTION VII LEARNING OBJECTIVES

Completing the exercises in this section of the workbook will prepare you to:

1. Manage patient anxiety and pain during dental hygiene treatment.
2. Provide a variety of dental hygiene treatment interventions.
3. Document clinical dental hygiene treatment.

COMPETENCIES FOR THE DENTAL HYGIENIST (APPENDIX A)

Competencies supported by the learning in Section VII

Core Competencies: C3, C4, C5, C7, C9, C10, C11, C12, C13

Health Promotion and Disease Prevention: HP1, HP2, HP4, HP5, HP6

Patient/Client Care: PC4, PC10, PC11, PC12, PC13

36

Anxiety and Pain Control

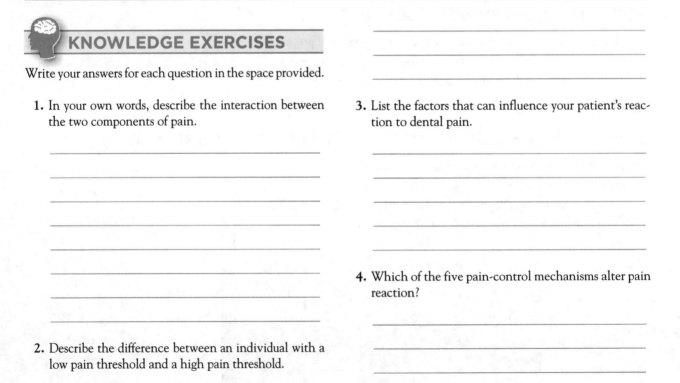

KNOWLEDGE EXERCISES

Write your answers for each question in the space provided.

1. In your own words, describe the interaction between the two components of pain.

_____

_____

_____

_____

_____

_____

2. Describe the difference between an individual with a low pain threshold and a high pain threshold.

_____

_____

_____

3. List the factors that can influence your patient's reaction to dental pain.

_____

_____

_____

_____

_____

4. Which of the five pain-control mechanisms alter pain reaction?

_____

_____

_____

_____

5. Which of the pain-control mechanisms relies for success on your ability to communicate with and educate your patient?

_____

_____

6. Figure 36-1 shows a nitrous oxide delivery system. Label the following components on the figure. It might be useful to use colored pencils (use green for oxygen and blue for nitrous oxide, of course!). Note that some components may not be easy to identify or locate on the figure, but do your best; then investigate or ask your instructor to find out if your idea was correct.

   - *Oxygen tank*
   - *Nitrous oxide tank (add a notation to identify the gas pressure)*
   - *Cylinder valves used to open and close each tank (Hint: There is one on each tank.)*
   - *Hoses that carry only oxygen gas*
   - *Hoses that carry only nitrous oxide gas*
   - *Hoses that can carry both nitrous oxide gas and oxygen*
   - *Regulator or reducing valve (location not discussed in the **textbook**)*
   - *Flow meter (location not discussed in the **textbook**) (Hint: The clinician uses this to control the level of each gas administered to the patient.)*
   - *On-demand valve (Hint: Probably located near the flow meter.)*
   - *Reservoir bag*
   - *Nasal hood, nose piece, or mask*
   - *Scavenger system*
   - *Areas where there are connectors (It is important to know where these are because you will regularly need to inspect and test them for potential leaks.)*

7. Conscious sedation, produced by administration of a combination of nitrous oxide and oxygen, is frequently used to reduce patient anxiety and perception of pain during short dental procedures that are expected to cause a low level of pain. Identify the two properties of nitrous oxide useful for reducing pain.

_____

_____

8. Why is nitrous oxide sedation especially useful for control of soft tissue discomfort during dental hygiene procedures?

_____

_____

9. What is the appropriate range for percentage of nitrous oxide during dental hygiene procedures?

_____

10. During administration of nitrous oxide analgesia, how much time is usually required for primary saturation of blood to occur?

_____

11. What is the minimum amount of oxygen flow that is maintained by the gas delivery system for patient safety?

_____

12. Describe diffusion hypoxia.

_____

_____

_____

Figure 36-1

13. How can oxygen hypoxia be prevented?

_____

_____

_____

14. List contraindications for the use of nitrous oxide during dental hygiene care.

_____

_____

_____

_____

_____

_____

_____

15. Attention to the details for providing an effective scavenging system, rigorous equipment maintenance, and the initiation of other methods for preventing overexposure are imperative when nitrous oxide is used during patient care. What are the potential health hazards for clinicians who are exposed to excessive levels of nitrous oxide?

_____

_____

_____

_____

_____

_____

_____

16. Without looking in the **textbook**, list the steps you will use to administer nitrous oxide–oxygen analgesic during patient care. For each step, when appropriate, indicate the time frame and the amount of oxygen or nitrous flow.

_____

_____

_____

_____

_____

_____

_____

_____

_____

_____

_____

_____

_____

_____

_____

17. In your own words, explain how the nitrous oxide gas is titrated during administration.

_____

_____

_____

_____

_____

_____

18. Identify at least three advantages and three disadvantages of using conscious sedation anesthesia (such as nitrous oxide) to reduce patient pain and anxiety during dental hygiene treatment.

- _Advantages:_

_____

_____

_____

_____

_____

- _Disadvantages:_

_____

_____

_____

_____

_____

_____

19. List three important components to document in your patient's progress notes after you administer nitrous oxide during dental hygiene treatment.

_____

_____

_____

20. Which of the five basic pain-control mechanisms alter pain perception?

_____

_____

_____

_____

_____

21. Describe how a nonopioid analgesic alters pain perception.

_____

_____

_____

22. List the indications for applying topical anesthetic to reduce your patient's perception of intraoral pain.

_____

_____

_____

_____

23. Identify the active ingredients available as noninjectable or topical anesthetic preparations and the amount of time that each provides anesthesia to the tissues.

_____

_____

_____

_____

_____

_____

_____

_____

24. Match each description below with the correct amide type of local anesthesia. Each type of anesthesia is used more than once; some descriptions apply to more than one type of anesthesia.

Type of Amide Anesthetic	Description
A. Articaine	____ Long-acting amide drug
B. Bupivacaine	____ Short- or medium-acting amide drug
C. Etidocaine	____ Citanest plain and Citanest forte
D. Lidocaine	____ Carbocaine, Polocaine, Isocaine
E. Mepivacaine	____ Duranest
F. Prilocaine	____ Marcaine
	____ Septocaine, Septanest, and Ultracaine
	____ Xylocaine, Octocaine, Lignospan
	____ Available in 1.8 mL of solution in cartridge
	____ Most widely used amide; also available as a topical
	____ Causes less vasodilation, so can be used without a vasoconstrictor
	____ Diffuses best through soft and hard tissues
	____ Provides extended period of analgesia to manage postcare pain
	____ Metabolic by-products can temporarily reduce the oxygen-carrying capacity of blood
	____ Potential drug interaction if patient is taking the drug cimetidine

25. Match each description below with the correct dental cartridge ingredient.

Dental Cartridge Ingredient	Description
A. Amide anesthetic	____ Creates isotonic match with the body
B. Antioxidant	____ Blocks the transfer of ions across the nerve membrane
C. Sodium chloride	____ Constricts blood vessels
D. Sterile water	____ Preservative for the vasoconstrictor
E. Vasoconstrictor	____ Diluting agent

26. Match each description below with the correct group of local anesthesia drugs. Each group is used more than once.

Local Anesthesia Drug Group	Description
A. Amide	____ Currently used only in topical anesthetics
B. Ester	____ Metabolized in blood plasma
	____ Low incidence of allergic reactions
	____ Less effective and shorter acting
	____ Higher incidence of allergic reactions
	____ Less effective and shorter acting
	____ Metabolized by the liver
	____ Causes vasodilation

27. Which ingredient in a topical anesthetic is most likely to cause an allergic reaction in your patient?

_____

_____

28. Which ingredient in topical anesthetic is the most likely to cause a toxic reaction in your patient?

_____

29. In your own words, describe the techniques and armamentarium used for administering noninjectable anesthesia.

_____

_____

_____

_____

_____

30. What techniques can be used to apply topical anesthesia to oral tissues?

_____

_____

31. Identify two vasoconstrictors commonly used in dental anesthetic and indicate the standard concentration of each one.

_____

_____

_____

_____

32. A vasoconstrictor offsets the vasodilating action of the local anesthetic. List reasons for including a vasoconstrictor in local anesthetic solution.

_____

_____

_____

_____

_____

_____

33. What preservative for the vasoconstrictor can cause a potential allergic reaction?

_____

_____

_____

34. What prescribed drugs can cause an adverse reaction when dental anesthetics with vasoconstrictors are used?

_____

_____

_____

_____

35. Name the drug that can be injected to reverse the effects of local anesthetic. What action reverses the effects?

_____

_____

_____

36. What are the sources of information you will use to assess your patient before providing local anesthetic?

_____

_____

_____

_____

_____

_____

37. What patient risk factors will you consider when selecting which local anesthetic solution to use during dental hygiene treatment?

_____

_____

_____

38. What medical conditions indicate the need for patient-specific evaluation and very careful consideration when determining local anesthesia use during dental hygiene treatment?

_____

_____

_____

_____

_____

_____

39. List the armamentarium you will assemble before providing local anesthesia.

_____

_____

_____

_____

_____

_____

_____

_____

40. Why do you position the patient with the head lower than the heart during a local anesthesia injection?

_____

41. What is prevented from happening when you aspirate before injecting local anesthesia solution?

_____

_____

42. In your own words, describe the procedure for aspiration using a conventional anesthetic syringe.

_____

_____

_____

43. The steps for syringe assembly are listed below. Some syringe components are printed in boldface; label each one on Figure 36-2.

Step 1: Pull back on the **thumb ring**.

Step 2: Insert the **cartridge** that contains the selected type of anesthetic. Identify the **rubber stopper** and the **diaphragm end** of the cartridge. Identify the **volume** of solution in the cartridge. Identify the **window** openings in the syringe that will allow you to view the cartridge during aspiration.

Figure 36-2

Step 3: Set the **harpoon** into the appropriate end of the cartridge and test for lock.

Step 4: Discard the **safety cap** from the **cartridge end** of the needle.

Step 5: With your fingers holding the **needle hub,** screw the needle securely onto the end of the syringe. Identify the **needle** that is used for injection. Indicate the available **lengths** and **diameters** of the needles that are used for injecting dental anesthetic.

In the detail view of the needle tip, identify the bevel of the needle and draw a line to indicate where the bone will be relative to the bevel when the needle is inserted for injection.

44. Describe what you will do if you see blood in the anesthetic cartridge when you aspirate while providing local anesthetic for your patient.

_____

_____

_____

_____

_____

_____

45. Identify the proper amount of time for depositing (injecting) a local anesthetic solution. Describe why the local anesthetic solution is deposited slowly.

_____

_____

_____

_____

46. What injections will ensure complete soft and hard tissue anesthesia for your patient when you are providing periodontal treatment for all of the teeth in the mandibular left quadrant.

_____

_____

_____

_____

47. Which injection will be needed to anesthetize the lingual tissue so that complete patient comfort is achieved during dental hygiene procedures in this same area of the mouth?

_____

_____

48. Use a colored pencil to mark Figure 36-3 to identify the areas that are anesthetized after an MSA injection on the right-hand side of the patient's mouth.

Figure 36-3

49. Use a colored pencil to mark Figure 36-3 to identify the area that is anesthetized after the ASA injection on the right-hand side of the patient's mouth.

50. What structure in the molar teeth is not completely anesthetized after a PSA injection?

_____

51. Which injections anesthetize only the terminal nerve endings for one individual tooth?

_____

_____

_____

52. It is imperative to be able to identify the type and the cause of any patient reaction quickly when you are providing local anesthesia. Match each description with the correct symptom. Some symptoms are used more than once; some descriptions apply to more than one type of symptom.

Symptom	Description
A. Adequate anesthesia	___ Anxiety reaction
B. Allergy	___ Can be the result of too rapid absorption of a drug into bloodstream
C. Epithelial desquamation	___ Can indicate that topical anesthetic was left in contact with the tissue for too long
D. Hematoma	___ Can result from reduced ability to eliminate or metabolize the local anesthesia drug
E. Overdose	
F. Paresthesia	___ Caused when a vein or artery is opened and leaks blood into the surrounding tissue
G. Psychogenic reaction	___ Experience of a profound effect for the duration of the procedure
H. Trismus	___ Extended duration of anesthesia effect
	___ Hypersensitive state that can result in exaggerated response to a subsequent exposure to local anesthesia drug
	___ Onset may range from a few seconds to many hours later
	___ Patients will sometimes report this reaction as an allergy to local anesthesia
	___ Response can range from mild to generalized life-threatening anaphylaxis
	___ Spasm of jaw muscle that restricts opening after injection
	___ Syncope and hyperventilation are the most common responses
	___ Tissue sloughing
	___ Toxic levels of local anesthesia drug are present in the bloodstream
	___ Prevention of these complications relies on the use of excellent injection technique
	___ This response can be made less likely if you use excellent patient communications skills and gentle administration techniques when you are injecting local anesthesia

✓ COMPETENCY EXERCISES

Apply information from the chapter and use critical thinking skills to complete the competency exercises. Write responses on paper or create electronic documents to submit your answers.

1. Today you are presenting your dental hygiene care plan for four-quadrant, initial therapy scaling and root planing to Mr. Shizoka. You will ask the patient to sign an informed consent form before you begin your treatment. Mr. Shizoka does not have much previous dental experience. When you were collecting assessment data for the care plan, he appeared to be very nervous. He asked lots of questions about what you were doing and stopped you frequently when you were trying to probe because he was concerned about whether he would feel pain.

Mr. Shizoka's medical history indicates that he has iron-deficiency anemia and takes a ferrous iron supplement daily. He has hypertension and takes an antihypertensive medication; however, he tells you that whenever he is highly stressed, he gets a headache. Write a dental hygiene diagnosis statement related to Mr. Shizoka's anxiety about receiving dental hygiene treatment.

2. In the dental hygiene care plan you have developed, you plan to use nitrous oxide–oxygen for pain and anxiety control during Mr. Shizoka's four scaling and root planing appointments. You have already explained to Mr. Shizoka what nitrous oxide–oxygen sedation is and how it works. Explain the advantages and disadvantages so that he can be completely informed about the use of this pain and anxiety control measure.

3. Mr. Shizoka agrees to try the nitrous oxide–oxygen sedation for at least his first dental hygiene appointment to see if he is comfortable with it. Use your institution's guidelines for writing in patient records to document that you have fully informed Mr. Shizoka and that he has agreed to the use of nitrous oxide analgesia during his dental hygiene treatment.

4. At his next appointment, you carefully titrate the nitrous oxide–oxygen combination for Mr. Shizoka, and he shows all the signs of ideal sedation. When you begin the injection of local anesthesia into the area where you will be providing care, Mr. Shizoka becomes agitated and starts moving his arms and legs. His rate of respiration increases significantly, he starts to sweat, and his eyes tear up. You immediately stop injecting the local anesthesia. He says he feels sick to his stomach and wants to sit up. Discuss two possibilities for what is happening in this scenario?

5. What will you do next in the situation that is described in question 4?

6. Use your institution's guidelines for writing in patient records to document what happened today at Mr. Shizoka's dental hygiene appointment.

7. Explain, in patient-appropriate language, how the noninjectable local anesthesia patch is administered.

EVERYDAY ETHICS

Before completing the learning exercises below, reread and reflect on the Everyday Ethics Scenario and Questions for Consideration in this chapter of the **textbook**. It may also be useful to review the Dental Hygiene Ethics discussion in Chapter 1, the Ethical Applications in the introduction pages for each section in the **textbook**, as well as the Codes of Ethics in **textbook** Appendices I–IV.

Individual Learning Activity

Imagine that you are the dental hygienist in this scenario. Answer each of the questions for consideration at the end of the scenario.

Collaborative Learning Activity

Answer each of the questions for consideration at the end of the scenario in the **textbook**. Compare what you wrote with answers developed by another classmate and discuss differences/similarities.

Factors to Teach the Patient

This scenario is related to the following factors listed in this chapter of the **textbook**:

▷ Be careful not to bite lip, cheek, or tongue while tissues are without normal sensations. Warn and watch children to prevent injury. Do not test anesthesia by biting the lip.

▷ Avoid chewing hard foods and avoid hot food and drinks until normal sensation has returned.

Because a scheduled patient did not arrive and you have some time free, you are asked to spend the time speaking to Miriam's mother. Miriam Carroll is 9 years old. She has many dental problems but is always cooperative during treatment. At Miriam's appointment today, Dr. Steve will extract three primary molar root tips, and both the maxillary and mandibular arches on the left-hand side of her mouth will be anesthetized for the extractions. This is the first time Miriam will experience the effects of local anesthesia.

Using the principles of motivation interviewing (see **workbook** Appendix D) as a guide, prepare a conversation that you might use to provide postoperative follow-up information to Miriam's mother.

MeSH TERMS

Use a combination of MeSH terms and other key words to develop an effective and efficient PubMed literature search strategy.

Anesthesia, dental	Vasoconstrictor agents
Mepivacaine	Bupivacaine
Amides	Epinephrine
Prilocaine	Lidocaine
Esters	Nitrous oxide

Instruments and Principles for Instrumentation

KNOWLEDGE EXERCISES

Write your answers for each question in the space provided.

The following questions help you look at each type of instrument from several perspectives. If possible, have real instruments available to look at as you are doing these exercises so you can thoroughly understand the instruments' similarities and differences and visualize their parts.

1. Locate and label each of the following parts on the instrument shown in Figure 37-1.

Figure 37-1

- *Blade*
- *Shank*
- *Lower shank*
- *Handle*
- *Serrated surface of the handle*

2. The instrument shown in Figure 37-1 has a relatively straight shank shape and is probably intended for use on _____ teeth.

3. Label the instruments shown in Figure 37-2.

Figure 37-2

- *Scaler*
- *Curet*

4. Label the following areas of both instruments shown in Figure 37-2.
   - *Pointed tip*
   - *Rounded toe (tip)*
   - *Cutting edges*
   - *Area of the cutting edge that is adapted to the tooth during scaling*

- *Face of the blade*
- *Terminal shank*

5. Match each description below to the letter that indicates the appropriate instrument shown in Figure 37-3 by writing the correct letter in the space provided.

_____ Area-specific curet

_____ Scaler

6. Label the following areas on the working ends of each of the instruments shown in Figure 37-3.

Figure 37-3

- *Rounded toe (tip)*
- *Pointed tip*
- *Face of the blade*
- *Cutting edges*
- *Area of the cutting edge that is adapted to the tooth when scaling*
- *Terminal shank*
- *Lateral surface and back of the blade*

7. Match each description below to the letter that indicates the appropriate instrument shown in Figure 37-4 by writing the correct letter in the space provided.

_____ Area-specific curet

_____ Universal curet

_____ Scaler

8. Label or mark the following areas on the cross section of working ends of each instrument shown in Figure 37-4.

Figure 37-4

- *Face of the blade*
- *Cutting edges*
- *Terminal shank*
- *Lateral surface(s)*
- *Back of the blade*

9. List the five basic principles for use of instruments.

_____

_____

_____

_____

_____

10. When you are activating your instruments during dental hygiene treatment, the proper modified pen grasp is controlled and firm, but not tight and rigid. What are the effects of a grasp that is too tight and rigid?

_____

_____

_____

_____

11. During instrumentation why must the instrument be rolled between the fingers?

_____

_____

_____

12. In your own words, explain how a power-driven scaler removes calculus and enhances debridement of bacteria in the sulcus or periodontal pocket.

_____

_____

_____

13. Label the following areas of a magnetostrictive insert shown in Figure 37-5.

- *O-Ring*
- *Point*
- *Magnetostrictive stack*
- *Tip*
- *Grip*

Figure 37-5

14. Explain cavitation.

_____

_____

_____

_____

15. List the steps used to prepare an ultrasonic unit.

_____

_____

_____

_____

_____

_____

16. Describe the contraindications to ultrasonic instrumentation.

_____

_____

_____

_____

_____

_____

_____

_____

17. What risk does an ultrasonic instrument present to the patient with a cardiac pacemaker?

_____

_____

_____

18. Your patient presents with a titanium implant abutment on tooth 22. You plan to use an ultrasonic scaler for this patient. How will be modify your treatment to accommodate this patient?

_____

_____

_____

19. Complete Infomap 37-1 with information from the **textbook** to help you compare the different types of power-driven scaling devices.

20. What factors can influence your risk for cumulative trauma injury and pain from incorrect use of instruments during dental hygiene procedures?

_____

_____

_____

_____

✓ COMPETENCY EXERCISES

Apply information from the chapter and use critical thinking skills to complete the competency exercises.

The only real way to become competent in the skills described in this chapter of the **textbook** is to practice. It is, of course, difficult to help you do that in a workbook format. But here are some exercises you can do on your own to help you become competent in identifying instruments and practicing the principles of instrumentation. If you'd like, work in small groups with two or three of your student colleagues. Using the information and descriptions in Chapter 37 in the **textbook**, group members can provide feedback about each person's instrument technique.

1. Gather together a variety of instruments and lay them out on a table in front of you. Examine them carefully and thoroughly, identifying the instrument parts, the types, and the adaptation characteristics (such as the angle of the shank) of each instrument you have available. Then practice picking up the instrument in the modified pen grasp, placing a fulcrum on the tip of the thumb of your nondominant hand, and adapting the blade of the instrument on your fingernail in the correct position for activation.

2. Examine each instrument to determine its characteristics—such as balance, shank length, fabrication materials, and shape and rigidity of the shank. Discuss the purpose and uses of each instrument. Think about

INFOMAP 37-1						
TYPE	FREQUENCY	MODE OF ACTION	TIP TYPE AND MOVEMENT	WATER USE	CONTRAINDICATIONS, PRECAUTIONS, AND RISK FACTORS FOR USE	PRINCIPLES OF INSTRUMENTATION AND TECHNIQUE FOR USE
Sonic scaler						
Ultrasonic magnetostrictive						
Ultrasonic piezoelectric						

area of the mouth the instrument is appropriate for, the technique the instrument is intended for (e.g., heavy calculus or root planing), and any other indications/contraindications for use that pertain to the instrument's design.

3. Examine each instrument to determine the correct cutting edge and area of the cutting edge most useful for calculus removal.

4. To develop your dexterity, practice each of the strength, stretching, writing, and instrument exercises described in the Section "Dexterity Development" of Chapter 37 in the **textbook**.

5. Sit comfortably in a chair that has no arms. Practice placing shoulders, arms, elbows, and wrists in a neutral position. While you are sitting there, practice each of the exercises in Figures 37-25, 37-27, and 37-28 in the **textbook**.

Factors to Teach the Patient

This scenario is related to the following factors listed in this chapter of the **textbook**:

▷ Why it is necessary to use a variety of instruments for scaling.

Today is your first scaling and root-planing appointment with Mr. Nicholas Diamond. When you open your sterilized instruments and line them up on the tray, Mr. Diamond expresses amazement at the number of them and comments on their different shapes.

Write a statement explaining to Mr. Diamond why you have so many different instruments on your tray. Use the conversation you create to educate a patient or friend who is not a student colleague.

EVERYDAY ETHICS

Before completing the learning exercises below, reread and reflect on the Everyday Ethics Scenario and Questions for Consideration in this chapter of the **textbook**. It may also be useful to review the Dental Hygiene Ethics discussion in Chapter 1, the Ethical Applications in the introduction pages for each section in the **textbook**, as well as the Codes of Ethics in **textbook** Appendices I–IV.

Individual Learning Activity

Imagine that you have observed what happened in the scenario, but are not one of the main characters involved in the situation. Write a reflective journal entry that:

- Describes how you might have reacted (as an observer—not as a participant),
- Expresses your personal feelings about what happened or identifies personal values that affect your reaction to the situation.

Discovery Activity

Ask a dental hygienist who has been practicing for a year or more to read the scenario. Provide them with a copy of the Code of Ethics as well. Share the responses you have made to answer each question and ask that person to discuss the situation with you. What insights did you have or what did you learn during this discussion?

MeSH TERMS

Use a combination of MeSH terms and other key words to develop an effective and efficient PubMed literature search strategy.

Dental instruments	Cumulative trauma
Dental prophylaxis	disorders
Dental scaling	Carpal tunnel syndrome
Root planing	Ultrasonics
Periodontal debridement	

CHAPTER 37 CROSSWORD PUZZLE

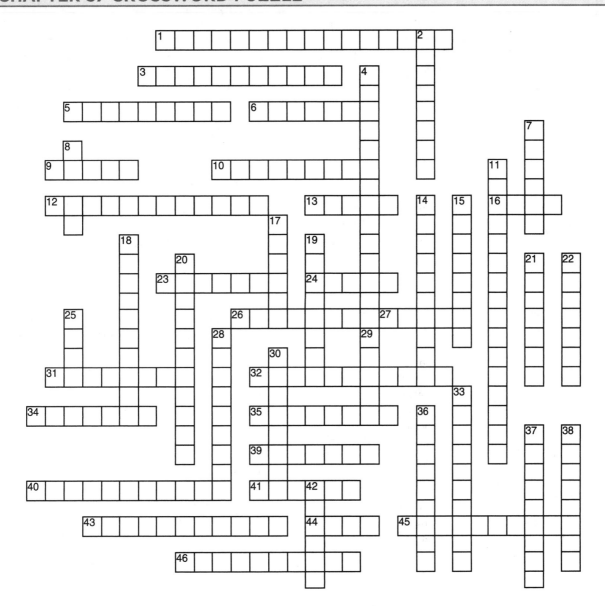

Puzzle Clues

Across

1. Inserts made of flat metal strips sandwiched together.

3. This type of instrument has paired working ends that may be either mirror image or complementary (two words).

5. The two cutting edges of this instrument meet at the point of the tip.

6. One of three types of strokes that can be applied against the tooth surface with an instrument; a diagonal stroke.

9. Term used to describe the cutting edge of an instrument that is a fine line, has no width, and does not reflect light.

10. Refers to a stroke that is dependent on the surface texture of the area being instrumented; lighter pressure is applied progressively as strokes continue and the surface becomes smooth (two words).

12. This type of lateral pressure when scaling contributes to burnishing of calculus.

13. A scaling instrument with a rounded working end; there are two types: universal and area-specific.

16. Term used to describe the cutting edge of an instrument that visually presents a rounded, shiny surface that reflects light.

23. The position of wrist, forearm, elbow, and shoulder that prevents occupational pain risk for dental hygienists.

24. The thick, stronger, less flexible instrument shank needed for the removal of heavy calculus deposits.

26. To smooth and polish the surface of calculus (usually with an instrument that is not sharp) instead of removing it completely with a well-sharpened instrument.

27. Type of scaler that operates on a frequency of 2,500–7,000 cps.

31. This thinner type of instrument shank may provide more tactile sensitivity and is used to remove fine calculus or for maintenance root debridement.

32. The type of instrument shank that is designed to help adapt the instrument to difficult-to-reach areas, such as the distal surfaces of molars (two words).

34. The combined push-and-pull stroke commonly used to activate a periodontal probe.

35. Refers to the size of the instrument handle; usually available in four sizes.

39. The pressure that is required of an instrument to the tooth during a scaling procedure.

40. Refers to the fine line where the face and the lateral surfaces of a well-sharpened dental instrument meet (two words).

41. Single, unbroken movement of the instrument as it is applied against the tooth surface.

43. Dental hygiene instrument that is usually held by the nondominant hand using a modified pen grasp (two words).

44. A type of scaling instrument that has multiple cutting edges lined up on a round, oval, or rectangular base.

45. Provides stabilization and control during instrumentation (two words).

46. Refers to the unique area of each instrument that is used to carry out the purpose and function of that instrument (two words).

Down

2. A working stroke that is parallel with the long axis of the tooth being treated.

4. Type of scaler that is activated by dimensional changes in crystals.

7. When you are using the modified pen grasp, the position of the instrument against this finger is extremely important to instrument control.

8. Connects the handle and the working end of a dental instrument.

11. The hand position that is used to hold a dental instrument (three words).

14. A working stroke that is applied parallel with the occlusal surface of the tooth being treated.

15. Refers to the use of a mirror to view an area of the mouth.

17. Refers to any scaling instrument with two cutting edges that meet in a point; can have a curved or straight blade.

18. Relationship between the working end of the instrument and the tooth surface being treated.

19. This type of instrument shank indicates the instrument is primarily used in anterior teeth.

20. A light pressure stroke that disrupts dental biofilm from the root surface of a previously root-planed tooth surface.

21. Stroke that applies definite, well-controlled pressure on the surface of a tooth; refers to instrumentation of a tooth to remove calculus.

22. The support upon which your scaling hand finger rests so that force can be exerted during the scaling procedure in order to remove calculus.

25. The type of stroke that is used when activating most scaling instruments.

28. This type of lateral pressure can result in gouging of the root surface, patient discomfort, and clinician fatigue.

29. Sharpened working end of a dental instrument.

30. Refers to the hand that is usually used for holding a scaling instrument during treatment.

33. The finger that establishes a fulcrum when using a modified pen grasp during instrumentation (two words).

36. The control, coordination, and strength needed to become proficient in the efficient and effective use of dental instruments.

37. A unit of energy equal to 1,000 cps.

38. Fluid agitation or turbulence that has ability to disrupt bacterial matrix.

42. The position of the blade of an area-specific Gracey curet.

Instrument Care and Sharpening

KNOWLEDGE EXERCISES

Write your answers for each question in the space provided.

The following questions help you look at each type of instrument from several perspectives. If possible, have real instruments available to look at as you are doing these exercises so you can thoroughly understand the instruments' similarities and differences and visualize their parts.

1. In your own words, explain the benefits of using carefully sharpened instruments during patient care.

_____

_____

_____

2. Describe the objective and purpose of sharpening the cutting edge of a dental instrument.

_____

_____

_____

_____

_____

_____

3. Two basic sharpening techniques include the moving _____ and the moving _____ techniques.

4. When sharpening curets and scalers, the visible angle at which the stone is placed relative to the face of the instrument is _____ degrees.

5. Without looking at the figure in the **textbook**, draw a straight line on Figure 38-1 to indicate how the face of the sharpening stone would be placed (and angled) to sharpen *each* of the cutting edges of each instrument shown. After you draw your lines and label each angle, use a protractor to measure those angles. If your diagram is not correct, erase your lines and redraw them using the protractor to help you place the angle of your sharpening stone correctly.

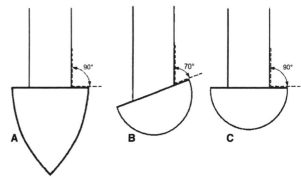

Figure 38-1

6. Imagine that you are using the moving-stone technique to sharpen the instruments shown in Figure 38-1. Draw an arrow to indicate the direction of the stroke in which you would apply the most pressure as you move the stone. (*Hint:* This is also the direction you would finish each area as you are sharpening.)

7. In your own words, describe how to care for a flat sharpening stone.

_____

_____

_____

_____

 COMPETENCY EXERCISES

Apply information from the chapter and use critical thinking skills to complete the competency exercises.

The only real way to become competent in the skills described in this chapter of the **textbook** is to practice. It is, of course, difficult to help you do that in a workbook format.

However, here are some exercises you can do on your own to help you become competent in identifying instruments and practicing the principles of instrument sharpening. If you'd like, work in small groups with two or three of your student colleagues. Using the information and descriptions in Chapter 38 in the **textbook**, group members can provide feedback about each person's instrument sharpening technique.

1. Gather together a variety of instruments and lay them out on a table in front of you. Examine them carefully and thoroughly to determine whether the cutting edge is sharp. Practice the correct placement of a sharpening stone to sharpen each instrument.

2. Explain the benefits of telling your patient you always make sure to use a "well-honed" instrument rather than a "sharpened" instrument during patient care.

 MeSH TERMS

Use a combination of MeSH terms and other key words to develop an effective and efficient PubMed literature search strategy.

Dental instruments   Root planing
Dental scaling

EVERYDAY ETHICS

Before completing the learning exercises below, reread and reflect on the Everyday Ethics Scenario and Questions for Consideration in this chapter of the **textbook**. It may also be useful to review the Dental Hygiene Ethics discussion in Chapter 1, the Ethical Applications in the introduction pages for each section in the **textbook**, as well as the Codes of Ethics in **textbook** Appendices I–IV.

Individual Learning Activity

Imagine that you have observed what happened in the scenario, but are not one of the main characters involved in the situation. Write a reflective journal entry that:

- Describes how you might have reacted (as an observer—not as a participant),
- Expresses your personal feelings about what happened, or
- Identifies personal values that affect your reaction to the situation.

Discovery Activity

Ask a dental hygienist who has been practicing for a year or more to read the scenario. Provide them with a copy of the Code of Ethics as well. Share the responses you have made to answer each question and ask that person to discuss the situation with you. What insights did you have or what did you learn during this discussion?

 Factors to Teach the Patient

This scenario is related to the following factors listed in this chapter of the **textbook**:

▷ Benefits of using a finely sharpened instrument for calculus removal.

▷ Harmful effects of using dull instruments.

Today is your first scaling and root-planing appointment with Mr. David Crawford. When you begin to check the cutting edges of each instrument before using them, he wants to know what you are looking for.

Write a statement explaining to Mr. Crawford why you always make sure each one of your instruments is well honed before you begin his treatment. Use the conversation you create to educate a patient or friend who is not a student colleague.

CHAPTER 38 CROSSWORD PUZZLE

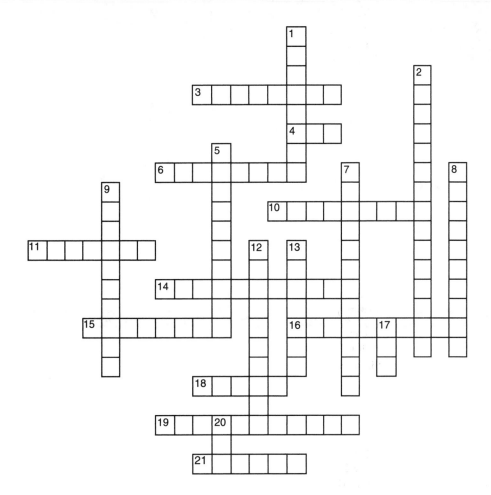

Puzzle Clues

Across

3. A fine grit natural sharpening stone.

4. The number of surfaces to be sharpened on a hoe scaler.

6. Minute particles on a sharpening stone that accomplish the work of grinding the instrument.

10. Examination of the cutting edge under a light to determine the sharpness of the cutting edge (two words).

11. This can happen when a dull scaler is passed over tenacious calculus in an attempt to remove the deposit.

14. When using this sharpening technique, the hand-holding instrument is stabilized against an immovable surface (two words).

15. Metal particles remaining on the edge of a newly sharpened instrument (two words).

16. You will feel this when a well-sharpened explorer or scaling instrument is pulled over the surface of a plastic testing stick.

18. A natural stone that comes in a variety of grits.

19. The fine line formed between the face and lateral surface of a dental hygiene scaling instrument (two words).

21. A more patient-friendly term for sharpening.

Down

1. A sharpening technique that does not use water or a lubricant (two words).

2. Sharpening technique that is recommended when sharpening with certain quarried stone sharpeners (two words).

5. A file scaler is sharpened with this flat sharpening instrument (two words).

7. Type of curet that is only sharpened on the longer cutting edge (two words).

8. Sharpening stones need to be _____ prior to use.

9. A ceramic aluminum oxide sharpening stone is this type.

12. Placing the stone at the correct _____ when sharpening ensures a fine, sharp edge.

13. A sharpening stone made from quarried mineral stones.

17. This rounded portion of the universal curet is sharpened along with the cutting edges on both sides of the face.

20. The number of surfaces to be sharpened on a sickle scaler.

Nonsurgical Periodontal Therapy and Adjunctive Therapy

 KNOWLEDGE EXERCISES

Write your answers for each question in the space provided.

1. List the components of nonsurgical periodontal therapy.

2. What are the therapeutic goals of nonsurgical periodontal treatment for the patient with early-to-moderate periodontitis?

3. What are the therapeutic goals of providing nonsurgical periodontal treatment for the patient with more advanced periodontal conditions?

4. Describe the aims and expected outcomes of providing complete and carefully performed nonsurgical periodontal therapy.

_____

_____

_____

_____

_____

5. Briefly describe the clinical end points that indicate successful nonsurgical periodontal instrumentation?

_____

_____

_____

_____

_____

6. What changes occur in the subgingival microflora after instrumentation procedures during periodontal debridement.

_____

_____

_____

_____

_____

_____

_____

_____

7. List situations that indicate the need to plan multiple appointments for completion of periodontal debridement procedures.

_____

_____

_____

_____

_____

8. In your own words, describe tissue conditioning.

_____

_____

_____

_____

_____

9. If multiple dental hygiene appointments are planned for nonsurgical periodontal therapy, when should you evaluate the success of your initial periodontal debridement?

_____

_____

_____

10. In your own words, briefly describe the process and rationale for a full-mouth disinfection.

_____

_____

_____

_____

_____

_____

11. Describe definitive nonsurgical periodontal therapy.

_____

_____

_____

_____

12. List the steps that will help you formulate your strategy for instrumentation when preparing to provide nonsurgical periodontal instrumentation.

_____

_____

_____

_____

_____

13. What will you look for during a visual examination of your patient's gingival tissues to help you formulate your strategy for instrumentation?

_____

_____

_____

14. Why will you perform a tactile subgingival examination, using a periodontal probe and explorer, before beginning periodontal instrumentation to remove calculus?

_____

_____

_____

15. Why is it important to have your patient's radiographs available for review during scaling and root-planing procedures?

_____

_____

_____

_____

16. What postoperative instructions will you provide for your patient following scaling and root-planing procedures?

_____

_____

_____

_____

_____

_____

_____

17. What factors are taken into account when determining a maintenance interval after completion of non-surgical periodontal treatment?

_____

_____

_____

_____

_____

_____

_____

_____

18. Identify some factors that affect which instruments you will select for calculus removal during an individual patient's nonsurgical care.

_____

_____

_____

_____

_____

19. List the factors and variables that make instrumentation of subgingival surfaces more complex.

_____

_____

_____

_____

_____

_____

_____

_____

_____

20. Some suggested steps for providing manual scaling are listed below. Put the list in the correct order (1 = first step; 10 = last step).

Order	Description
_____	Select the correct cutting edge of the instrument.
_____	Stabilize your hand, using a finger rest.
_____	Adapt the toe of the cutting edge of the instrument against the tooth surface.
_____	Use smooth, overlapping, light pressured finishing strokes that provide maximum sensitivity to minute irregularities of the tooth surface.
_____	Apply sufficient (moderate-to-heavy) lateral pressure for calculus removal.
_____	Angle the instrument blade for insertion to the base of the periodontal pocket.
_____	Activate the instrument, maintaining the angulation and adaptation of the cutting edge evenly during the stroke.
_____	Pick up the instrument using a light-modified pen grasp.
_____	Repeat in overlapping, channeled strokes to remove all calculus.
_____	Apply light lateral pressure for instrument insertion and confirmation of soft tissue attachment.

21. What is the purpose of making scaling strokes in overlapping channels during subgingival scaling.

_____

_____

22. In your own words, explain micro-ultrasonics.

_____

_____

_____

23. List the indications for use of an endoscope during periodontal debridement.

_____

_____

_____

_____

24. Briefly describe the use of lasers for nonsurgical periodontal therapy.

_____

_____

_____

_____

_____

25. What factors are taken into consideration to determine a continuing care interval once a patient has completed initial therapy?

_____

_____

_____

_____

_____

_____

26. List two ways in which pharmacologic agents are used as adjuncts to scaling and root planing for treatment of periodontal disease.

_____

_____

27. Explain how the appropriate systemically delivered antibiotic is selected.

_____

_____

_____

28. List two objectives of antimicrobial therapy.

_____

_____

_____

29. Sometimes individuals do not respond to initial therapy. What conditions might be reasons for using systemic antibiotics?

_____

_____

_____

_____

_____

_____

_____

30. List at least four factors that contribute to the success of antimicrobial materials placed directly in an infected periodontal pocket.

_____

_____

_____

_____

31. Match the active ingredient of the local delivery antimicrobial (first column) to the trademark name of the drug (second column).

Active Ingredient	Trademark Name
_____ Chlorhexidine gluconate	A. Arestin
_____ Doxycycline hyclate	B. Atridox
_____ Minocycline HCl	C. PerioChip

32. Describe and compare two antibacterial agents used for direct placement in infected periodontal pockets.

_____

_____

_____

_____

_____

_____

33. Locally delivered antibiotic therapy is contraindicated for patients who are sensitive to _____ and for women who are pregnant and breastfeeding.

34. List some potential reasons for recurrence or progression of periodontal disease following treatment.

_____

_____

_____

_____

_____

_____

_____

_____

✓ COMPETENCY EXERCISES

Apply information from the chapter and use critical thinking skills to complete the competency exercises. Write responses on paper or create electronic documents to submit your answers.

The only real way to become competent in the skills described in this chapter of the **textbook** is to practice. It is, of course, difficult to help you do that in a workbook format. One way to enhance your competency in instrumentation skills is to work with a partner to provide feedback for each other during clinical exercises. Exercise 1 below provides one scenario for you to consider. As you work with student colleagues, you will find many more opportunities to explain and provide feedback on each other's instrumentation skills.

1. You are watching your student colleague, Mary Neely, while she is performing nonsurgical periodontal therapy. You have been designated as her mentor colleague, and your task for today is to give her verbal feedback about all areas of her clinical performance and instrumentation techniques while she is providing patient care. Tomorrow she will observe you providing patient care and will have feedback for you.

While you are observing Mary, you notice that as she is scaling in the maxillary posterior areas she is having some trouble placing a comfortable fulcrum during her activation stroke. You also observe that as she activates the instrument, her wrist motion seems to move the instrument handle from side to side and her hand pivots back and forth on her finger rest.

Explain what this type of hand motion might indicate about the angle of the blade of the instrument against the surface of the tooth down inside the periodontal pocket. Explain what Mary is doing incorrectly and how she might change the motion of her hand to increase her ability to remove calculus. (*Hint:* You can practice moving your instrument on a typodont or model to help you visualize what you are trying to describe.)

2. Describe how advanced instrumentation strategies can enhance outcomes of treatment for patients with advanced periodontal disease.

3. Explain why it is important to be extremely careful to control the pressure with which you express the liquid when using a cannula to insert antimicrobials into a periodontal pocket.

4. Develop an infomap to help you compare information about the type and amount of active ingredient or agent that is delivered to the sulcus, delivery methods, placement procedures, and care and storage of each of the different types of local delivery antimicrobials.

To make this a discovery exercise, gather samples of each of the products that are described in the **textbook** and use the packaging information to complete the infomap.

To enhance your ability to make evidence-based decisions for planning patient care, refer Chapter 2 in the **textbook** and the list of MeSH terms to help you complete a review of the current literature about one or more of the local delivery systems described in this chapter.

5. You are filling out the patient record for Bruce Wilden after his appointment. Today, you placed one cartridge of minocycline in a 6-mm pocket on the mesiolingual surface of tooth #3 and another one in a 7-mm pocket on the mesial surface of tooth #5. You educated Mr. Wilden about the self-care

regimens he will follow for the next few days, and you scheduled an appointment for follow-up procedures. Using your institution's guidelines for writing in patient records, document Mr. Wilden's appointment procedures.

Factors to Teach the Patient

This scenario is related to the following factors listed in this chapter of the **textbook**:

▷ The rationale for reevaluation following the completion of scaling and root planing.

At the last appointment in a multiple-appointment series, during which you have provided quadrant-by-quadrant scaling and root planing for Mr. Davis, you remind him to schedule a treatment evaluation appointment in 3–4 weeks with the front desk manager on his way out. He complains that he really does not want to come to see you one more time this year and he feels that a recall visit 6 months from now will be sufficient.

Use the principles of motivational interviewing (see **workbook** Appendix D) as a guide to prepare a conversation that you will use to explain the need for final evaluation prior to determining an appropriate recall interval. Use the conversation you create to educate a patient or friend. Then modify your conversation based on what you learned from their feedback.

MeSH TERMS

Use a combination of MeSH terms and other key words to develop an effective and efficient PubMed literature search strategy.

Periodontal debridement	Chlorhexidine
Root planing	Doxycycline
Subgingival curettage	Minocycline
Dental instruments	Endoscopy
Anti-infective agents	

EVERYDAY ETHICS

Before completing the learning exercises below, reread and reflect on the Everyday Ethics Scenario and Questions for Consideration in this chapter of the **textbook**. It may also be useful to review the Dental Hygiene Ethics discussion in Chapter 1, the Ethical Applications in the introduction pages for each section in the **textbook**, as well as the Codes of Ethics in **textbook** Appendices I–IV.

Collaborative Learning Activity

Work with another student colleague to role-play the scenario. The goal of this exercise is for you and your colleague to work though the alternative actions in order to come to consensus on a solution or response that is acceptable to both of you.

Discovery Activity

Ask a dental hygienist who has been practicing for a year or more to read the scenario. Provide them with a copy of the Code of Ethics as well. Share the responses you have made to answer each question and ask that person to discuss the situation with you. What insights did you have or what did you learn during this discussion?

CHAPTER 39 CROSSWORD PUZZLE

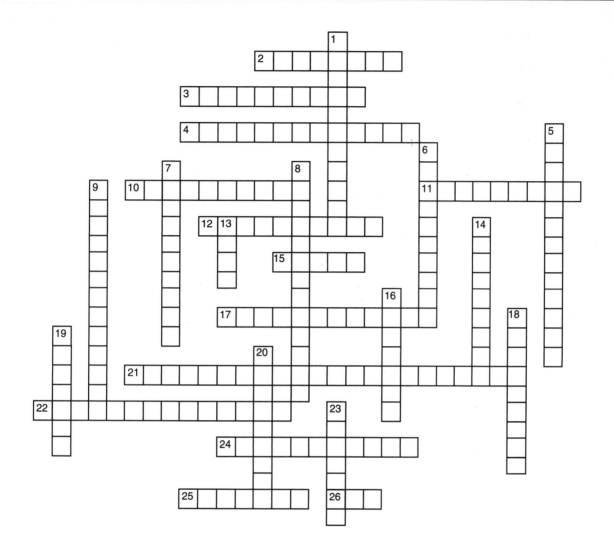

Puzzle Clues

Across

2. Method of delivering antibiotics to the infected area through blood circulation.

3. Not responding to usual treatment.

4. Can be broken down by a biologic process, such as by bacterial or enzymatic reaction.

10. The last step of calculus removal in which the clinician uses an explorer to determine the outcome of treatment.

11. The area between the roots of a multirooted tooth.

12. An agent produced by or obtained from microorganisms that can kill other microorganisms or inhibit their growth.

15. The amount of lateral pressure used during assessment procedures and instrument insertion.

17. Treatment by means of a chemical or pharmaceutical agent.

21. Disruption and removal of biofilm, endotoxins, and calculus from root surfaces (two words).

22. A second infection usually resistant to treatment of a first infection.

24. Definitive periodontal treatment that removes altered cementum or contaminated surface dentin from the root surface of a tooth (two words).

25. Scaling technique that uses overlapping strokes to ensure complete removal of calculus from a tooth or root surface.

26. Type of attachment that describes the union of tissues with a root surface that has been deprived of its original attachment apparatus.

Down

1. Removal of dental biofilm and calculus.

5. Antimicrobial rinse recommended after nonsurgical periodontal therapy is provided for advanced periodontitis or acute gingival infections; can be used as a preprocedural rinse to reduce microorganisms.

6 Not responding to treatment.

7. Presence of bacteria in the blood.

8. Therapy that uses chemical or pharmaceutical agents for the control or destruction of microorganisms.

9. Available for absorption by the body.

13. Acronym for dental biofilm removal and control, supragingival scaling, tooth debridement, and adjunctive treatments used to restore periodontal health.

14. A device used to visualize below the gingival margin for diagnosis and instrumentation.

16. Pressure applied during instrumentation.

18. Method of delivering minocycline hydrochloride directly into periodontal pocket.

19. Tubular end of an instrument used to introduce antimicrobial medication directly into the periodontal pocket.

20. Lipopolysaccharide complex found in the cell wall of many gram-negative microorganisms; toxic to human tissue.

23. The instrumentation of the crown or root surfaces of a tooth to remove calculus.

Sutures and Dressings

40

LEARNING OBJECTIVES

Upon successful completion of these exercises, you will be able to:

1. Identify and define the key terms and concepts related to sutures and periodontal dressings.

2. Identify the components/materials used for sutures and periodontal dressings.

3. Explain the procedures for placement and removal of sutures and periodontal dressings.

4. Discuss the rationale for and provide posttreatment instructions to patients with periodontal dressings.

5. Identify the components of appropriate documentation for surgical treatment, and suture and dressing placement and removal.

KNOWLEDGE EXERCISES

Write your answers for each question in the space provided.

1. List three functions of postsurgical suture placement.

_____

_____

_____

2. Which type of suture is capable of causing adverse tissue reaction?

_____

_____

3. What type of intraoral sutures must be removed by a dentist or dental hygienist within a specific period of time?

_____

4. Many types of suturing needles are available. What three factors influence selection of a specific type?

_____

_____

5. Which part of the needle is grasped by a needle holder during the suturing procedure?

_____

_____

6. List at least three requirements of an acceptable surgical suture needle.

_____

_____

_____

7. Describe the main reason why suture knots are tied on the facial surface of the alveolar ridge and tied with a 2- to 3-mm suture tail.

_____

_____

_____

8. How long should removable sutures be left in place?

_____

9. When removing a suture, it is necessary to raise the knot and hold it with a slight tension, slightly depress the tissue with the back of the scissors blade, and cut the suture in the part that was previously buried in the tissue. In your own words, describe why this procedure is followed.

_____

_____

_____

_____

10. Describe the purposes of using a periodontal dressing.

_____

_____

_____

_____

11. Describe the characteristics of an acceptable dressing material.

_____

_____

_____

_____

_____

_____

_____

12. List three disadvantages of zinc oxide with eugenol dressing material.

_____

_____

_____

13. List three advantages of chemical-cured dressings.

_____

_____

_____

14. List the characteristics of a well-placed dressing.

_____

_____

_____

_____

_____

_____

_____

_____

15. Describe the benefit of using a collagen dressing.

_____

_____

_____

_____

16. How long is a surgical dressing typically left in place?

_____

17. Identify a necessary component of the patient dismissal process following the placement of a periodontal dressing.

_____

_____

18. List the components of the detailed documentation required following suture removal.

_____

_____

_____

_____

_____

19. Following the removal of sutures or dressing, when should the return appointment to observe the surgical area be scheduled?

_____

_____

_____

✓ COMPETENCY EXERCISES

Apply information from the chapter and use critical thinking skills to complete the competency exercises. Write responses on paper or create electronic documents to submit your answers.

1. Mrs. Belinda Hawkins had periodontal surgery about 10 days ago. She is scheduled with you this afternoon for suture removal. List and explain the purpose of all the items and instruments you will need to set up in your treatment room to prepare for her postsurgical dressing and suture removal appointment.

2. After you seat Mrs. Hawkins and update her medical history, you examine the surgical areas and find out that the dressing is completely intact on the maxillary arch but that the dressing on the mandibular arch has partly broken off and the sutures are uncovered. One suture appears as though it may be partially imbedded in the dressing material. You note that all areas are fairly free of debris, and the surrounding mucosal tissue looks healthy. Describe the procedure you will use for removing the periodontal dressings.

3. Explain why you need to place each suture on a gauze sponge for postprocedural counting.

4. You gently rinse and examine Mrs. Hawkins' mouth. All areas appear to be healing well, with only slight redness in the area of tooth 30 where the suture had been embedded in the dressing. Explain follow-up bacterial biofilm control procedures to Mrs. Hawkins.

5. Write a progress note to document Mrs. Hawkins' suture removal procedure. Follow your institution's guidelines for writing in patient records.

? QUESTIONS PATIENTS ASK

What sources of information can you identify that will help you answer your patient's questions in this scenario?

When you greet Mrs. Hawkins in the reception room and walk with her back to your treatment room for her suture removal appointment, she is clearly nervous about the impending procedure. She asks, "Will it hurt? Will there be any bleeding?"

🖥 MeSH TERMS

Use a combination of MeSH terms and other key words to develop an effective and efficient PubMed literature search strategy.

Periodontal dressings   Sutures
Eugenol

EVERYDAY ETHICS

Before completing the learning exercises below, reread and reflect on the Everyday Ethics Scenario and Questions for Consideration in this chapter of the **textbook**. It may also be useful to review the Dental Hygiene Ethics discussion in Chapter 1, the Ethical Applications in the introduction pages for each section in the **textbook**, as well as the Codes of Ethics in **textbook** Appendices I–IV.

Individual Learning Activity

Imagine that you are the dental hygienist in this scenario. Answer each of the questions for consideration at the end of the scenario.

Discovery Activity

Ask a friend or relative who is not involved in health care to read the scenario and discuss it with you from the perspective of a "patient" who receives services within the healthcare system. Discuss what you learned from the concerns, insights, or difference in perspective that person expressed.

Factors to Teach the Patient

This scenario is related to the following factors listed in this chapter of the **textbook**:

▷ Explanations for the items in Table 40-2 in the **textbook**.

▷ Care of the mouth during the period after surgical treatment while wearing a periodontal dressing.

▷ That tobacco use is detrimental and delays healing.

Because you provided initial therapy care for Mr. Bruce Barramundi, you are very interested in observing when he is scheduled for periodontal surgery. After the surgical procedure is complete and the sutures and dressings are placed, you are asked to give him the printed instructions for posttreatment care you created based on Table 40-2 in the **textbook**.

You know that compliance with recommendations is always better if you provide verbal instructions as well as written. Besides, there are several factors that you think are important to emphasize. You know that Mr. Barramundi is still smoking, even though you have had a conversation about this risk factor. You also know that he has a very vigorous toothbrushing style and is always working very hard to make sure every tiny area of dental biofilm is completely removed.

Use the patient instructions for posttreatment care (Table 40-2 in the **textbook**) and the principles of motivational interviewing (see **workbook** Appendix D) as a guide to prepare an outline for a verbal reinforcement of posttreatment instructions for Mr. Barramundi.

Use the conversation you create to role-play this situation with a fellow student. If you are the patient in the role-play, be sure to ask questions. If you are the dental hygienist, try to anticipate questions and answer them in your explanation.

CHAPTER 40 WORD SEARCH PUZZLE

```
Z  T  Y  U  U  S  S  L  I  N  G  J  R  Z  R  E  P
R  V  E  X  E  U  A  P  C  M  B  G  Q  A  A  L  E
T  H  J  P  U  R  P  P  P  O  I  D  V  L  U  B  R
C  V  T  M  Y  N  X  R  R  N  A  Y  M  N  O  A  I
Q  I  R  I  P  S  E  D  T  O  U  P  C  I  A  B  O
C  J  R  G  R  S  E  E  C  F  T  D  T  E  C  R  C
J  X  X  K  S  R  R  G  T  I  E  E  N  X  O  O  A
N  B  C  U  M  D  N  E  J  L  V  T  C  C  N  S  R
J  K  R  O  E  I  K  T  X  A  V  P  H  T  T  B  E
K  E  L  N  S  N  R  E  X  M  S  U  G  N  I  A  Z
W  D  T  S  A  O  H  G  F  E  E  R  P  F  N  V  Q
N  A  E  L  P  F  J  T  I  N  B  R  E  T  U  A  E
L  R  B  V  N  Y  R  J  H  T  O  E  Q  F  O  J  G
D  P  K  Y  Z  Y  F  S  Q  O  J  T  Z  M  U  L  A
G  Y  S  T  E  R  I  L  I  T  Y  N  I  N  S  D  W
S  I  S  L  Y  O  R  D  Y  H  X  I  P  O  A  P  S
D  N  S  I  S  A  T  S  O  M  E  H  F  F  W  M  N
```

Puzzle Clues

1. Suture that is broken down by body enzymes or by water.
2. Suturing procedure that forms loops on one side of an incision and a series of stitches directly over the incision; also called a continuous lock.
3. Shaping of the peripheries of a dressing by manual manipulation of the tissue adjacent to the borders to duplicate the contour and size of the vestibule (two words).
4. Approximate the edges of a wound with no overlap.
5. Suture that is an uninterrupted series of stitches tied at one or both ends.
6. Material used to cover or protect a wound; also called a pack.
7. Termination of bleeding by mechanical or chemical means.
8. Process in which water penetrates and causes breakdown of a suture.
9. Suture that joins flaps on both the lingual and the facial sides of the dental arch.
10. Single-strand suture.
11. Paste–gel type of chemical-cured dressing; a brand name.
12. Type of dressing used to control bleeding.
13. Type of dressing that shields an area from injury or trauma.
14. Suture used when the flap is only one side; also called a suspension suture.
15. Important characteristic of a suture or needle for preventing infection.
16. Stitch or series of stitches made to secure apposition of the edges of a surgical or traumatic wound.
17. Eyeless end of a needle that allows suture material and needle to act as one unit.
18. Presence of potentially pathogenic microorganisms.

41

Dentinal Hypersensitivity

LEARNING OBJECTIVES

Upon successful completion of these exercises, you will be able to:

1. Identify and define the key terms and concepts related to dentin hypersensitivity.

2. Discuss the etiology of hypersensitivity and the hydrodynamic theory of pain transmission.

3. Identify factors that influence desensitization.

4. Identify pain characteristics and determine and document potential differential diagnoses.

5. Plan dental hygiene interventions to manage dentin hypersensitivity.

KNOWLEDGE EXERCISES

Write your answers for each question in the space provided.

1. In your own words, define *hypersensitivity*.

2. The highest prevalence of hypersensitivity is found in _____. Incidence and severity usually _____ in older folks due to the occurrence of natural mechanisms of desensitization.

3. In your own words, list the types of stimuli that can elicit hypersensitivity pain reaction.

4. List at least three *patient* behaviors that can trigger a hypersensitivity pain response.

5. What condition precedes the development of dentinal hypersensitivity?

6. Describe the role of dentinal tubules in the development of hypersensitivity.

7. There are very many factors that contribute to gingival recession, subsequent dentin exposure, and potential dentin hypersensitivity. Name as many as you can before looking in the **textbook** to check your answer.

_____

_____

_____

_____

_____

_____

_____

8. In about _____ % of teeth, the enamel and the cementum do not meet, leaving an area of exposed dentin.

9. What factors contribute to erosion on an exposed root surface?

_____

_____

_____

10. In your own words, describe *abfraction*.

_____

_____

_____

11. Which natural desensitization mechanism is related to narrowing of the inside wall of the dentin tubules?

_____

12. A smear layer can reduce dentin sensitivity by blocking the dentin tubules. What causes a smear layer?

_____

_____

_____

_____

13. Explain why a patient may notice sensitivity following the removal of heavy deposits of calculus during a dental hygiene appointment.

_____

_____

14. Pain perception is subjective. What does that statement mean?

_____

_____

_____

15. List the data collected by interview as you assess your patient's dental history of hypersensitivity.

_____

_____

_____

_____

16. Identify two patient response–related diagnostic tests that can be used to determine location and severity of tooth pain.

_____

_____

17. Without looking at the **textbook** (you won't always have it with you when you are interviewing a patient), identify at least three trigger questions you can ask your patient about tooth pain.

_____

_____

_____

_____

18. You can use a VRS to rate the level of pain your patient is feeling. If your patient describes her tooth-related pain as a "level 3," what does she mean?

_____

_____

19. Identify the clinical examination techniques and diagnostic tests that can be used to differentiate among the variety of potential causes for dental pain.

_____

_____

_____

_____

20. What are the two basic goals for treatment of dental hypersensitivity?

_____

_____

21. Treatment options offered to the patient should begin with the most _____ and least _____ measures.

22. What self-care measures can you suggest to your patient to help reduce dentin hypersensitivity?

_____

_____

_____

_____

_____

_____

23. List at least five factors that you will take into consideration when selecting a desensitizing agent.

_____

_____

_____

_____

_____

24. Briefly explain how the therapeutic ingredient in most desensitizing agents work.

_____

_____

25. List as many as you can of the therapeutic ingredients available to improve dental hypersensitivity.

_____

_____

_____

_____

_____

26. List two means of physically covering exposed dentinal tubules at the CEJ.

_____

_____

_____

_____

27. How is a laser used to treat hypersensitivity?

_____

_____

28. What dental hygiene procedures can increase potential pain related to hypersensitivity?

_____

_____

_____

_____

✓ COMPETENCY EXERCISES

Apply information from the chapter and use critical thinking skills to complete the competency exercises. Write responses on paper or create electronic documents to submit your answers.

1. Explain how abfraction differs from abrasion.

2. Using patient-appropriate language, describe the hydrodynamic theory.

3. Compare and contrast the two different subjective pain assessment scales (the VAS and the VRS) identified in Box 41-2 in the **textbook**. Why would you use both of them together for patient assessment?

4. Mr. Mustafa's chief complaint is a frequently occurring, sharply painful sensation on the right-hand side of his mouth. The pain often occurs when he grinds his teeth together during stressful moments at work. He says sometimes that area of his mouth causes pain when he drinks very cold water or chews on cold foods or hard, crunchy foods.

Dr. Bedron, who is busy with another patient and cannot take time to examine Mr. Mustafa today, asks you to assess Mr. Mustafa's complaint and document your findings and differential diagnosis in the patient record for him to read at the appointment Mr. Mustafa has scheduled with him next week. Your intraoral examination discovers many areas of deep recession along the facial cervical margins, toothbrush abrasion along the facial surfaces of all his molar teeth, and numerous large MOD restorations that were placed a very long time ago. Several of the restorations are beginning to break down, but you do not find any current large carious lesions.

You know that Dr. Bedron will need to do a very thorough clinical examination and question your patient carefully before he can diagnose the problem. But, using the information you have here and your school's guidelines for writing progress notes, document your differential diagnosis for conditions may potentially be causing Mr. Mustafa's tooth pain. Support your selections using the information in Table 41-1 in the **textbook**.

EVERYDAY ETHICS

Before completing the learning exercises below, reread and reflect on the Everyday Ethics Scenario and Questions for Consideration in this chapter of the **textbook**. It may also be useful to review the Dental Hygiene Ethics discussion in Chapter 1, the Ethical Applications in the introduction pages for each section in the **textbook**, as well as the Codes of Ethics in **textbook** Appendices I–IV.

Individual Learning Activities

Imagine that you are the dental hygienist in this scenario. Answer each of the questions for consideration at the end of the scenario.

Imagine the scenario from the patient's perspective. How might the patient's response to the questions following the scenario be different from those of the dental hygienist involved?

Factors to Teach the Patient

This scenario is related to the following factors listed in this chapter of the **textbook**:

▷ Contributing factors for dentin hypersensitivity.

▷ Appropriate oral hygiene self-care techniques, such as using a soft toothbrush and avoiding vigorous brushing, which may contribute to gingival recession and subsequent abrasion of root surface.

▷ Toothbrushing is not recommended immediately following consumption of acidic foods or beverages.

You are at your desk writing out a dental hygiene care plan for Mrs. Jernigan. Her chief symptom of tooth pain has been diagnosed by Dr. Hockwater as dentin hypersensitivity. Mrs. Jernigan is scheduled with you later this week for education and counseling. This is the first patient you have counseled regarding the management of dentin hypersensitivity, and you want to be thorough.

Use the principles of motivational interviewing (see **workbook** Appendix D) as a guide to create a conversation and to role-play this situation with a fellow student.

QUESTIONS PATIENTS ASK

What sources of information can you identify that will help you answer your patient's questions in this scenario?

Some patients express concerns related to a friend's experiences. "My friend bleached her teeth and said that it caused sensitivity. Should I avoid bleaching my teeth?"

A patient may express concern over the diagnosis of hypersensitivity for a specific area. "How do you know that I have sensitivity and not a cavity?" Many patients will want to understand more completely how the desensitizing agents will work to help their problem. "How soon after I start using sensitivity toothpaste will I notice an improvement in my hypersensitivity? Will I need to use a desensitizing product forever? Will I ever be able to have ice in my summer drinks again? Should I drink my morning orange juice before or after I brush my teeth?"

MeSH TERMS

Use a combination of MeSH terms and other key words to develop an effective and efficient PubMed literature search strategy.

Dentin	Smear layer
Dentin sensitivity	Pain perception
Dentin desensitizing agents	Pain threshold
	Pain measurement
Fluorides	Tooth abrasion
Dentin permeability	Gingival recession
Dentinal fluid	

Extrinsic Stain Removal

KNOWLEDGE EXERCISES

Write your answers for each question in the space provided.

1. What is the purpose of coronal polishing?

2. List the potential negative effects of polishing.

3. Identify actions you can take and polishing techniques you can use to minimize the negative effects of polishing.

4. Which abrasives commonly used in dental cleaning and polishing agents have a Mohs hardness value that indicates that they are less likely to scratch your patient's exposed tooth surfaces?

5. What characteristics and application principles affect the abrasive action of polishing agents?

- *Characteristics of abrasive particles:*

  _____

  _____

  _____

  _____

- *Application principles:*

  _____

  _____

  _____

6. In your own words, explain the difference between cleaning and polishing agents.

_____

_____

_____

7. What is the rotation speed of a low-speed handpiece?

_____

_____

8. Describe the kinds of prophylaxis angle attachments (polishing cups) available for you to use when polishing stain in different areas of the tooth.

_____

_____

_____

_____

_____

_____

_____

9. In your own words, describe the procedure used for applying the polishing agent to an area of stained enamel.

_____

_____

_____

_____

_____

_____

_____

_____

_____

_____

10. How is a bristle brush used?

_____

_____

_____

_____

_____

_____

11. How can stain be removed from proximal surfaces of teeth?

_____

_____

_____

12. What special care is required when using finishing strips to remove stain from proximal surfaces of anterior teeth?

_____

_____

_____

_____

_____

13. How does an air-powder polisher work?

_____

_____

_____

_____

_____

14. List the advantages of air-powder polishing.

_____

_____

_____

15. In your own words, describe the techniques you will use for reducing your exposure to aerosolized spray and for protecting both your patient and yourself when polishing, especially when using an air-powder polisher.

_____

_____

_____

_____

_____

_____

_____

_____

_____

_____

_____

16. What are the indications for polishing?

_____

_____

_____

_____

_____

17. List the clinical findings that indicate you should _not_ polish your patient's teeth during the dental hygiene appointment.

_____

_____

_____

_____

_____

_____

_____

_____

_____

_____

_____

_____

18. What is tribology?

_____

_____

19. What is a three-body abrasive polishing agent?

_____

_____

_____

_____

_____

20. What is the most common cause of aerosol production when using air-powder polishing?

_____

21. Describe potentially negative effects and sequelae of incorrectly directing the handpiece nozzle during air-powder polishing.

_____

_____

_____

_____

_____

_____

22. How can the clinician prevent potential injury while using the air-powder polisher?

_____

_____

_____

_____

_____

_____

COMPETENCY EXERCISES

Apply information from the chapter and use critical thinking skills to complete the competency exercises. Write responses on paper or create electronic documents to submit your answers.

1. What is the difference between polishing and abrasion? In what ways can you produce one but not the other when you remove stain from your patient's teeth?

2. Winston Nottingham always brings you a small packet of tea from England when he comes in for his regular periodontal maintenance appointment. He drinks tea every day, and you usually notice staining on the lingual surfaces of his maxillary and mandibular anterior teeth and on a few lingual proximal surfaces of the lower premolars. He has significant recession, especially on the facial surfaces on his lower molars and the facial and lingual surfaces of his maxillary molars owing to previous history of periodontal infection.

3. Write a dental hygiene diagnosis statement identifying Mr. Nottingham's condition in relation to the stain and the recession.

4. What dental hygiene interventions are appropriate for addressing Mr. Nottingham's problem?

5. Using your institution's guidelines for writing in patient records, document the procedure you used to remove the tea stain from Mr. Nottingham's teeth.

6. Mr. Nottingham's son, Will, who is 12 years old, is also your patient. He is in the office for a regularly scheduled 6-month prophylaxis appointment. You are glad he has returned as scheduled, because there are several areas of demineralization that you are monitoring. Will also has significant areas of dental stain because he drinks tea every morning with his parents. You point out the areas of stain to him and you mention that you must polish quite a few areas in his mouth.

While you are preparing to polish his teeth, Will picks up the container of polishing paste and notices that it contains fluoride. He points that out to you and wants to know why he must also undergo the "icky" fluoride treatment after you finish polishing. He wants to know why you can't just polish all of the areas of his teeth and then skip the regular fluoride treatment completely. Discuss why the use of a fluoride-containing polishing paste is not a replacement for a conventional topical application of fluoride.

Factors to Teach the Patient

This scenario is related to the following factors listed in this chapter of the **textbook**:

▷ How dental biofilm and stains form on the teeth and their replacements.

As noted in the Everyday Ethics case study for this chapter in the **textbook**, Carol explained to Mr. Jackson that colorings from food and drink can stain both natural teeth and the cosmetic restorations he had placed a year ago. Carol encouraged him to cut back on drinking tea, reinforced his role in stain prevention, and stressed the benefits to his appearance of compliance.

Apply the principles of motivational interviewing (see **workbook** Appendix D) to prepare an outline for a conversation for discussing the concept of stain formation with Mr. Jackson. Use the outline you create as the starting point to educate a patient or friend (not a student colleague) about stain formation.

MeSH TERMS

Use a combination of MeSH terms and other key words to develop an effective and efficient PubMed literature search strategy.

Dental equipment	Silicon dioxide
Dental polishing	Aerosols
Calcium carbonate	Bacteremia

EVERYDAY ETHICS

Before completing the learning exercises below, reread and reflect on the Everyday Ethics Scenario and Questions for Consideration in this chapter of the **textbook**. It may also be useful to review the Dental Hygiene Ethics discussion in Chapter 1, the Ethical Applications in the introduction pages for each section in the **textbook**, as well as the Codes of Ethics in **textbook** Appendices I–IV.

Individual Learning Activity

Identify a situation you have experienced that presents a similar ethical dilemma. Write about what you would do differently now than you did at the time the incident happened—support your discussion with concepts from the dental hygiene codes of ethics.

Discovery Activity

Ask a friend or relative who is not involved in health care to read the scenario and discuss it with you from the perspective of a "patient" who receives services within the healthcare system. Discuss what you learned from the concerns, insights, or difference in perspective that person expressed.

Tooth Bleaching

LEARNING OBJECTIVES

Upon successful completion of these exercises, you will be able to:

1. Identify and define the key terms and concepts related to tooth bleaching.

2. Compare the types of procedures, and discuss the processes of tooth bleaching systems.

3. Discuss the risks and potential side effects of bleaching.

4. Identify the indications and contraindications for dental bleaching treatment.

KNOWLEDGE EXERCISES

1. What is the difference between bleaching and whitening?

_____

_____

_____

_____

2. External tooth bleaching/whitening procedures can be used for both _____ and _____ teeth.

3. Describe the process for bleaching nonvital teeth.

_____

_____

_____

4. What ingredients are used for bleaching nonvital teeth?

_____

_____

5. Describe the mechanism of bleaching vital teeth.

_____

_____

_____

_____

_____

_____

6. Explain the action of each of the two active ingredients used in bleaching systems for vital teeth.

_____

_____

_____

7. Explain the difference in working time for each of the two active ingredients used in bleaching systems for vital teeth.

_____

_____

_____

_____

8. How long does hydrogen peroxide continue to work on the vital tooth after placement?

_____

9. How long does carbamide peroxide continue to work on the vital tooth after placement?

_____

10. List and describe the purpose of additional ingredients used in bleaching systems.

Ingredient(s)	Purpose

11. Identify the safety concerns or effects of bleaching associated with each of the following factors.

Factor	Safety Concerns/ Effects of Bleaching
Tooth structure	
Oral soft tissue	
Restorative materials	
Systemic effects	

12. Which vital tooth conditions would respond favorably to tooth bleaching?

_____

13. Which vital tooth conditions do not respond favorably to tooth bleaching?

_____

_____

14. What tooth conditions indicate need for a dental intervention prior to tooth bleaching?

_____

_____

_____

15. Describe effective methods for reducing sensitivity related to bleaching.

_____

_____

_____

_____

_____

16. What factors can influence the final outcome of tooth bleaching treatment?

_____

_____

_____

_____

17. Explain why vital teeth appear whiter immediately after completion of a tooth bleaching procedure.

_____

_____

_____

18. What are the potential reversible side effects of bleaching?

_____

_____

_____

19. Identify potential irreversible effects of bleaching on tooth structure.

_____

_____

_____

_____

20. List methods used for vital tooth bleaching.

_____

_____

_____

_____

_____

_____

 COMPETENCY EXERCISES

1. Although many of your patients will desire to have their teeth whitened, each one must be assessed carefully to determine the safety and appropriateness of this dental procedure. Identify contraindications for tooth bleaching. As you answer this question, take into consideration all of the factors you will assess in relation to each of the various types of tooth bleaching systems that are available.

2. Nell Katsipis is a new patient. Right after you seat her in the dental chair, she points to a darkened front tooth and tells you that the tooth had a root canal about 5 years ago. She wants to know why the over-the-counter tooth-whitening product she has applied almost made it look worse. How will you answer her question?

3. As you continue to talk with Nell, you mention that there is a procedure to whiten a nonvital tooth. She gets excited about that possibility and wants to know how the procedure is done. Even though you would like to get started with her complete history assessment and oral examination first, you know that it is important to at least provide a brief answer to her question. How will you explain the procedure to her?

4. During your assessment, you determine there are numerous demineralized areas on the surfaces of Nell's teeth, and you suspect these are probably due to overuse of the whitening products. What interventions will you include in her care plan to address the issue?

 DISCOVERY EXERCISES

Go to the American Dental Association website at http://www.ada.org/ and type the word "whitening" into the search box to find the latest ADA information about whitening products.

Systematic reviews offer the clinician the most reliable research and information. Using the MeSH terms, conduct a literature search by using the following link to PubMed: http://www.ncbi.nlm.nih.gov/pubmed.

Choose clinical queries; then enter the terms in the search box. Learn about the most recent systematic reviews of tooth-whitening products.

? QUESTIONS PATIENTS ASK

What sources of information can you identify that will help you answer your patient's questions in this scenario?

"Which bleaching/whitening method is best?" "How white will my teeth actually get?" "Should I whiten my teeth before or after you place those new fillings in my front teeth?" "Can I have my teeth bleached in the office now and then use an over-the-counter product to keep them white?"

 MeSH TERMS

Use a combination of MeSH terms and other key words to develop an effective and efficient PubMed literature search strategy.

Esthetics, dental	Dentin sensitivity
Tooth bleaching	Enamel microabrasion
Tooth bleaching agents	

EVERYDAY ETHICS

Before completing the learning exercises below, reread and reflect on the Everyday Ethics Scenario and Questions for Consideration in this chapter of the **textbook**. It may also be useful to review the Dental Hygiene Ethics discussion in Chapter 1, the Ethical Applications in the introduction pages for each section in the **textbook**, as well as the Codes of Ethics in **textbook** Appendices I–IV.

Individual Learning Activity

Imagine that you are the dental hygienist in this scenario. Answer each of the questions for consideration at the end of the scenario.

Discovery Activity

Ask a friend or relative who is not involved in health care to read the scenario and discuss it with you from the perspective of a "patient" who receives services within the healthcare system. Discuss what you learned from the concerns, insights, or difference in perspective that person expressed.

Factors to Teach the Patient

This scenario is related to the following factors listed in this chapter of the **textbook**:

Using the principles of motivational interviewing (see **workbook** Appendix D) as a guide, write a conversation you could use to obtain informed consent for a light-activated, in-office tooth-bleaching procedure. Use your conversation to educate a patient or a friend, and then modify it based on what you learned from the interaction.

This scenario is related to the following factors:

▷ In-office whitening may produce more sensitivity than over-the-counter and at-home products.

▷ In most cases, whitening must be periodically repeated to maintain desired tooth color.

▷ Existing tooth-colored restorations will not change color, and therefore may not match and may need to be replaced after whitening.

Implementation: Treatment

Chapters 36–43

COMPETENCY EXERCISES

Apply information from the chapters and use critical thinking skills to complete the competency exercises. Write responses on paper or create electronic documents to submit your answers.

SECTION VII—PATIENT ASSESSMENT SUMMARY				
Patient Name: *Aidan O'Connor*		Age: *21*	Gender: M	☑ Initial Therapy
				☐ Maintenance
Provider Name: *D.H. Student*		Date: *Today*		☐ Re-evaluation

Chief Complaint:

I came home from college this weekend and my mother made this appointment for me. I can't believe how much my teeth and gums are hurting. This upper right tooth—I think it is one of the molars—has just been throbbing for the past 2 weeks. And my mouth tastes terrible, but I can't even brush my teeth because my gums hurt so much!

Assessment Findings

Health History

- No medical visits for 2 years—no current medications
- High-stress levels related to upcoming end-of-term exams
- Tobacco use: 1 pack per day for 1 year—mostly while studying
- Alcohol use: usually only one alcoholic drink daily –however, on questioning, he admits to occasional excess in alcohol use as a stress reduction measure
- ASA classification-I, ADL level-0

At Risk For:

Social and Dental History

- Had regular dental care as a child; most recent visit was 2 years ago
- Denies neglect of regular daily oral hygiene measures except for the past week or so when mouth has been hurting
- Sips high sucrose, carbonated beverage while studying

At Risk For:

Dental Examination

- Generalized visible oral biofilm and debris in all areas of mouth
- Generalized visible calculus
- Generalized erythematic and sloughing gingival tissue; craterlike defects in lower anterior and lower left premolar area
- No visible decay; no restorations; intact dental sealants detectable on #14 and #19. Broken sealant remnants on #3 and #30

Periodontal Diagnosis/Case Type and Status:

DENTAL HYGIENE DIAGNOSIS statements related to TREATMENT interventions

Problem	Clinical Treatment Interventions

PLANNED INTERVENTIONS

(to arrest or control disease and regenerate, restore, or maintain health)

Clinical Treatment Interventions

At Risk For:

Caries Management Risk Assessment (CAMBRA) level:

☐ Low   ☐ Moderate   ☐ High   ☐ Extreme

Review Section VII Patient Assessment Summary for Aidan O'Connor to help you answer questions #1–3. The template included with his assessment summary will provide spaces for you to record your answers for these questions.

1. Complete the blank "At Risk For," "Periodontal Diagnosis," and "CAMBRA" sections of the assessment form as best you can with the information in the patient assessment.

2. Write at least three dental hygiene diagnosis statements for Aidan's dental hygiene care plan that are related to clinical treatment interventions that are within the scope of dental hygiene practice.

3. List clinical treatment interventions you will plan to help arrest or control disease and regenerate, restore, or maintain oral health in Aidan's mouth.

4. Describe the dental hygiene instruments and procedures you will select and use when you are providing dental hygiene care for each of the following patients. Discuss the rationale for your selections.

   - Mrs. Louise Gaiter presents with heavy, tenacious ledges of subgingival calculus in all areas of her mouth. In most areas of her mouth, you have recorded 3- to 5-mm pocket probing depths, but in several molar areas, there is calculus to the base of 7- to 9-mm pocket probing depths. Her gingival tissues are keratinized from long-term tobacco use.

   - Mr. Randall Forbes presents with spiny or nodular areas of calculus on surfaces just beneath the proximal contact areas of almost all of his teeth. His gingival tissues were bleeding heavily as you recorded probing depths during your assessment.

   - Mrs. Amelia Pritchert, who has had previous periodontal surgery, presents for her continuing care appointment with some areas of slight calculus and no probing depths deeper than 3 mm. But you have recorded 3–4 mm of gingival recession in most of the areas of her mouth.

   - Ms. Claudia Exeter drinks tea. She has very slight supragingival calculus in a few areas of her mouth but has a generalized moderate extrinsic stain on most of her tooth surfaces.

   - Amal, who is 8 years old, presents with slight lower anterior calculus, generalized dental biofilm, and moderate gingivitis with bleeding on probing in all areas of his mouth.

   - Mr. Robert Galen presents with slight generalized supragingival and subgingival calculus. He has a dental implant to replace tooth #38.

DISCOVERY EXERCISES

1. Spend time searching the Internet to find manufacturer and/or product websites that provide information about instruments and local anesthesia–related products, such as syringes, cartridges, and needle-safety devices. Create a "Webliography" (similar to an annotated bibliography) that contains a list of web addresses (URLs) for sites providing information about specific dental hygiene–related products; include a brief description of the information each website contains.

2. Use the product information you find to compare current dental hygiene instruments in terms of availability, handle size, design, and price.

3. Search the literature to locate the most current evidence to support the use of a specific dental hygiene therapy, such as root planing, selective polishing, ultrasonic scaling, tooth whitening, or placement of local-delivery antibiotics during the treatment of periodontal disease. Write a brief report on your findings.

4. Search the American Dental Hygienists' Association website (www.adha.org) to find information about which states in the United States allow provision of local anesthesia within the scope of dental hygiene practice. Describe how the ability to provide pain control during dental hygiene procedures can affect the success of the patient's treatment.

5. Research to find out which treatment interventions described in this section of the **textbook** are legal within the dental hygiene scope of practice.

6. Conduct a review of literature to determine:

- Types of topical anesthesia that can be applied to an abraded or incompletely healed area.
- Types of water-based gel that can be used to soften crusted sutures.

 FOR YOUR PORTFOLIO

1. Include a Webliography you create about any topic related to dental hygiene care (see Discovery Exercise 1).

2. A brief written report (make sure to cite your references accurately) about the information you gathered during your literature search for Discovery Exercise 3 would provide excellent documentation of your ability to use outside sources to find current information about dental hygiene care.

3. Include a variety of patient care plans you have developed to highlight your expertise at planning patient-specific clinical interventions for your patients.

Evaluation

SECTION VIII LEARNING OBJECTIVES

Completing the exercises in this section of the workbook will prepare you to:

1. Identify the key concepts in evaluating the outcomes of dental hygiene interventions.

2. Apply outcomes of assessment findings to plan maintenance care.

3. Document patient outcomes and recommendations for follow-up and continuing care.

COMPETENCIES FOR THE DENTAL HYGIENIST (APPENDIX A)

Competencies supported by the learning in Section VIII

    Core Competencies: C3, C4, C5, C6, C7, C9, C10, C11, C12, C13

    Health Promotion and Disease Prevention: HP2, HP4, HP5, HP6

    Patient Care: PC1, PC2, PC3, PC4, PC11, PC12, PC13

44

Principles of Evaluation

KNOWLEDGE EXERCISES

Write your answers for each question in the space provided.

1. State the purpose of evaluating treatment outcomes at the end of a sequence of dental hygiene interventions.

2. State the purpose of ongoing evaluation during each appointment of a multi-appointment treatment sequence.

3. What steps will you take to evaluate the dental hygiene care you provide for each patient?

4. List three ways to evaluate posttreatment outcomes.

5. List five to seven procedures you might assess during an immediate process evaluation.

6. List the factors that determine need for retreatment, referral, or maintenance interval.

_____

_____

_____

_____

7. What is interview evaluation?

_____

_____

_____

8. What is the reason for comparison of pre- and post-treatment assessment findings?

_____

_____

9. List the six categories that provide guidance for adhering to the ADHA standards for clinical dental hygiene practice.

_____

_____

_____

_____

_____

_____

10. List three sources for determining standard of care during a legal dispute.

_____

_____

_____

_____

_____

_____

11. What is the purpose for ongoing self-assessment and personal reflection regarding professional skills and knowledge in dental hygiene practice?

_____

_____

_____

_____

12. Unscramble the following words help you learn about the skills you can develop for reflective dental hygiene practice.
- kcabdeef

_____

- notiflecer

_____

- fwesrsa-lseaen

_____

- yanslais (this one is critical)

_____

- notleavuai

_____

13. Define three steps that can be used to direct reflective thinking and self-assessment about everyday occurrences related to dental hygiene practice.

_____

_____

_____

_____

✓ COMPETENCY EXERCISES

Apply information from the chapter and use critical thinking skills to complete the competency exercises. Write responses on paper or create electronic documents to submit your answers.

1. Explain the concept of professional standards of care. Discuss the role dental hygiene standards of care can play in ongoing self-assessment and reflective dental hygiene practice.

2. Ms. Olivia Qaba has just moved to your town and is scheduled today as a new patient in your clinic. Dr. Kish briefly examines her, and then you spend the rest of the appointment collecting thorough assessment data and providing the dental hygiene clinical interventions and education required to meet her needs.

When dental hygiene care is complete, you evaluate treatment outcomes. When you are planning maintenance care for Ms. Qaba (or for any patient), Dr. Kish requires that you consult with him to decide the appropriate continuing care interval for each case. Because Dr.

Kish has only briefly examined Ms. Qaba prior to your treatment, he is unlikely to know as much about her as you do after your interaction with her during the series of dental hygiene appointments. What important knowledge do you bring to recommending a continuing care interval for your patient that Dr. Kish may not know after his brief examination? (*Hint: Think about this question particularly in terms of the indicators you will use to measure the success of your dental hygiene interventions related to health behaviors*).

DISCOVERY EXERCISES

Initiate the practice of reflective self-assessment of your professional approach to dental hygiene care by starting a *"Critical Incident"* journal. Plan to write in the journal at least once every week until you graduate. Each week, select a situation related to your dental hygiene education that poses a question for you, causes you confusion, or is in some way meaningful for your professional development. Follow the three steps and use example questions from Table 44-2 in this chapter of the **textbook** to write a brief (no more than one to two pages) journal entry that describes what happened, analyzes why it was important for your learning or professional practice, and outlines additional learning or further steps that will help you enhance your professionalism, clinical skills, or knowledge.

Factors to Teach the Patient

This scenario is related to the following factors listed in this chapter of the **textbook**:

▷ The need for evaluation to establish the basis for "next step" treatment and maintenance decisions.

▷ How outcomes from dental hygiene interventions are used to determine further treatment needs and maintenance interval.

Salima, the dental hygienist in the Everyday Ethics scenario for this chapter, knows she must educate her patient, Mrs. Midoun, during this appointment about the need to evaluate the outcomes of dental hygiene treatment. Use the motivational interviewing principles found in **workbook** Appendix D to outline an approach Salima can use as she provides information about the need for outcomes assessment for her patient.

MeSH TERMS

Use a combination of MeSH terms and other key words to develop an effective and efficient PubMed literature search strategy.

Outcome assessment (health care)	Analysis
	Self-assessment
Patient outcome assessment	Feedback
Treatment outcome	Standard of care
	Practice guideline
Data collection	Guideline adherence

EVERYDAY ETHICS

Before completing the learning exercises below, reread and reflect on the Everyday Ethics Scenario and Questions for Consideration in this chapter of the **textbook**. It may also be useful to review the Dental Hygiene Ethics discussion in Chapter 1, the Ethical Applications in the introduction pages for each section in the **textbook**, as well as the Codes of Ethics in **textbook** Appendices I–IV.

Collaborative Learning Activity

Answer each of the questions for consideration at the end of the scenario in the **textbook**. Compare what you wrote with answers developed by another classmate and discuss differences/similarities.

Discovery Activity

Ask a dental hygienist who has been practicing for a year or more to read the scenario. Provide them with a copy of the Code of Ethics as well. Share the responses you have made to answer each question and ask that person to discuss the situation with you. What insights did you have or what did you learn during this discussion?

Continuing Care

 KNOWLEDGE EXERCISES

Write your answers for each question in the space provided.

1. If a disease does not respond to routine therapy, the disease is considered to be resistant, or _____.

2. The concept of continuing dental hygiene care is introduced to the patient in the initial dental hygiene care plan. Identify the purposes of a periodontal maintenance program for patients who successfully complete initial therapy.

_____

_____

_____

_____

_____

_____

3. List the factors you will consider when deciding upon a continuing care appointment interval that meets your patient's needs.

_____

_____

_____

_____

_____

_____

_____

_____

_____

_____

4. Identify assessment procedures and dental hygiene interventions that are commonly provided during a continuing care dental hygiene appointment.

- *Assessment procedures:*

_____

_____

_____

_____

_____

- *Dental hygiene interventions:*

_____

_____

_____

_____

_____

5. What factors contribute to the recurrence of peri-odontal disease?

_____

_____

_____

_____

6. You and the attending general dentist will decide together if there is a need to refer your patient to a periodontist for specialized periodontal therapy. Under what conditions might you refer a new patient directly to a periodontist?

_____

_____

_____

7. What criteria are used to determine referral when you evaluate treatment outcomes during a periodontal maintenance appointment after you have provided the initial therapy?

_____

_____

_____

_____

_____

_____

8. List the factors to consider when scheduling a patient's continuing care interval.

_____

_____

_____

_____

_____

9. A dental clinic continuing care plan can be set up using a card-file system or a computer-assisted approach. Identify two administrative methods for implementing the scheduling plan and scheduling patient appointments.

_____

_____

✔ COMPETENCY EXERCISES

Apply information from the chapter and use critical thinking skills to complete the competency exercises. Write responses on paper or create electronic documents to submit your answers.

1. Many factors contribute to the success of periodontal therapy and the remission or recurrence of periodontal disease.
- For which factors are the dental hygienist's actions particularly important in arresting disease?
- How does patient compliance affect the recurrence of periodontal disease?
- What risk factors for recurrence of periodontal disease are not easily modifiable by dental hygiene interventions?
- How do all of these factors interplay when making decisions regarding the frequency of individualized patient maintenance appointments?

2. Follow your school guidelines to write a progress note documenting maintenance interval recommendations for Mrs. Qaba. (See the Factors to Teach the Patient exercise for this chapter for more information.)

🔍 DISCOVERY EXERCISES

Before you do this exercise, take a moment to read Chapter 2 in the **textbook**. Then read a bit about Ms. Qaba, in the Factors to Teach the Patient exercise. Develop a PICO question related to determining an appropriate periodontal maintenance interval for Ms. Qaba. Use the PICO question you develop to find evidence in the dental literature to support your maintenance-interval recommendations.

EVERYDAY ETHICS

Before completing the learning exercises below, reread and reflect on the Everyday Ethics Scenario and Questions for Consideration in this chapter of the **textbook**. It may also be useful to review the Dental Hygiene Ethics discussion in Chapter 1, the Ethical Applications in the introduction pages for each section in the **textbook**, as well as the Codes of Ethics in **textbook** Appendices I–IV.

Individual Learning Activity

Imagine that you are the dental hygienist in this scenario. Answer each of the questions for consideration at the end of the scenario.

Collaborative Learning Activity

Work with another student colleague to role-play the scenario. The goal of this exercise is for you and your colleague to work though the alternative actions in order to come to consensus on a solution or response that is acceptable to both of you.

Factors to Teach the Patient

This scenario is related to the following factors listed in this chapter of the **textbook**:

▷ Purposes of follow-up and continuing care or maintenance appointments.

▷ Importance of keeping all maintenance appointments.

Together, you and Dr. Kish decide that a 3-month maintenance interval is appropriate for Ms. Qaba (first introduced in the Competency Exercise in Chapter 44). One reason for this decision is that even though her tissues are healthy right now, she is HIV positive and has a history of significant bone loss from past periodontal infection. You know from her dental history that she has previously been scheduled for 3-month periodontal maintenance, but Ms. Qaba states that she is not sure there is much point to having her teeth cleaned so often. She says that she was really hoping to stretch the interval to 6 months because she no longer has dental insurance.

Use a motivational interviewing approach (see **workbook** Appendix D) to write a statement about how you will explain your maintenance-interval recommendation to Ms. Qaba. Make sure to include a discussion of the literature articles you located when you did the aforementioned discovery exercise.

MeSH TERMS

Use a combination of MeSH terms and other key words to develop an effective and efficient PubMed literature search strategy.

Comprehensive dental care

Outcome assessment (health care)

Treatment outcome

Treatment failure

Standard of care

Practice guideline

Patient compliance

Evaluation

Chapters 44–45

 COMPETENCY EXERCISES

Apply information from the chapter and use critical thinking skills to complete the competency exercises. Write responses on paper or create electronic documents to submit your answers.

Read Section VIII Patient Assessment Summary to help you answer questions #1 and #2.

1. According to the documentation in her reevaluation section of her care plan, Charen Woodmacher has been referred to the periodontist for specialized care, even though her tissue health has improved because of the dental hygiene treatment she received. Explain why.

2. Even though Charen has been referred to the periodontist, the care plan recommends that a 6-month continuing care appointment is scheduled with the general practice dentist. Explain why. (*Hint*: It may be helpful to look at the pretreatment assessment data as you think about this question.)

 DISCOVERY EXERCISES

1. Investigate and describe the recall system used in your school clinic. What is your role as a student in making the system work and for making sure that complete oral health continuing care is scheduled and delivered as needed for the patients you provide care for in your clinic?

2. As an exercise in self-evaluation, imagine that you are a clinical instructor assigned to evaluate your patient care and provide feedback at the end of a patient appointment. Take a few moments at the end of one or more patient appointments to complete the same evaluation form your instructor would use to evaluate your progress. Compare your own self-evaluation score with the score and feedback that is actually provided by your instructor for the same patient. How will differences you discover between the two evaluations redirect future self-evaluation of your clinical skills?

 FOR YOUR PORTFOLIO

Maintain a reflective journal by writing "critical incident" entries related to patient care experiences over several weeks or months during your education. Organize the individual journal entries by broad topic areas; for example, ethical issues, healthcare knowledge, clinical skills, evaluating patient care, motivating patient behavior change, and so on. When you have collected several journal entries related to one topic, you can "reflect on your reflection." This action can enhance your understanding of your professional self and your ability to self-evaluate by analyzing and reflecting about what you have learned over time.

SECTION VIII—PATIENT ASSESSMENT SUMMARY

Patient Name: *Charen Woodmacher*   Age: *15*   Gender: F   ☐ Initial Therapy

                                                                                 ☐ Maintenance

Provider Name: *D.H. Student*   Date: *Today*   ☑ Re-evaluation

Chief Complaint:

Pt presents for re-evaluation following the completion of a series of quadrant scaling and root planing appointments with significant oral health educational interventions provided at each appointment.

RE-EVALUATION FINDINGS

Retreat ☐   Refer ☑   **Continuing care interval**: *6 months recall appointment (in general practice office)*

Description of posttreatment outcomes:

Resolution of carious lesion on tooth #30 (root canal completed, appointment for crown scheduled within 1 month). Patient appears to be more motivated in self-care practices and biofilm levels are significantly reduced. Generalized probing depths are reduced to 3 mm and tissue health improved: reduction in erythema, bulbous appearance, and generalized bleeding. However, 6- to 8-mm pockets, with bleeding on probing, have not resolved in lower anterior sextant and in molar areas.

Referral *to physician for complete medical work-up*

Referral *to periodontist for assessment of specialized periodontal treatment needs*

*Assessment Findings from Charen Woodmacher's Pretreatment Assessment
Provided here for Additional Information*

Health History

- Recent diagnosis of bulimia—currently undergoing psychological assessment and treatment
- Iron-deficiency anemia
- Contraceptive pills
- Daily iron supplement
- ASA classification-II
- ADL level-0

At Risk For:

- Enamel erosion
- Increased susceptibility to dental caries
- Increased gingival response to oral biofilm

Social and Dental History

- Regular dental care until 2 years ago when she started refusing to come to the dentist
- Good general knowledge, but admits to recent general neglect of oral hygiene
- Had orthodontic bands until 6 months ago, but all appliances were removed and treatment was discontinued

At Risk For:

- Increased susceptibility to dental caries
- Demineralization
- Periodontal infection

Dental Examination

- Deep caries no. 30 with abscess visible on radiograph
- Evidence of lingual erosion on maxillary incisors
- General biofilm accumulation
- Heavy calculus in all areas
- Generalized erythema, bulbous papilla, and bleeding on probing
- Generalized 4-mm with 6- to 8-mm pockets in mandibular anterior sextant and on #3 mesial, #14 mesial and distal, and #18 mesial

At Risk For:

- Oral pain
- Dental caries
- Gingival or periodontal infection/abscess

SECTION VIII SUMMARY PUZZLE CLUES

```
E R E F V A F B Q R R Q A G C D J E R M M I L I
K V C Q E R V E U G V F G T J H A Y Z I C C C C
M S R B Z K E W E H R U I E S X O E V B P R G O
X Y O E G H J F R D V S F S V C F P J T G I T N
I R T J N X H C L L B K U E Z O T E O R T T C T
K V C B V X Y I O E Y A G G P L A V U R G I K I
S S A J D A P N N T C V C C C O C I T N W C S N
G R F O Z E I B K G R T T K N I T I C R Y A G U
B B K D P R E B O O K N I K T C I S O T G L J I
A R S D L G U E N C E G P V U S L U M P T I M N
G M I D I K G K J M Q V F B E G E E E B T N S G
U J R P G N O Z S E G P Q X T P D W G H G C Q C
A T D J I B P S X S G A E W C V R V Y H I I E A
J E P O T K E E T T E T Y O J O K A Q X R D U R
N Z G W S S B H H Q V V M B L I G W C B H E K E
W N T L S T H N U P C P A E U X V O T T N N O E
O I O A B M P Z Y T L A V L K V Z B V X I T V A
P M X H Q Q W Z F I H I A E U T T U P D H C U Y
J P Q H E P G J A J T E O I W A M H F A K M E I
F A F I L U E N J A R G A C W Y T T T V J J T
N C B B M J C O M T K L I C Z M C I V A U H X Y
P T M S W E I M K U S I S Y L A N A O N R H R S
W X K B H I U W M O S O N J B O K B I N X D U T
P T O T W S W B Y R O T C A R F E R U Y O S D N
```

Puzzle Clues

1. Standard #5 in the ADHA Standards for Clinical Dental Hygiene Practice.

2. A reflective-practice journaling approach that is useful in guiding clinicians to assess and to document learning from their actions and responses during clinical situations (two words).

3. A characteristic, habit, or predisposing condition taken into consideration when planning for the patient's maintenance interval following the evaluation of initial treatment outcomes (two words).

4. Information collected during the evaluation procedure.

5. Long-term maintenance phase of dental hygiene care (two words).

6. Evaluated following the completion of dental hygiene treatment and patient education.

7. Providing communication about the outcome of dental hygiene treatment.

8. The "so what" component of reflection and self-assessment.

9. Perceptive self-awareness, judgment, critical analysis and synthesis of information, and application of new knowledge are key skills practitioners need for (two words).

10. This step in the dental hygiene process of care has many of the same components as the evaluation step.

11. A type of evaluation that assesses long-term effectiveness of dental hygiene care in achieving health goals.

12. The method of administering a patient's maintenance plan by scheduling the next appointment before a patient leaves the current appointment.

13. Refers to the patient's health behavior actions that are in accordance with the clinician's recommendations.

14. Type of evaluation; determines whether goals stated in the patient's care plan have been met.

15. Not responding to therapy.

16. Type of evaluation; provided at all appointments during a patient's treatment sequence.

17. Type of evaluation; checking of root surfaces with an explorer to assess for residual calculus or other iatrogenic factors.

Patients with Special Needs

SECTION IX LEARNING OBJECTIVES

Completing the exercises in this section of the workbook will prepare you to:

1. Identify the treatment and education modifications necessary to meet the needs of individuals with physical, mental, and medical conditions or limitations.

2. Plan and provide dental hygiene care for individuals with special needs in both traditional and nontraditional practice settings.

3. Document all aspects of dental hygiene care.

COMPETENCIES FOR THE DENTAL HYGIENIST

All competencies listed in the *ADEA Competencies for Entry into the Profession of Dental Hygiene* **(Appendix A) are supported by the learning in Section IX.**

46

The Pregnant Patient and Infant

KNOWLEDGE EXERCISES

Write your answers for each question in the space provided.

1. Dental hygiene care is an integral and essential part of your pregnant patient's _____ care.

2. One-third of a pregnancy, a 3-month period, is referred to as _____.

3. What is a teratogenic effect?

_____

_____

4. Name an antibiotic that has the well-known effect of staining the infant's teeth if taken by the pregnant mother after 4 months of gestation.

_____

5. List three oral findings common during pregnancy.

_____

_____

_____

6. In your own words, describe the clinical appearance and significance of a pregnancy epulis.

_____

_____

_____

_____

_____

_____

7. What recommendations can the dental hygienist provide for the patient with a pregnancy-related condition that is a risk factor for demineralization and acid erosion of teeth?

_____

_____

_____

_____

_____

_____

8. Identify reasons why some women have more problems with gingivitis during pregnancy.

_____

_____

_____
_____
_____
_____

9. List three signs you might observe in your pregnant patient that would make you suspect depression.

_____
_____
_____

10. Visualizing a timeline can often help put information into perspective. Use the timeline to identify the oral/facial feature developing in the fetus during the approximate time indicated by each of the lettered segments.

Facial Development Gestation Timeline

A. _____

B. _____

C. _____

D. _____

E. By this time (8th week), a(n) _____ is apparent in the developing fetus.

F. By this time (12th week), a(n) _____ is apparent in the developing fetus.

11. What are the possible adverse effects on the fetus when a woman uses tobacco, alcohol, or other substances of abuse during pregnancy?

_____
_____
_____

12. What is supine hypotensive syndrome?

_____
_____
_____
_____
_____

13. List the symptoms of supine hypotensive syndrome.

_____
_____

14. What preventive measure will you provide for a pregnant patient to prevent the symptoms of supine hypotensive syndrome?

_____
_____
_____

15. How does anticipatory guidance aid a parent?

_____
_____
_____

16. List as many topics as you can think of that are appropriate to include in oral health education you provide for a patient who is a new mother or mother-to-be.

_____
_____
_____
_____
_____
_____
_____
_____
_____

17. Describe the position that provides the most effective visual access for examining an infant's oral tissues.

_____
_____
_____
_____

18. List the risk factors for early childhood caries.

_____
_____
_____
_____
_____

19. Describe vertical transmission.

_____

_____

_____

 COMPETENCY EXERCISES

Apply information from the chapter and use critical thinking skills to complete the competency exercises. Write responses on paper or create electronic documents to submit your answers.

1. Mrs. Jill Mason, who is in her late second trimester of a healthy pregnancy, presents for her dental hygiene appointment with a toothache and a swelling on the right-hand side of her mandible. The dentist orders a single periapical radiograph of the area. Mrs. Mason is concerned about the effect of the radiation on her developing baby. Using all the information available to you in Chapters 46 and 15 to describe the educational approach, protective measures, and radiographic techniques, you will use to relieve her fears and maximize safety for her and the baby.

2. Using the format for writing progress notes that is used in your school, document the patient position adaption used during Mrs. Mason's treatment.

Read the Chapter 46 Patient Assessment Summary for Mrs. White to help you answer the following questions.

3. Mrs. White mentions she frequently experiences nausea, gagging, and vomiting, followed by an unpleasant taste. You realize from looking at the patient assessment data collected during her previous appointment that she is at risk for several additional oral problems. Identify the possible oral problems, and provide three self-care measures that will minimize their oral effects.

4. Using the dental hygiene diagnosis format, identify a cause or factor that could result in increased risk for dental caries during the course of Mrs. White's pregnancy.

5. Write a goal for the problem identified in the dental hygiene diagnosis in question 4. Include a time frame for meeting the goal. How will you measure whether your patient met the goal?

6. Write one goal for Mrs. White's dental hygiene care plan to address the need to provide anticipatory guidance related to the oral care needs of her soon-to-be-born infant.

 QUESTIONS PATIENTS ASK

What sources of information can you identify to help you answer your patient's questions in this scenario?

"Because of my nausea, I have to eat frequent small snacks. I usually nibble on granola bars—those are healthy snacks, aren't they?" "I heard that pregnancy takes calcium away from my teeth, so is that why I seem to be getting more cavities?" "Should I just wait until after the baby is born to have my fillings done?" "Is it safe to use a mouthwash while I am pregnant?"

 MeSH TERMS

Use a combination of MeSH terms and other key words to develop an effective and efficient PubMed literature search strategy.

Pregnancy	Infant
Pregnancy trimester, first	Infant, newborn
Pregnancy trimester, second	Breast feeding
Pregnancy trimester, third	Bottle feeding
Pregnancy outcomes	Natal teeth
Dental care for children	Tooth, deciduous
	Tooth eruption

EVERYDAY ETHICS

Before completing the learning exercises below, reread and reflect on the Everyday Ethics Scenario and Questions for Consideration in this chapter of the **textbook**. It may also be useful to review the Dental Hygiene Ethics discussion in Chapter 1, the Ethical Applications in the introduction pages for each section in the **textbook**, as well as the Codes of Ethics in **textbook** Appendices I–IV.

Collaborative Learning Activity

Answer each of the questions for consideration at the end of the scenario in the **textbook**. Compare what you wrote with answers developed by another classmate and discuss differences/similarities.

Discovery Activity

Ask a friend or relative who is not involved in health care to read the scenario and discuss it with you from the perspective of a "patient" who receives services within the healthcare system. Discuss what you learned from the concerns, insights, or difference in perspective that person expressed.

Factors to Teach the Patient

This scenario is related to the following factors listed in this chapter of the **textbook**:

▷ The relationship of oral health of the mother to the general health of the fetus and newborn.

▷ The serious effects of tobacco and other drugs on the health of the fetus, the infant, and the child.

▷ Reasons for limiting fermentable carbohydrate intake and maintaining a healthy diet from the fruit, vegetable, grain, meat and meat alternatives, and dairy food groups.

Using the example Patient Assessment Summary for Mrs. White, your answers to the questions about her in the competency exercises for this chapter, and the principles of motivational interviewing (see **workbook** Appendix D) as a guide, prepare an outline for a conversation that you might use to educate Mrs. White regarding one of the problems identified in the dental hygiene diagnosis. Use the conversation to educate a patient or friend, and then modify it based on what you learned by using the outline.

CHAPTER 46 —PATIENT ASSESSMENT SUMMARY

Patient Name: *Mrs. Diane White*   Age: *27*   Gender: F   ☐ Initial Therapy
                                                                             ☑ Maintenance
Provider Name: *D.H. Student*   Date: *Today*   ☐ Re-evaluation

Chief Complaint:

Presents for routine maintenance appointment. Gum tissues bleed when brushing and flossing.

Assessment Findings

Health History

- First trimester of first pregnancy; experiences significant nausea daily and occasional morning vomiting
- Husband smokes cigarettes in house and car; patient does not smoke
- ASA Classification-II and ADL level-0

At Risk For:

- Enamel erosion and increased dental caries risk
- Infant at risk for second-hand smoke exposure

Social and Dental History

- Nine months since previous recall appointment; missed her 6-month appointment
- Infrequent flossing
- Uses bottled water with no fluoride content; smell of fluoridated toothpaste makes her feel nauseated
- Frequent high-carbohydrate snacks (graham crackers) to help control nausea

At Risk For:

- Increased risk for periodontal disease
- Increased caries risk and risk for enamel erosion
- Increased caries risk

Dental Examination

- No current cavitated lesions; a small number of occlusal surface restorations are all in good repair
- Moderate biofilm along cervical margins and on proximal surfaces
- Generalized 4-mm probing depths; no radiographic indication of bone loss
- Generalized red, bulbous tissue and generalized bleeding on probing

At Risk For:

- Increased risk for caries and periodontal infection
- Oral infection, increased risk for periodontal/gingival infection
- Increased risk for periodontal/gingival infection and pyogenic granuloma

Periodontal Diagnosis/Case Type and Status

- Gingivitis

Caries Management Risk Assessment (CAMBRA) Level:

- ☐ Low ☑ Moderate ☐ High ☐ Extreme

The Pediatric Patient

 KNOWLEDGE EXERCISES

Write your answers for each question in the space provided.

1. Match each characteristic on the right (as described in this chapter of the **textbook**) with the most appropriate age category on the left. Each age category can be matched to more than one characteristic.

Age Category	Characteristic
A. Toddler	____ Lift the lip to examine anterior teeth
B. Preschool child	____ All permanent dentition
C. School-age child	____ Avoid using negative words
D. Adolescent	____ Usually have mixed dentition
	____ Able to become an active, cooperative participant during the dental visit
	____ Conversations become more mature and links past actions to present events

Age Category	Characteristic
	____ Increased need for privacy and desire for independence
	____ Can dress self and begin to brush own teeth with supervision
	____ First dental visit
	____ Risk-taking behaviors more likely to begin
	____ Most are capable of sitting in the dental chair
	____ Use tiny "smear" of toothpaste on brush
	____ Begin use of pea-sized amount of toothpaste spread across surface of brush
	____ Crying during oral examination is normal
	____ Important to begin periodontal assessment at this age
	____ Reliance on friends and influenced by peers

2. In your own words, briefly describe why it is imperative to establish a dental home and a regular schedule of preventive visits for a child patient.

_____

_____

_____

_____

_____

3. Excellent _____ communication skills will aid in gaining the confidence and cooperation of a child patient.

4. Explain how child-friendly dental terms are used during dental hygiene treatment for a young child.

_____

_____

_____

5. In your own words, describe the best way for a dental hygienist to access and examine the oral cavity of child patient who is not old enough or cooperative enough to sit in the dental chair for an oral examination.

_____

_____

_____

_____

6. Why is a periodontal assessment necessary for the school-age through adolescent child patient?

_____

_____

7. _____ fluctuations can increase the adolescent patient's risk for biofilm-induced gingivitis.

8. The type of dental hygiene services provided for a child patient depends on the child's _____ and_____.

9. The need to take dental radiographs of the pediatric dental patient is determined by the _____ guidelines and the dentist's professional judgment about the patient's needs.

10. A recommendation for fluoride supplementation is considered when the child's exposure to fluoride is _____.

11. Dental sealants are recommended for the child patient when _____ or _____ are noted during caries risk assessment.

12. Syrup, gum, or lozenges with _____ can be recommended for the child with a moderate or high caries risk.

13. Briefly list the four principles of caries risk assessment.

_____

_____

_____

_____

14. In your own words, briefly explain the balance of risk factors and protective factors in determining a child's level of caries risk.

_____

_____

_____

15. List the criteria used to determine a high-caries risk classification for a child patient.

_____

_____

_____

_____

_____

16. _____ lesions, as well as cavitated carious lesions, are considered indicative of ECC or S-ECC.

17. Identify the two most important factors that predispose to ECC.

_____

_____

18. How much toothpaste is appropriate for parents to place on the toothbrush of a 4-year-old?

_____

_____

19. Identify at least three topic areas appropriate to address during anticipatory guidance educational interventions for the parents of a 4-year-old.

_____

_____

_____

20. Identify at least three topic areas appropriate to address during anticipatory guidance educational interventions for a 13-year-old patient and parents.

_____

_____

_____

✓ COMPETENCY EXERCISES

Apply information from the chapter and use critical thinking skills to complete the competency exercises. Write responses on paper or create electronic documents to submit your answers.

1. You are conducting an oral health education class for a mother's group at the community center near your house as part of a community service project. The mother of a darling 18-month-old girl asks you how many more teeth her child will get. Explain the development and eruption patterns of primary teeth.

2. Explain to this young mother why healthy primary teeth are important for the growth and development of a healthy permanent dentition.

3. In your own words, define *early childhood caries* as if you were explaining the concept to a parent.

4. Select one of the pediatric age groups identified in the chapter. Explain how knowledge of expected developmental milestones and the child's actual developmental level can assist you to provide dental hygiene care or self-care instruction for that child.

5. Make up three terms/names for dental equipment or instruments (different from those mentioned in the **textbook**) that you might use to explain what is happening during a dental visit to an anxious preschooler. For extra fun, share your names with those of your student colleagues.

6. Angela Flores, 3 years old, sits quietly in the dental chair for several minutes while you speak with her mother. She allows you to tilt the chair into a supine position, but begins to cry as soon as you approach her mouth with your mirror and explorer. She continues to cry and reach for her mother even after you explain all the fun games you will play together while you count her teeth. Outline an appropriate response to this situation.

7. Describe some ways in which a parent might prevent the transfer *Streptococcus mutans* from her mouth to her child's mouth.

Factors to Teach the Patient

This scenario is related to the following factors listed in this chapter of the **textbook**:

▷ How the bacteria that cause dental caries can be transferred to a baby's mouth from parents or other family members.

▷ How fluoride makes enamel stronger and more resistant to the bacteria that cause dental caries.

▷ Methods to prevent dental caries from developing in a young child's mouth.

▷ How feeding methods and snacking patterns can contribute to dental caries.

▷ How the parent can examine the infant/child's mouth and what to look for during the examination.

Mr. and Mrs. Jacobson are in your treatment room with their son, Eric, who is 2.5 years old. The dentist has diagnosed incipient early childhood caries based on observations made during her examination. You have been asked to educate these very concerned parents about how and why this is happening to their son and what can be done to arrest the decay process and prevent further problems.

Use the principles of motivational interviewing (see **workbook** Appendix D) as a guide to outline a conversation you might have with the Jacobson's. Compare your conversation with a student colleague's to identify any missing information.

MeSH TERMS

Use a combination of MeSH terms and other key words to develop an effective and efficient PubMed literature search strategy.

Dental care for children	Tooth eruption
Pediatric dentistry	Tooth, deciduous
Child	Dentition, mixed
Adolescent	Dentition, permanent

EVERYDAY ETHICS

Before completing the learning exercises below, reread and reflect on the Everyday Ethics Scenario and Questions for Consideration in this chapter of the **textbook**. It may also be useful to review the Dental Hygiene Ethics discussion in Chapter 1, the Ethical Applications in the introduction pages for each section in the **textbook**, as well as the Codes of Ethics in **textbook** Appendices I–IV.

Individual Learning Activity

Imagine that you have observed what happened in the scenario, but are not one of the main characters involved in the situation. Write a reflective journal entry that:

- Describes how you might have reacted (as an observer—not as a participant),

- Expresses your personal feelings about what happened, or

- Identifies personal values that affect your reaction to the situation.

Discovery Activity

Ask a dental hygienist who has been practicing for a year or more to read the scenario. Provide them with a copy of the Code of Ethics as well. Share the responses you have made to answer each question and ask that person to discuss the situation with you. What insights did you have or what did you learn during this discussion?

48

The Older Adult Patient

KNOWLEDGE EXERCISES

Write your answers for each question in the space provided.

1. In your own words, define the following terms related to aging.
   - *Aging:*

   - *Gerontology:*

   - *Biologic age:*

   - *Chronological age:*

2. There are two common classifications used to define individuals from older adult populations: age-related and function-related. These two systems used together can help provide an accurate description of your aging patients. List the categories for each of these classifications.

   - *Age-related classifications:*

   - *Function-related classifications:*

3. Differentiate between the terms *primary aging* and *secondary aging.*

4. For each of the following body systems, describe at least two changes that occur due to primary aging.

- *Musculoskeletal system:*

_____

_____

_____

- *Cardiovascular system:*

_____

_____

- *Respiratory system:*

_____

_____

- *Gastrointestinal system:*

_____

_____

- *Central nervous system:*

_____

- *Peripheral nervous system:*

_____

- *Sensory system:*

_____

_____

_____

_____

_____

- *Endocrine system:*

_____

_____

- *Immune system:*

_____

_____

_____

5. An older adult may react differently to disease than your younger patients. Identify the differences mentioned in the **textbook**.

_____

_____

_____

_____

_____

6. What risk factor related to chronic diseases is associated with increased risk for dental caries in older adult patients?

_____

_____

_____

7. List some of the most common chronic diseases associated with aging.

_____

_____

_____

_____

8. Identify two psychosocial conditions that can be of concern when treating older adult patients.

_____

_____

9. In your own words, define the term *dementia*.

_____

_____

_____

10. In your own words, briefly summarize what you learned about Alzheimer disease.

_____

_____

_____

_____

_____

_____

_____

_____

_____

_____

_____

11. List the two types of Alzheimer disease.

_____

_____

12. What is osteoarthritis?

_____

_____

_____

13. List the risk factors for osteoporosis.

_____

_____

_____

_____

_____

_____

_____

_____

_____

_____

_____

14. Your older patient with osteoporosis is considered to be at greater risk for periodontal bone loss. Describe the relationship of osteoporosis to oral bone loss and list the mutual risk factors that relate to osteoporosis and periodontal disease.

_____

_____

_____

_____

_____

15. What medication, commonly prescribed for individuals with osteoporosis, is a contraindication for dental surgery?

_____

_____

16. Identify the age-associated oral conditions described by each of the following statements.

Difficulty swallowing:

_____

_____

_____

Oral lesion that appears as skinfolds with fissuring at the corner of the mouth; not specifically an age-related lesion but is frequently seen among older persons:

_____

_____

Burning, smooth, shiny, bald tongue with atrophied papillae; related to nutritional deficiencies:

_____

_____

Deep red or bluish nodular masses commonly found during an intraoral examination of older individuals on either side of the midline on the ventral surface of the tongue:

_____

_____

Oral condition often noted in older adults related to pathologic states, drug-induced changes, or radiation-induced degeneration of salivary glands:

_____

_____

Dental disease occurring in older folks related to cementum exposed by periodontal infections and often to xerostomia:

_____

_____

17. A dry, purse-string opening of your older patient's lips may make wide opening difficult during dental hygiene treatment. What causes this condition?

_____

_____

_____

18. In your own words, describe common age-related atrophic changes to oral mucosa.

_____

_____

_____

_____

19. In your own words, briefly explain the oral effects of xerostomia.

_____

_____

_____

_____

_____

_____

20. Identify the risk factors for oral candidiasis that may be present in your older patient.

_____

_____

_____

_____

_____

_____

21. Identify risk factors that may contribute to root caries in older adults.

_____

_____

_____

_____

_____

22. Periodontal findings reflect the patterns of health and disease over the years of your older patient's life. Describe the range of tissue changes that may be noted when examining an older patient.

_____

_____

_____

_____

_____

_____

_____

_____

_____

_____

23. Identify barriers that can negatively impact access to dental hygiene care for an older individual.

_____

_____

_____

_____

24. Older patients often use more prescription drugs and more over-the-counter medications than other age groups. List the ways you can be sure you know what drugs your patient is taking so you make appropriate decisions when you plan dental hygiene care.

_____

_____

_____

_____

_____

_____

_____

_____

25. List factors likely to occur in your older patient that can contribute to accumulation and retention of dental biofilm and increased difficulty in removal.

_____

_____

_____

_____

26. Describe specific biofilm removal methods and techniques you can recommend for an older patient.

_____

_____

_____

27. What factors can contribute to dietary and nutritional deficiencies in your older patients?

_____

_____

_____

_____

_____

_____

_____

_____

_____

_____

_____

_____

✓ COMPETENCY EXERCISES

Apply information from the chapter and use critical thinking skills to complete the competency exercises. Write responses on paper or create electronic documents to submit your answers.

1. Explain why an older patient's slowness to master new oral hygiene techniques does not necessarily mean an inability to learn.

2. Develop an infomap (table) that briefly describes the characteristics of each of the progressive stages of Alzheimer disease and make a list of the types of patient care modifications or dental hygiene management considerations appropriate for each stage.

3. Today your patient is Marie Tonawonda, age 89 years. Refer to her patient assessment summary as you complete the following exercises.

   Ms. Tonawonda has been a patient in your clinic for many, many years, and she comes in every 4 months, like clockwork, for her periodontal maintenance appointments. Her father was a dentist, and she was his dental assistant when she was a young girl, so she loves to talk about the changes she has observed in dentistry.

As her nephew, Stan, escorts her slowly into your treatment room, you notice that, although she greets you cheerfully as usual, she is becoming increasingly frail. As Stan helps with a health history update, he mentions that his aunt has recently been placed on an antidepressant by her physician. Stan visits his aunt in her home nearly daily and recently noticed that she hasn't been eating regular meals. There has been other evidence that Ms. Tonawonda has been decreasingly able to provide her own daily self-care, and Stan says that, even when he reminds her, she does not always remember to brush her teeth or comb her hair every day.

Stan states that he will continue to bring her in for her regular dental care and that Ms. Tonawonda's insurance will continue to cover the cost of any dental needs she has.

While your dental assistant is taking radiographs of Ms. Tonawonda's teeth, you begin to jot down notes for her dental hygiene care plan. You suddenly remember the OSCAR assessment approach to identifying the needs of older individuals (see Table 22-2 in the **textbook**). Complete an OSCAR assessment to identify factors of concern for Ms. Tonawonda.

4. Using the assessment data from Ms. Tonawonda's patient assessment summary, your OSCAR assessment notes, and the information in Chapter 48 of the **textbook**, write three dental hygiene diagnoses statements for Ms. Tonawonda's care plan.

5. Because Ms. Tonawonda's cognitive abilities are declining, her need for education and oral hygiene instruction are very different from that of most of your other patients. Ms. Tonawonda will need ways to receive reminders for daily oral care. Using your school's format for writing progress notes, document the education and home care instructions you will provide during today's appointment.

CHAPTER 48—PATIENT ASSESSMENT SUMMARY

Patient Name: *Marie Tonawonda*   Age: *89*   Gender: F   ☐ Initial Therapy

☑ Maintenance

Provider Name: *D.H. Student*   Date: *Today*   ☐ Re-evaluation

Chief Complaint: *Her nephew states: "I brought her in today for her regular cleaning appointment."*

Assessment Findings

Health History

- Taking calcium-channel blocker for hypertension and sublingual nitroglycerine tablet as needed for occasional angina
- Recent antidepressant prescription
- Osteoporosis—exhibits curvature of upper back
- Increasing mental confusion and cognitive disability
- Decreased visual acuity even when corrected with glasses
- Wears a hearing aid
- ASA Classification-II and ADL level-2

At Risk For:

Social and Dental History

- History of dental visits every 4 months
- Recent increase in sucrose intake (described by nephew)
- High dental literacy—but recent cognitive decrease
- Assisted with daily care by her nephew who has little dental knowledge

At Risk For:

Dental Examination

- Xerostomia
- Generalized recession: 3–5 mm
- Generalized 3- to 4-mm probing depths; generalized slight bleeding at gingival margins
- Several class 1 and class II furcations in molar areas
- Very few restorations—all in good condition

At Risk For:

Periodontal Diagnosis/Case Type and Status

- History of generalized, controlled chronic periodontitis with recent increase in marginal gingivitis

Caries Management Risk Assessment (CAMBRA) Level:
☐ Low ☐ Moderate ☑ High ☐ Extreme

QUESTIONS PATIENTS ASK

What sources of information can you identify that will help you answer your patient's question in this scenario?

A healthy, functionally independent 70-year-old patient asks you if, at her age, she should consider dental implants for the molar teeth that were recently extracted. How will you respond?

MeSH TERMS

Use a combination of MeSH terms and other key words to develop an effective and efficient PubMed literature search strategy.

Dental care for aged
Health services for the aged
Geriatric dentistry
Geriatrics

Aged
Aged, 80 and over
Frail elderly
Aging
Ageism

EVERYDAY ETHICS

Before completing the learning exercises below, reread and reflect on the Everyday Ethics Scenario and Questions for Consideration in this chapter of the **textbook**. It may also be useful to review the Dental Hygiene Ethics discussion in Chapter 1, the Ethical Applications in the introduction pages for each section in the **textbook**, as well as the Codes of Ethics in **textbook** Appendices I–IV.

Collaborative Learning Activity

Work with another student colleague to role-play the scenario. The goal of this exercise is for you and your colleague to work through the alternative actions in order to come to consensus on a solution or response that is acceptable to both of you.

Discovery Activity

Ask a friend or relative who is not involved in health care to read the scenario and discuss it with you from the perspective of a "patient" who receives services within the healthcare system. Discuss what you learned from the concerns, insights, or difference in perspective that person expressed.

Factors to Teach the Patient

This scenario is related to the following factors listed in this chapter of the **textbook**:

▷ That dentition can last a lifetime.

▷ The value of a well-balanced diet.

▷ Importance of drinking fluoridated water.

You have recently learned that Marie Tonawonda (introduced in the Competency Exercises) has been moved to an extended-care facility. Her nephew, Stan, comes in for his regular appointment and thanks you again for all the information you provided when Ms. Tonawonda was in for her appointment. He reaffirms his commitment to maintaining his aunt's oral health.

He mentions his concern about your instructions to limit Ms. Tonawonda's exposure to high-sucrose foods. In order to increase nutritional intake, the residents at the Sunshine Residence Home seem to have access to food at any time they desire and, unfortunately, that includes availability of cookies all the time. Stan has encouraged the staff to provide support for his aunt's efforts at limiting sweets and conducting daily brushing and flossing, but he isn't sure his wishes are being met.

You decide that you will investigate the possibility of volunteering to provide staff in-service presentations about oral health to the caregivers at the extended-care facility. Develop an outline of the topics you would cover in these presentations.

The Patient with a Cleft Lip and/or Palate

LEARNING OBJECTIVES

Upon successful completion of these exercises, you will be able to:

1. Identify and define the key terms and concepts related to oral/facial clefts.
2. Identify the prenatal risk factors and developmental time frame for oral/facial clefts.
3. Describe the treatment for oral/facial clefts.
4. Use knowledge of the oral, physical, and personal characteristics of the patient to plan and document dental hygiene care and oral hygiene instructions.

KNOWLEDGE EXERCISES

Write your answers for each question in the space provided.

1. Describe the direction of the formation/fusion of the lip and palatal structures during development.

2. During which embryonic weeks does the palate develop?

3. Which class of cleft is identified as a submucous, imperfect muscle union cleft across the soft palate, producing an incomplete closure of the pharynx?

4. How is a class 3 craniofacial cleft defined?

5. Which classes of facial cleft involve lack of fusion in the premaxilla?

6. List three environmental risk factors for craniofacial clefts.

7. List three common characteristics that can affect the teeth of a patient with a craniofacial cleft.

8. List the three categories of professionals who contribute to the treatment of an individual with cleft lip and/or palate.

9. The dental hygienist is a member of the _____ team of specialists who care for individuals with a cleft lip and/or palate.

10. Select one of the dental specialties in which clinicians may provide care for a patient with a cleft and describe that practitioner's role in the treatment of the patient.

_____

_____

_____

_____

11. Ideally, treatment of a craniofacial cleft is begun before the infant is 6 months old. What is the purpose for such early intervention?

_____

_____

_____

12. What are the goals of surgical treatment for cleft lip and palate?

_____

_____

_____

_____

_____

13. In your own words, describe the benefits a dental prosthesis can provide for a patient with a cleft lip and palate.

_____

_____

_____

_____

_____

_____

✓ COMPETENCY EXERCISES

Apply information from the chapter and use critical thinking skills to complete the competency exercises. Write responses on paper or create electronic documents to submit your answers.

1. Discuss why lack of prenatal care is considered a risk factor for cleft lip and/or palate.

2. Describe characteristics that may make it difficult to communicate with an individual who has an incomplete palatal closure.

3. Adam Horconcitos, a 12-year-old, has recently come to America from Honduras to live with Mr. and Mrs. Mehlisch, his American adoptive parents. Adam has a class 5 unilateral (left side) facial cleft that was not treated when he was an infant. He is scheduled for his first surgical procedure in about 3 weeks. You are a member of Adam's care team, and you are seeing him today for the first time to evaluate his oral status.

The only dental visits Adam has had previously were about 2 years ago with a prosthodontist in Honduras. The doctor fabricated an appliance to provide for some closure of the palatal opening to enhance Adam's ability to swallow and speak.

When you talk with Adam and Mr. and Mrs. Mehlisch before the boy's examination, you find that Adam speaks fairly good English, because he went to an American school in his own country. He is a handsome, personable, and likable young man; however, he is really very shy and frequently hides his mouth and nose behind his hand as he speaks to you. His voice has a kind of nasal sound, but his hearing is normal, and with a bit of concentration, you can understand him fairly well. Adam does not have any major health problems, except for a susceptibility to frequent sore throats and ear infections.

Adam did not enjoy a good dental experience during the fabrication of his prosthesis or during his recent visits with the oral surgeon to plan his surgical care. He is extremely fearful of anyone or anything that comes near his mouth. In spite of that, he is wearing the prosthetic appliance every day, and it seems to be working well for him.

You are successful in using all of your most comforting patient management techniques, and you convince Adam to allow his mouth to be examined. During your examination, you discover that he has a mixed dentition with five primary molars still being retained, significant malocclusions, and two missing anterior teeth in the area of the cleft. His level of dental caries is fortunately quite low—only one small cavity in a deciduous molar that is already loose. You conclude, from a discussion with Mrs. Mehlisch, that Adam's snacking habits are not highly cariogenic.

His gingival health, however, is another matter. He won't usually let anyone touch his mouth, and he doesn't like to have a toothbrush near his mouth even when he does it himself. You find extensive biofilm accumulation on his teeth, gums, and tongue as well as on the prosthodontic appliance he wears. His mother complains that his breath is often very bad. His gums bleed extremely easily when they are touched.

Using the information in the case description above and a copy of the Dental Hygiene Care Plan template in **workbook** Appendix B, write an individualized dental hygiene care plan for Adam.

4. Using your school's format for writing progress notes, document the assessment visit for Adam's permanent record.

MeSH TERMS

Use a combination of MeSH terms and other key words to develop an effective and efficient PubMed literature search strategy.

Cleft lip   Cleft soft palate

Cleft palate   Palatal obturators

EVERYDAY ETHICS

Before completing the learning exercises below, reread and reflect on the Everyday Ethics Scenario and Questions for Consideration in this chapter of the **textbook**. It may also be useful to review the Dental Hygiene Ethics discussion in Chapter 1, the Ethical Applications in the introduction pages for each section in the **textbook**, as well as the Codes of Ethics in **textbook** Appendices I–IV.

Individual Learning Activities

Imagine that you are the dental hygienist in this scenario. Answer each of the questions for consideration at the end of the scenario.

Identify a situation you have experienced that presents a similar ethical dilemma. Write about what you would do differently now than you did at the time the incident happened—support your discussion with concepts from the dental hygiene codes of ethics.

Factors to Teach the Patient

This scenario is related to the following factors listed in this chapter of the **textbook**:

▷ Parental anticipatory guidance (see Chapters 47 and 48 of the **textbook**).

Today your patient is Mrs. Diane White. You have been providing dental hygiene care for her since she was in her first trimester of pregnancy. About 3 months ago, her little girl was born with a class 3 cleft palate. Although the child is well cared for by an interdisciplinary team of healthcare workers at the local hospital, Mrs. White notes that there is no dental hygienist on the team. She asks you for advice in providing oral care for her child as she grows.

Use information about cleft palate (see Chapter 49 in the **textbook**) and what you have learned about parental anticipatory guidance (in Chapters 47 and 48 in the **textbook**) and the motivational interviewing approach (see **workbook** Appendix D) to role-play this situation with a fellow student. If you are Mrs. White in the role-play, be sure to ask questions. If you are the dental hygienist, try to anticipate questions and answer them in your explanation.

CHAPTER 49 CROSSWORD PUZZLE

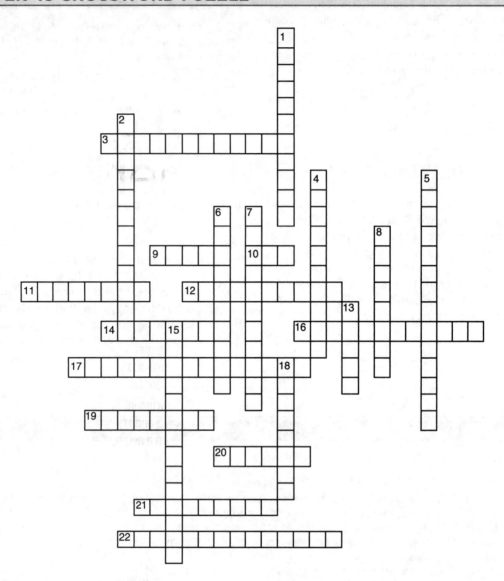

Puzzle Clues

Across

3. Pertaining to the part of the skull that encloses the brain and the face.

9. A unilateral or bilateral congenital facial fissure.

10. One source of the bone used for an autogenous bone graft.

11. A type of graft placed before the eruption of maxillary teeth at a cleft site to create a normal architecture through which the teeth can erupt.

12. Replaces or improves function of any absent part of the human body.

14. Combination of symptoms commonly occurring together.

16. The process of acquiring fitness for the first time; associated with persons who have acquired disabilities.

17. One important member of the interdisciplinary team who will treat the patient with a cleft lip and/or palate (two words).

19. Tissue transplanted and expected to become a part of the host tissue.

20. When this normal process does not happen during development, a facial cleft can result.

21. A prosthesis designed to cover the cleft of a hard palate.

22. This insufficiency affects closure of the opening between the mouth and nose in speech, resulting in a nasal-sounding voice.

Down

1. Plastic surgery of the nose.

2. Bilateral cleft lip separates this from its normal fusion with the entire maxilla.

4. Present at and existing from the time of birth.

5. Pertaining to or arising through the action of many factors.

6. Pertaining to the function of the skeletal system and its associated functions.

7. An agent, such as drugs of abuse during the first trimester of a pregnancy, that can increase risk for cleft lip and palate.

8. Genetic transmission of traits from parents to offspring.

13. A term describing a cleft of the uvula.

15. The process of restoring a person's abilities to the maximum possible fitness.

18. A combination of symptoms either resulting from a single cause or occurring commonly together as to form a distinct clinical picture.

The Patient with a Neurodevelopmental Disorder

 KNOWLEDGE EXERCISES

Write your answers for each question in the space provided.

1. List examples of neurodevelopmental disorders that are usually first diagnosed before or during adolescence.

2. List the five interrelated dimensions that contribute to testing the functioning level of an individual with an intellectual disorder.

3. In your own words, briefly summarize the characteristics for each classification of intellectual functioning that will impact the dental hygienist's approach to providing oral health education and oral hygiene instruction.

- *Mild:*

_____

_____

_____

_____

_____

- *Moderate:*

_____

_____

_____

_____

_____

- *Severe:*

_____

_____

_____

_____

- *Profound:*

_____

_____

_____

_____

4. Identify four categories of risk factors for intellectual disability.

_____

_____

_____

_____

5. What behavior-related factors during pregnancy may result in an infant with an intellectual disorder?

_____

_____

_____

_____

6. What can happen during the infant's birth that can lead to an intellectual disorder?

_____

_____

_____

_____

_____

7. What two early childhood situations can lead to intellectual disorders?

_____

_____

_____

8. Identify characteristic physical features or anomalies you might observe when performing an extraoral examination for your patient with an intellectual disorder.

_____

_____

_____

_____

_____

9. List five intraoral findings common in individuals with intellectual disorders.

_____

_____

_____

_____

_____

10. List five characteristics that can help you identify an individual with Down syndrome.

_____

_____

_____

_____

_____

11. Most individuals with Down syndrome have pleasant personalities. Identify three personal characteristics that make these individuals likable and easy to be around.

_____

_____

_____

12. Why do patients with Down syndrome often present for dental treatment with very cracked and dried lips?

_____

_____

13. Identify physical/medical health problems commonly found in individuals with Down syndrome that require special consideration or modifications during dental hygiene treatment.

_____

_____

_____

_____

_____

14. Describe fragile X syndrome.

_____

_____

_____

15. Describe four physical characteristics of a patient with fragile X syndrome.

_____

_____

_____

_____

16. List five common oral findings associated with fragile X syndrome.

_____

_____

_____

_____

_____

17. Briefly describe the characteristics that distinguish each of the five variations of autism spectrum disorder.

_____

_____

_____

_____

_____

_____

_____

_____

_____

18. In your own words, briefly summarize three main characteristics you are likely to observe during a dental hygiene appointment with your patient who has been diagnosed with an autism spectrum disorder.

_____

_____

_____

_____

19. Describe two types of treatment used to manage symptoms and increase the ability of the patient with autism to live a normal life.

_____

_____

20. Identify specific actions you can initiate during dental hygiene appointments to help your patient with an autistic spectrum disorder or any other neurodevelopmental disorder to learn how to cooperate.

_____

_____

_____

_____

_____

✓ COMPETENCY EXERCISES

Apply information from the chapter and use critical thinking skills to complete the competency exercises. Write responses on paper or create electronic documents to submit your answers.

1. Next week you will be starting a new part-time position as the dental hygienist for 50 resident patients in a small private residential facility. You will go once a week to work with Dr. Sally Roderick, the dentist who has been providing dental care at the residence for 25 years. The individuals living in the residence are classified as having severe or profound intellectual disorder. You are excited about the opportunity to work with Dr. Roderick and to learn about this population, which you have only read about in your **textbook**.

   To prepare for this new challenge, create a list of planning measures you can take and modifications you can make to your usual treatment procedures so you can increase your effectiveness when providing dental hygiene care for these patients.

2. On the first day at the residential center, you find that Dr. Roderick has done very well providing patients with restorative care, but not much attention has been paid to dental hygiene care and education. The patient in your clinic chair right now is Bonne. She is 22 years old and is classified as having a profound intellectual disability.

   One of the nurse's aides, who is her regular caregiver, helps you place Bonne in the papoose board and sits by the side of the dental chair to help when she can. You have some difficulty examining Bonne's mouth, but you can readily see that she has extensive biofilm buildup and significant amounts of calculus in all areas of her mouth.

   You know that it will take more than one appointment to assess Bonne's dental hygiene needs thoroughly and to make a full plan for care. However, Dr. Roderick asks you to write up a formal dental hygiene care plan

for what you will accomplish in the next three or four appointments so the plan can be recorded in Bonne's medical record. You know that you must plan enough time for the complete assessment you need to accomplish before you can fully understand Bonne's oral condition. You must also plan to educate the aide for daily biofilm control.

Use the Dental Hygiene Care Plan Template in **workbook** Appendix B to develop a formal, written care plan for clinical procedures and educational interventions you will provide during the four appointments you will schedule in the next few weeks for Bonne and her caregiver.

3. Today when you saw Bonne in the clinic, you reviewed her medical history, provided a limited intraoral assessment examination, and developed a written care plan. Use your institution's guidelines for writing in patient records to document these procedures.

 MeSH TERMS

Use a combination of MeSH terms and other key words to develop an effective and efficient PubMed literature search strategy.

Intellectual disability	Asperger syndrome
Developmental disabilities	Autistic disorder
	Down syndrome
Dental care for disabled	Tic disorders
Child development disorders, pervasive	Language disorders

 EVERYDAY ETHICS

Before completing the learning exercises below, reread and reflect on the Everyday Ethics Scenario and Questions for Consideration in this chapter of the **textbook**. It may also be useful to review the Dental Hygiene Ethics discussion in Chapter 1, the Ethical Applications in the introduction pages for each section in the **textbook**, as well as the Codes of Ethics in **textbook** Appendices I–IV.

Individual Learning Activity

Imagine that you have observed what happened in the scenario, but are not one of the main characters involved in the situation. Write a reflective journal entry that:

- Describes how you might have reacted (as an observer–not as a participant),
- Expresses your personal feelings about what happened, or
- Identifies personal values that affect your reaction to the situation.

Collaborative Learning Activity

Answer each of the questions for consideration at the end of the scenario in the **textbook**. Compare what you wrote with answers developed by another classmate and discuss differences/similarities.

Factors to Teach the Patient

This scenario is related to the following factors listed in this chapter of the **textbook**:

For the patient:

▷ How to perform oral self-care procedures.

▷ Why assistance from others is an important supplement to the patient's own efforts.

▷ How to use and show cooperation skills.

For the caregiver:

▷ Why a total preventive program is important.

▷ How to incorporate behavior modification into oral care procedures.

▷ The importance of repeating "show–tell–do" instructions often.

Use information in Chapter 50 in the **textbook** and the motivational interviewing approach (see **workbook** Appendix D) to develop a conversation you will use to provide oral hygiene instructions for a patient who is classified with a moderate intellectual disability. Include the patient's caregiver as you discuss strategies for daily oral care.

Use the conversation you create to role-play this situation with a fellow student. If you are the patient or the caregiver in the role-play, be sure to ask questions. If you are the dental hygienist, try to anticipate questions and answer them in your explanation. Modify your conversation based on what you learned.

CHAPTER 50 CROSSWORD PUZZLE

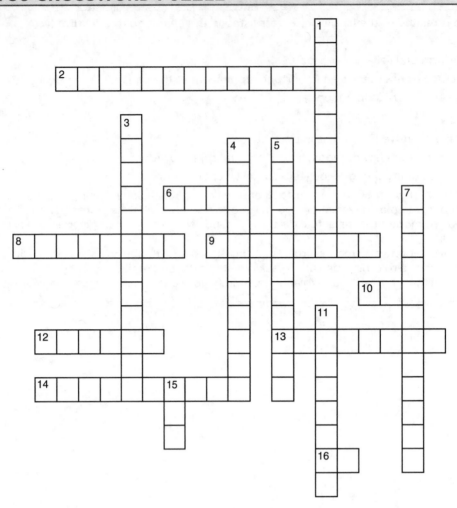

Puzzle Clues

Across

2. Unusually small head.

6. An autism spectrum disorder that occurs only in girls; characterized by repetitive hand movements.

8. An autistic spectrum disorder characterized mainly by impairment in social interactions.

9. Category of intellectual function in which the individual could most likely attend to personal oral care with some reminders from a caregiver.

10. Most common single-gene cause of autism spectrum disorder (acronym).

12. Developmental disorder affecting communication and social interaction.

13. Classification of intellectual function for which the individual would most likely need to have all daily oral hygiene measures provided by a caregiver.

14. A vertical fold of skin on either side of the nose; a normal characteristic of persons of some races that is also associated with Down syndrome.

16. Score derived from standardized tests used to assess intellectual ability.

Down

1. Abnormality in morphologic development.

3. Very large tongue.

4. Indicative of a particular disease or syndrome.

5. Movement disorder that is repetitive, nonfunctional motor behavior that interferes with normal activities.

7. Trisomy 21 syndrome (two words).

11. Refers to coexisting medical conditions.

15. Sudden nonrhythmic motor movement or vocal sound.

The Patient with a Disability

LEARNING OBJECTIVES

Upon successful completion of these exercises, you will be able to:

1. Identify and define the key terms and concepts related to individuals with disabilities.

2. Identify oral conditions caused by or resulting from disabling conditions.

3. Describe the procedures and factors that contribute to safe and successful dental hygiene treatment for individuals with disabilities.

4. Identify the factors that affect interpersonal communication and patient education.

5. Describe the factors that enhance the prevention of oral disease for individuals with disabilities and their caregivers.

6. Plan and document adaptations that enhance dental hygiene care for a patient with a sensory impairment.

KNOWLEDGE EXERCISES

Write your answers for each question in the space provided.

1. Briefly describe the components included in the two main sections of the World Health Organization International Classifications of Functioning, Disability, and Health.

Part 1: Functioning and disability

_____

_____

_____

_____

_____

_____

Part 2: Contextual factors

_____

_____

_____

_____

_____

_____

2. In what way does the ADA define the responsibility of the dental practitioner in meeting the needs of a patient with a hearing or vision impairment?

_____

_____

_____

_____

_____

3. In your own words, define *visual impairment*.

_____

4. Explain the term *legally blind*.

_____

_____

_____

_____

5. _____ during pregnancy is the cause of at least half of the blindness in children.

6. In your own words, define *glaucoma*.

_____

_____

_____

_____

7. Define the term *deaf*.

_____

_____

8. What descriptive phrase is sometimes used for a patient who cannot hear as well as someone with normal hearing?

_____

_____

9. Describe a cochlear implant.

_____

_____

_____

_____

10. In your own words, define *a barrier-free dental treatment facility*.

_____

_____

11. How wide must outdoor walkways and indoor passageways be to accommodate a wheelchair?

_____

12. An appropriately constructed wheelchair ramp entrance has a handrail and a gentle slope that rises _____ for every _____ in length.

13. Lightweight doors with lever handles must open at least _____ wide for a wheelchair to pass through.

14. A dental chair that is accessible for wheelchair transfers can be lowered to at least _____ from the floor.

15. List three areas of risk assessment to consider when treating a patient with a disability.

_____

_____

_____

_____

16. List common oral findings in patients with a disability that can be a source of increased risk for oral disease.

_____

_____

_____

_____

_____

_____

_____

_____

_____

17. List common oral effects related to drug therapies used to treat patients with disabilities.

_____

_____

_____

_____

_____

18. List the components of an oral disease prevention and control program for a patient with a disability.

_____

_____

_____

19. To plan oral hygiene instructions for your patient with a disability, it is important for you to understand the ability of your patient to perform daily living and self-care skills such as toothbrushing. Briefly describe the functioning ability for each ADL/IADL level.

- *ADL/IADL level 0:*

  _____

  _____

- *ADL/IADL levels 1 and 2:*

  _____

  _____

- *ADL/IADL level 3:*

  _____

  _____

20. What is the dental hygienist's role in providing oral hygiene instructions for an individual who is identified as having a moderate- or low-functioning level?

   _____

   _____

   _____

21. When should you recommend that the use of a dentifrice be limited or eliminated from the oral care regimen of a patient with a disability?

   _____

   _____

   _____

22. What recommendations can you make so a patient who cannot use a dentifrice receives the benefits of fluoride?

   _____

   _____

   _____

   _____

23. Self-care aids can make a difference in the ability of a patient or caregiver to maximize effectiveness of oral care. List the general prerequisites of a good oral self-care aid.

   _____

   _____

   _____

   _____

24. Identify three general modifications that can be made to a toothbrush handle to enhance the ability of a patient with a disability to provide oral self-care.

   _____

   _____

   _____

25. What factors will you take into consideration when recommending the use of a power-assisted toothbrush for a patient with a disability?

   _____

   _____

   _____

26. Briefly describe modifications that can be made to help a patient with a disability care for a removable dental prosthesis.

   _____

   _____

   _____

27. In your own words, describe the position a caregiver can use to be most effective when providing daily oral care for a person with disabilities.

   _____

   _____

   _____

   _____

   _____

28. List factors to take into consideration when planning dietary recommendations for your patient with a disability.

   _____

   _____

   _____

   _____

   _____

29. In your own words, summarize precautions you can take and patient care modifications you can make to ensure safety and comfort for your patient with a disability.

   _____

   _____

   _____

   _____

_____

_____

_____

_____

_____

30. Unless an extreme cognitive impairment has been identified, communication related to dental hygiene care is always addressed first to _____.

31. For you to plan dental hygiene care that takes all of the needs of your patient with a disability into consideration, it is essential to gather as much information as possible before the first appointment. Identify three individuals (or groups) who can provide the needed information.

_____

_____

_____

_____

32. List factors to consider when scheduling appointments for an individual with a disability.

_____

_____

_____

_____

33. List factors that contribute to safety and comfortable positioning or stabilization of your patient with a disability while he or she is in the dental chair.

_____

_____

_____

_____

34. What precautions are required if protective stabilization is considered?

_____

_____

_____

_____

_____

_____

_____

35. Describe a technique for safely stabilizing a patient's head during dental hygiene treatment.

_____

_____

36. List the types of aids that can be used to stabilize the patient's mouth while providing dental hygiene treatment or during daily oral care provided by caregivers.

_____

_____

37. List precautions to observe if you are using a mouth prop.

_____

_____

_____

38. Briefly explain some actions the dental hygienist can take to assure understanding when providing oral hygiene instructions for the patient with a visual impairment.

_____

_____

_____

39. Why do you always speak to patients who have a significant visual impairment each time before you enter or leave the room and each time before you touch them during dental hygiene treatment?

_____

_____

40. In your own words, what is ASL?

_____

_____

_____

41. If your patient is speech reading, what can you do to enhance his or her understanding during oral hygiene instructions?

_____

_____

_____

_____

_____

_____

_____

_____

_____

42. List three basic types of wheelchair transfers.

_____

_____

_____

43. What is the first thing you should do before starting a wheelchair transfer?

_____

_____

44. Who can give you advice in how best to help during a wheelchair transfer?

_____

45. List three factors that take special consideration during a wheelchair transfer.

_____

_____

_____

46. Describe the position of the wheelchair with respect to the position of the dental chair when transferring your patient from the wheelchair to the dental chair.

- _Mobile transfer:_

_____

_____

- _Immobile transfer:_

_____

_____

_____

- _Sliding board transfer:_

_____

_____

_____

47. It makes sense, when transferring your patient back to the wheelchair after treatment, to position the seat of the dental chair slightly _____ than the seat of the wheelchair.

48. If you are helping your patient with a mobile transfer from a wheelchair to the dental chair, where are your patient's arms and hands?

_____

_____

_____

49. Describe the position of the first aide's hands/arms when two people are helping with an immobile patient transfer.

_____

_____

50. What is the responsibility of the second assistant during an immobile patient transfer?

_____

_____

51. What is your role when seating a patient with a walker, crutches, or a cane in the dental chair?

_____

_____

_____

_____

52. What are the best ways to evaluate the success of an in-service program?

_____

_____

53. List at least four additional oral care/disease prevention topics or techniques to teach during staff in-service training.

_____

_____

_____

_____

_____

_____

_____

✓ COMPETENCY EXERCISES

Apply information from the chapter and use critical thinking skills to complete the competency exercises. Write responses on paper or create electronic documents to submit your answers.

1. In your own words, explain the relationship between the terms impairment, disability, and handicap.

2. To avoid confusion, it is imperative to ask direct questions concerning the type and severity of your patient's disability. In your own words, list some basic categories of information to obtain from a patient with a disability or the caregiver that will assist in patient management.

3. In your own words, identify at least three objectives for providing quality dental and dental hygiene care for individuals with disabilities.

4. Steve McKnight is your patient with cerebral palsy. He is charming and witty. He works for a company that develops voice technology for computers. He has significant physical impairments associated with his condition and moves about with difficulty, using crutches and special leg braces to walk. He is fiercely independent, preferring to manage as many tasks as possible on his own.

   Steve moves his hands with difficulty and cannot grasp small objects very well. He feeds himself using specially adapted utensils. When you talk to him about his daily oral care, he mentions that he used a power-driven toothbrush for a while but that it was heavy and, when it started to vibrate, he could barely hold it up to his mouth. He sighs and says that he really wishes he could find a regular toothbrush that he could hold on to without dropping it in the sink all the time.

   Find appropriate materials and make a device to adapt a toothbrush and floss handle that would help Steve continue to be independent in his daily oral care. Share your design with your classmates. Does your design meet the general prerequisites for a self-care aid as described in the **textbook**?

5. You have completed Mr. Corkman's dental hygiene treatment for today, and you direct him down to Jenny, the appointment manager, so he can schedule his next visit while you clean and disinfect the treatment room for your next patient. When he gets to the end of the hallway, you hear him say, "Delighted to meet you, Benny!" in a very loud voice. You observe him at the front desk for a bit and then walk up to him and remind him that he turned his hearing aid off when you were using the ultrasonic scaler during his treatment. What did you observe to indicate Mr. Corkman had forgotten to turn it on again?

6. Your next patient, Damian, arrives with a huge golden retriever guide dog he calls Harrison. You are a bit flustered and you hold out your hand to greet Damian without first letting him know you have come into the room with him. He bumps into you as he turns to return your greeting and you realize Damian is almost totally blind. You aren't quite sure what to do next. You cover your distress by complimenting him on the beauty of his dog and bending down to hug the dog.

   You gently take Harrison by the collar and lead him down the hall to the door of your treatment room. Damian follows you and his dog into the room. You raise the chair up a bit higher, so the seat is just above the level of Damian's knees and you turn him around and gently ease him back until he is sitting against the edge of the dental chair. You tell him you will place the dog out in the hall where there is significantly more room. He seems uneasy about that, but you reassure him that no one will be going by to step on the dog, as your treatment room is the last one down the hall.

   As you return to the room, Damian pushes himself up and back into the chair, turns, and slides his feet up on the footrest. You wince as his head just misses the dental light, but he doesn't hit it and you breathe a sigh of relief. You notice the time is running out for your appointment, so you quickly update his health history (no significant findings), lower the chair, and then tell Damian to grab hold of the armrests before you tilt him back. You complete your oral assessment and begin scaling.

   Later, after polishing his teeth, you squirt lots of water so he can rinse his mouth. Damian raises himself from the chair, swallows twice, and then apologizes and asks for a cup to rinse. After you help him rinse with a cup, you are feeling that this appointment has been very stressful for both of you, and you would love to have a quiet minute to recover your calm. As Damian gets out of the dental chair, you walk out into the hallway to bring Harrison back in to him.

   What could you have done differently to manage Damian's care in a way that reduces both his stress and your own during this appointment?

EVERYDAY ETHICS

Before completing the learning exercises below, reread and reflect on the Everyday Ethics Scenario and Questions for Consideration in this chapter of the **textbook**. It may also be useful to review the Dental Hygiene Ethics discussion in Chapter 1, the Ethical Applications in the introduction pages for each section in the **textbook**, as well as the Codes of Ethics in **textbook** Appendices I–IV.

Individual Learning Activity

Imagine that you are the dental hygienist in this scenario. Answer each of the questions for consideration at the end of the scenario.

Collaborative Activity

Answer each of the questions for consideration at the end of the scenario in the **textbook**. Compare what you wrote with answers developed by another classmate and discuss differences/similarities.

Factors to Teach the Patient

This scenario is related to the following factors listed in this chapter of the **textbook**:

▷ Practice a healthy lifestyle, including a healthy diet.

Use the information about a healthy diet in Chapter 33, the principles of anticipatory guidance (Chapter 47), and a motivational interviewing approach (see **workbook** Appendix D) to write a conversation educating the mother of a 4-year-old child who has a disability about the general concepts of maintaining a tooth healthy diet.

DISCOVERY EXERCISE

Explore the Americans with Disabilities Act website at http://www.ada.gov.

MeSH TERMS

Use a combination of MeSH terms and other key words to develop an effective and efficient PubMed literature search strategy.

Amputees
Cataracts
Communication aids for disabled
Dental care for disabled
Developmental disabilities
Diabetic retinopathy
Disabled children
Disabled persons
Glaucoma
Hearing aids
Hearing disorders
Hearing impaired persons

Hearing loss
Intellectual disability
Macular degeneration
Mentally disabled persons
Mentally ill persons
Retinopathy of prematurity
Self-help devices
Tinnitus
Vision disorders
Vision, low
Visually impaired persons
Wheelchairs

CHAPTER 51 CROSSWORD PUZZLE

Puzzle Clues

Across

2. An aid that can be used to help transfer an individual from a wheelchair to the dental chair and back again (two words).

5. Enables a person to read by touch.

6. A dental treatment room that is not wheelchair-accessible is an example of this kind of barrier that can hinder access to oral care.

10. Language use to emphasize the individual, not the disability (two words).

12. The need for longer appointment time—and the dental professional's need to be reimbursed for providing that time—can constitute this type of barrier that limits oral care options for an individual with a disability.

16. Opacity of the lens of the eye.

18. Padding and other body stabilization methods used to facilitate patient comfort and safety.

19. The Americans with Disabilities Act, not the American Dental Association!

20. Refers to a disability of indefinite duration with an onset before the age of 18.

21. Accessible; obstacles to passage or communication have been removed (two words).

Down

1. Education program about some specific topic, such as oral care for individuals with disabilities, that is provided for parents, teachers, volunteers, nurses, or other health professionals (without the hyphen).

3. Surgical implant that enables healing.

4. Refers to the restriction that results from an impairment.

7. A term that refers to several techniques for moving a person from a wheelchair to a dental chair and back.

8. Dental professionals who do not feel adequately trained to provide safe treatment is an example of this type of barrier to care for individuals with a disability.

9. Person who performs or helps to perform daily life activities.

11. The individual responsible for making decisions if a person is declared incapacitated in a legal process; requires written proof for decision making.

13. Two chronic diseases present.

14. Type of disability associated with a person's ability to understand or use one's native language.

15. Refers to dental hygiene care delivered with the help of a dental assistant (two words).

17. Level of function identified by an ADL/IADL level of 0.

Neurologic Disorders and Stroke

LEARNING OBJECTIVES

Upon successful completion of these exercises, you will be able to:

1. Describe the characteristics, complications, occurrence, and medical treatment of a variety of neurologic disorders.

2. Identify the oral factors and findings related to neurologic disorders.

3. Plan and document modifications for dental hygiene care based on assessment of needs that are specific to a patient's physical impairment.

KNOWLEDGE EXERCISES

Write your answers for each question in the space provided.

1. For each definition provided below, identify the correct term or concept related to movement or sensory–motor impairment.

   a. Loss of voluntary motion. _____

   b. Immobility due to direct union between parts. _____

   c. Defect in expression by or comprehension of speech, writing, or signs. _____

   d. Cell death activated by a biochemical reaction. _____

   e. Wasting or decrease in size of muscle fibers. _____

   f. Abnormal slowness of movements. _____

   g. Destruction of brain substance because of intracerebral hemorrhage, thrombosis, embolism, or vascular insufficiency; also called stroke. (acronym) _____

   h. Ulcer that usually occurs over a bony prominence as a result of prolonged, excessive pressure from body weight. _____

   i. Visual perception of two images of a single object. _____

   j. Muscle impairment that causes verbal impairment. _____

   k. Difficulty in swallowing. _____

   l. Excess of cholesterol in the blood. _____

   m. Raised triglyceride blood level. _____

   n. Deficiency in blood flow caused by obstruction of a blood vessel. _____

   o. Abnormal convexity in the curvature of the thoracic spine (viewed from the side). _____

   p. Orthopedic appliance that supports, aligns, prevents, corrects deformities, or improves function of a part of the body. _____

   q. Surgical excision or destruction of part of the globus pallidus in the basal ganglia to prevent symptoms of Parkinsonism. _____

   r. Loss or impairment of motor function in a body part. _____

   s. Complete paralysis of one side of the body. _____

   t. Incomplete paralysis of one side of the body. _____

   u. Abnormal sensation, such as burning, prickling, tingling. _____

v. Passage between two natural channels; to bypass or drain an area. _____

w. Shunt created between a cerebral ventricle and a cardiac atrium by means of a plastic tube. _____

x. Shunt created between a cerebral ventricle and the peritoneum by means of a plastic tube. _____

y. Excessive secretion of saliva. _____

z. Brief episode of cerebral ischemia that results in no permanent neurologic damage. (acronym) _____

2. List three types of neurologic disorders associated with physical disability.

_____

_____

_____

3. Describe the sensorimotor effects of the following lesions.
   • *Complete spinal cord injury lesion:*

   _____

   _____

   • *Incomplete spinal cord injury lesion:*

   _____

   _____

4. Identify the appropriate descriptive term and the number of vertebrae associated with each of the following letters.

   C: _____ _____
   T: _____ _____
   L: _____ _____

5. A patient's level of disability depends on the level of the spinal cord injury. Paralysis occurs in the limbs and muscle groups innervated by nerve fibers extending at and below the injured vertebrae. Individuals who are most likely to need adaptive measures for daily oral healthcare procedures are those with a spinal cord injury above _____.

6. Paralysis of limbs, the need for wheelchair use, and potential complications associated with a high spinal cord injury can require that you be prepared to modify standard patient care techniques. Identify modifications you might make during dental hygiene treatment to accommodate your patient's comfort and safety.

   _____

   _____

_____

_____

_____

_____

_____

_____

_____

_____

_____

7. What causes a decubitus ulcer and how can you help prevent this condition during dental hygiene treatment of a patient with paralysis?

   _____

   _____

   _____

   _____

   _____

   _____

8. Describe the correct response to hyperreflexia?

   _____

   _____

   _____

   _____

   _____

   _____

   _____

9. Mouth-held appliances can aid many patients who have upper body disabilities in performing a variety of basic procedures that contribute to independence. List the criteria for an adequate oral orthosis.

   _____

   _____

   _____

   _____

   _____

   _____

10. In your own words, define three different etiologic factors that cause a CVA (or stroke).

_____

_____

_____

11. What is a TIA?

_____

_____

_____

12. What conditions increase an individual's risk for CVA?

_____

_____

_____

_____

_____

_____

_____

_____

13. Which patient assessment technique, commonly used by dental hygienists, can provide information that may indicate your patient's increased risk for CVA.

_____

_____

14. Describe signs and symptoms commonly observed in a patient with a history of CVA.

_____

_____

_____

_____

15. What is _aphasia?_

_____

_____

16. If your patient has a history of CVA damage to the right-hand side of the brain, that patient would exhibit _____-side hemiplegia, have difficulty with action requiring _____, and would likely behave in a(n) _____ manner.

17. If your patient has a history of CVA damage to the left-hand side of the brain, that patient would exhibit _____-side hemiplegia, have difficulty with _____ communication, and would likely behave in a(n) _____ manner.

18. Complete Infomaps 52-1 and 52-2 with just enough basic information to help you identify and differentiate among the listed developmental and acquired disabling conditions.

19. What percent of patients with cerebral palsy also have brain damage that causes intellectual or cognitive impairment?

_____

20. What additional disabling conditions can sometimes accompany a diagnosis of cerebral palsy?

_____

_____

_____

INFOMAP 52-1	DEVELOPMENTAL CONDITIONS (ONSET BEFORE AGE 18)		
CONDITION	CAUSE/ OCCURRENCE	BASIC CHARACTERISTICS	CONSIDERATIONS FOR DENTAL HYGIENE CARE
Cerebral palsy			
Muscular dystrophy, Duchenne			
Muscular dystrophy, facioscapulohumeral			
Myelomeningocele			

INFOMAP 52-2	ACQUIRED IMPAIRMENT (ONSET AFTER AGE 18)		
CONDITION	CAUSE, OCCURRENCE, PATHOLOGY	BASIC CHARACTERISTICS	CONSIDERATIONS FOR DENTAL HYGIENE CARE
Bell's palsy			
Multiple sclerosis			
ALS			
Myasthenia gravis			
Parkinson's disease			
Scleroderma, progressive systemic sclerosis			
PPS			

21. What oral characteristics are associated with cerebral palsy?

_____

_____

_____

_____

_____

_____

_____

_____

22. What symptoms of muscular dystrophy can directly affect your patient's oral health status?

_____

_____

_____

23. Describe the categories used to identify types of multiple sclerosis.

_____

_____

_____

_____

_____

_____

_____

24. ALS is also sometimes called _____.

25. Describe early/onset symptoms for each of the two types of ALS.

_____

_____

_____

_____

26. Both myasthenia gravis and scleroderma are disabling conditions that have special significance for dental professionals. Why?

_____

_____

_____

_____

_____

_____

_____

27. Care is taken when raising the dental chair after treatment of your patient with Parkinson disease who is being treated with dopamine replenishment medications, because of the possibility of _____.

28. Osteoarthritis is a chronic degenerative joint disease common in individuals who are _____.

29. Describe the location and progression of osteoarthritis symptoms.

_____

_____

_____

_____

_____

_____

30. Describe osteoarthritis symptoms that can occur in the temporomandibular joint.

_____

_____

31. What modifications to standard treatment techniques can you use to increase the comfort of your patient who has arthritic involvement of the temporomandibular joint while you are providing dental hygiene treatment?

_____

_____

_____

_____

_____

_____

_____

✓ COMPETENCY EXERCISES

Apply information from the chapter and use critical thinking skills to complete the competency exercises. Write responses on paper or create electronic documents to submit your answers.

Read the Chapter 52 Patient Assessment Summary to help you answer questions #1 through #3.

1. Anitha Jones presents for an initial visit dental hygiene appointment. Laura, Anitha's new caregiver, introduces herself as she assists you in transferring Anitha to the dental chair. While you are helping transfer Anitha to the dental chair, you note that she cannot control the constant disorganized movements of her arms, legs, and head. When you mistakenly startle her by reaching quickly to move the dental light out of the way, this uncontrolled movement becomes intensified. Anitha's hand flings out and bumps into the instrument tray, scattering instruments all over the floor. Anitha's face muscles are in constant motion; she drools and breathes through her mouth. Describe steps you will take to determine modifications in your usual patient care procedures that will help to keep both you and Anitha safe and comfortable during dental hygiene treatment.

2. When she is trying to communicate, it takes Anitha a long time to say anything and you cannot understand her very well. What communication strategies will help you successfully determine answers to the questions you need to ask in order to complete your patient assessment?

3. As you complete assessment data, you realize that Anitha has enjoyed regular professional and personal dental care throughout her life. A caregiver has always provided daily oral biofilm removal. Laura admits to having very little dental knowledge, but she very much wants to learn how to keep Anitha's mouth as healthy as the previous caregiver has done. Use the assessment summary data for Anitha and a copy of the Dental Hygiene Care Plan template (see **workbook** Appendix B) or the care-plan form used by your school clinic to complete a dental hygiene care plan for Anitha that includes appropriate education for Laura.

4. Mr. O'Brien, who has been recovering for about 9 months since experiencing a CVA, has been receiving physical and occupational therapy to help him learn how to use his left hand to do what he used to do with his, now partially paralyzed, right hand and arm. He is very proud of his growing independence and slowly tells you about how he can now comb his own hair and brush his own teeth. While you are performing an oral examination, you note that his biofilm control is very poor and that there is a bolus of leftover food pocketed in his right cheek. The paralyzed muscles on that side of his face have affected his ability to self-clean and even to detect the food that is pouching there after he eats.

   • Explain how you can counsel Mr. O'Brien about his oral health needs and encourage him to let his wife help him clean his mouth, especially on the paralyzed side, while still respecting his desire to independently care for his own personal needs.

CHAPTER 52—PATIENT ASSESSMENT SUMMARY

Patient Name: *Ms. Anitha Jones*   Age: *30*   Gender: F   ☑ Initial Therapy

☐ Maintenance

Provider Name: *D.H. Student*   Date: *Today*   ☐ Re-evaluation

Chief Complaint:

Patient has recently moved into the area. She presents for routine 3-month maintenance and new patient examination.

Assessment Findings

Health History   **At Risk For:**

- Medical diagnosis of cerebral palsy
- Spasticity, athetosis, facial movements
- No intellectual or cognitive disability
- Takes antiseizure medication once per day, but caregiver who accompanies her to the appointment is not sure what it is
- ASA Classification-III
- ADL level-3

Social and Dental History   **At Risk For:**

- Previous history of excellent professional dental care
- Personal dental literacy is high
- New caregiver with low dental knowledge

Dental Examination   **At Risk For:**

- Difficulty controlling jaw and face movements during examination
- Bruxism; incisal attrition, and history of anterior fractures
- Evidence of past lip and cheek-biting trauma
- Mouth breathing; slight anterior gingivitis
- Increased gag reflex
- Current posterior restorations in good repair
- Healthy periodontal tissues; probing depths <3 mm

EVERYDAY ETHICS

Before completing the learning exercises below, reread and reflect on the Everyday Ethics Scenario and Questions for Consideration in this chapter of the **textbook**. It may also be useful to review the Dental Hygiene Ethics discussion in Chapter 1, the Ethical Applications in the introduction pages for each section in the **textbook**, as well as the Codes of Ethics in **textbook** Appendices I–IV.

Cooperative Learning Activity

Answer each of the questions for consideration at the end of the scenario in the **textbook**. Compare what you wrote with answers developed by another classmate and discuss differences/similarities.

Discovery Activity

Investigate the practice act in your state to determine the legal issues involved as the dental hygienist in this scenario contemplates what action to take.

Factors to Teach the Patient

This scenario is related to the following factors listed in this chapter of the **textbook**:

▷ That daily, thorough biofilm removal is particularly necessary to reduce the occurrence of oral disease.

▷ That regular maintenance appointments are important to promote oral health.

▷ Why maintaining periodontal health has added value for teeth used as abutments for a mouth-held implement.

▷ How to clean and maintain the mouth-held implement.

▷ The need to maintain teeth in order to tolerate a mouth-held aid.

Once a month, your employer, Dr. Tom Buckner, and his entire dental team provide care in the little dental clinic inside a nearby assisted-living residence. Your next patient, Terry Biensfield, 25 years old, sustained a level C5 spinal cord injury in a motorcycle accident several years ago. He has worked hard in his physical therapy sessions to maximize his level of function in activities of daily living by using adaptive aids. You have taught him how to brush his own teeth using a modified, long-handled toothbrush attached to one hand, but he still needs some caregiver support and reminders that he must complete his daily oral care routine.

Last month, Dr. Buckner and the physical therapist devised a mouthstick appliance that allows Terry to use a computer. Terry has been practicing with the computer every day, when he participates in an online discussion for people with spinal cord injuries. He now has lots of new ideas for ways he can use his mouth-stick to be more independent and creative in his daily life.

Use a motivational interviewing approach (see **workbook** Appendix D) to write a statement explaining to Terry how important it is for him to maintain an optimum level of oral health so his teeth can continue to support the use of the mouthstick.

MeSH TERMS

Use a combination of MeSH terms and other key words to develop an effective and efficient PubMed literature search strategy.

Dental care for disabled
Neuromuscular diseases
Parkinson's disease
Ischemia
Ischemic attack, transient
Paralysis
Postpoliomyelitis
   syndrome
Bell's palsy
Meningomyelocele
Cerebral palsy (many
   specific types are also
   listed as MeSH terms)
Muscular dystrophies

Muscular dystrophies,
   limb-girdle
Muscular dystrophy,
   Duchenne
Muscular dystrophy,
   Emery-Dreifuss
Muscular dystrophy,
   facioscapulohumeral
Muscular dystrophy,
   oculopharyngeal
Arthritis
   Arthritis, rheumatoid
   Osteoarthritis

The Patient with an Endocrine Condition

KNOWLEDGE EXERCISES

Write your answers for each question in the space provided.

1. Hormones, which together with the nervous system maintain body homeostasis, are excreted by _____ and transported to body cells or other glands by _____.

2. In your own words, describe the purpose of the endocrine system.

_____

_____

3. In your own words, describe a hormone.

_____

_____

_____

4. List the vital functions that hormones regulate.

_____

_____

_____

_____

5. List the major endocrine glands and briefly describe the function of each.

_____

_____

_____

_____

_____

_____

_____

_____

6. Both _____ and _____ of a hormone can affect a patient's physical and mental status.

7. Cyclic menstruation is regulated by fluctuations in estrogen and progesterone and, with some variations and irregularities, is usually about 28 days in length. In your own words, explain how the levels of each of these two hormones vary relative to menstruation and ovulation during the menstrual cycle. (*Hint*: Describe Figure 53-2 in the **textbook**.)

_____

_____

_____

_____

_____

_____

_____

_____

8. Some women experience discomfort for several days preceding the beginning of their menstrual flow. If your patient mentions that she is feeling the effects of premenstrual symptoms, what is she likely to be experiencing?

_____

_____

_____

_____

_____

9. If your patient is experiencing irregularity or other problems with her menstrual cycle, a careful assessment and review of her health history is imperative, because she can also be experiencing other _____ problems.

10. List the side effects of oral contraceptives that will be of concern when you are providing dental hygiene care for your patient.

_____

_____

_____

_____

_____

11. Summarize the effects of puberty-linked hormone increases on the physical development of both males and females.

_____

_____

_____

_____

12. Match the statement (first column) with the gland (second column). Letters representing glands may be used more than once.

Statement	Gland
___ The anterior lobe serves as the master gland of the body.	A. Adrenals
___ These glands are located on the kidneys.	B. Gonads
___ Levothyroxine is a medication used to treat disorders of this gland.	C. Hypothalamus
___ The hormone of this gland regulates calcium, phosphorus, and vitamin D levels in the blood and bone.	D. Pancreas
___ Cushing syndrome is caused by an increase in cortisol secreted by this gland.	E. Parathyroid
___ Humoral factors hormones are produced by this gland.	F. Pineal
___ The hormone of this gland regulates blood glucose.	G. Pituitary
___ Grave disease is associated with this gland.	H. Thymus
___ This gland secretes melatonin.	I. Thyroid
___ The hormones of these glands influence puberty.	
___ An adenoma is the most common form of tumor of this gland.	
___ This gland controls hormone production in the pituitary gland.	
___ A lack of hormone produced by this gland is related to Hashimoto disease.	
___ Addison disease is associated with this gland.	

13. Most adverse oral changes related to menopause can be prevented or diminished with adequate nutrition and thorough daily oral hygiene care. List the oral changes that can be associated with menopause.

_____

_____

_____

_____

_____

14. Too high or too low of a hormone level can cause a variety of uncomfortable signs and symptoms. Contrast and compare the general characteristics of hypothyroidism and hyperthyroidism. In other words, what are the differences between the signs and symptoms of hypothyroidism as compared to hyperthyroidism?

Hypothyroidism	Hyperthyroidism

15. An adrenal crisis is associated with _____.

16. List the signs and symptoms of adrenal crisis.

_____

_____

_____

_____

_____

_____

_____

_____

_____

_____

_____

17. Which gland is associated with myxedema?

_____

_____

18. What is the cause of myxedema?

_____

_____

19. What are the signs of myxedema?

_____

20. List the patient management considerations for a patient who presents with hypoadrenalism.

_____

_____

_____

_____

_____

_____

_____

_____

_____

_____

_____

✓ COMPETENCY EXERCISES

Apply information from the chapter and use critical thinking skills to complete the competency exercises. Write responses on paper or create electronic documents to submit your answers.

Georgina Steele, a woman in her late 40s, was last seen 6 months ago. Today, when you entered the reception area, you noticed that Georgina's appearance seemed different. She was significantly heavier than you remembered and appeared flustered. You made a mental note to investigate the weight gain during the health history update. She also was wearing a heavy winter sweater even though it was August.

As you escorted her to the treatment room, you offered to hang her sweater, but she preferred to keep it on due to the air conditioning. It was too cold for her, even though the office temperature was 72 degrees. Her last visit with her physician was 13 months ago. Georgina expressed concern and frustration with her recent weight gain over the last few months. She didn't think her eating patterns had changed significantly and was now being extra diligent about her eating habits. She mentioned to you that she felt tired all the time and suffered from muscle cramps and even pain most days, regardless of her level of physical activity. She told you that at work she is often feeling confused and overwhelmed by the work project, something that had never happened before. She was not taking any prescription medication, but occasionally took 200 mg of ibuprofen because of the pain in her legs and arms. But this provided little relief, so she was coping the best she could by trying to stay busy. Vital signs were taken. Her BP, temperature, and respirations were normal, but her pulse rate was 55.

As you began the extraoral examination, you noticed that the facial skin appeared rather dry. Georgina stated that she had been trying different moisturizers with little improvement. As you palpated the neck/throat region, you sensed an enlargement in her thyroid gland which was not present 6 months ago. It was not tender. All other extra-oral findings were normal.

Intraorally, the tissues seemed dry. Most of the left buccal mucosa had a pattern of lacy white lines covering the tissue. Georgina reported no discomfort in the tissues, other than the dryness. Her periodontal status remained unchanged (slight localized gingivitis) and no new areas of decay were evident.

1. What are the adverse medical and oral signs and symptoms discovered during the examination?
2. Based on the findings of your examination and interview with the patient, what do you suspect could be causing these changes in appearance and behavior? What are the differential diagnoses based on the findings of this examination?
3. What are your recommendations for Georgina?
4. In outline form, devise a plan for discussing the findings with Georgina.

EVERYDAY ETHICS

Before completing the learning exercises below, reread and reflect on the Everyday Ethics Scenario and Questions for Consideration in this chapter of the **textbook**. It may also be useful to review the Dental Hygiene Ethics discussion in Chapter 1, the Ethical Applications in the introduction pages for each section in the **textbook**, as well as the Codes of Ethics in **textbook** Appendices I–IV.

Individual Learning Activity

Imagine that you are the dental hygienist in this scenario. Answer each of the questions for consideration at the end of the scenario.

Collaborative Learning Activity

Work with another student colleague to role-play the scenario. The goal of this exercise is for you and your colleague to work though the alternative actions in order to come to consensus on a solution or response that is acceptable to both of you.

Factors to Teach the Patient

This scenario is related to the following factors listed in this chapter of the **textbook**:

▷ The impact of menopause on oral health.
▷ The benefits of fluoride throughout life.
▷ The importance of nutrition, exercise, and sleep for good health.

Today is the first time you are providing dental hygiene care for Rosalee Ayers, aged 55 years. She arrives late and mentions that because she is under high stress these days and hasn't been eating or sleeping very well, she overslept this morning. Rosalee is a high-powered businesswoman who takes great pride in her youthful appearance and her healthy lifestyle. As you update her health history, you note that she has received regular dental hygiene care for the last 15 years. Her general health status is very good, and she takes no medications. A notation in her record states that she is in menopause; her menses ceased 1 year ago.

When you begin your oral examination, Rosalee mentions that because of the oral hygiene instruction she has received at this clinic, she has always brushed and flossed every day. Lately, however, she has noticed that her mouth frequently feels really dry, and sometimes she feels a burning sensation on her tongue, palate, and inside her lips.

Your assessment findings indicate that her biofilm levels are very low, there are very few dental restorations, and there are no current carious lesions.

Her oral tissues are generally very healthy looking. Periodontal pocket depths are all less than 3 mm. Past periodontal charts have recorded generalized 2- to 3-mm recession in all premolar and molar areas, but there are no changes in the level of recession when you do your periodontal charting today.

After your assessment is complete, you write a brief care plan and, because of your patient's increased risk for root caries, you include a recommendation for fluoride treatment.

When you discuss your care plan with Rosalee, she chuckles and says, "Look, I'm not a kid any more. What on earth do I need a fluoride treatment for?"

Use a motivational interviewing approach found in **workbook** Appendix D as a guide to develop a conversation to use when you are talking with Rosalee about the value of fluoride treatments.

MeSH TERMS

Use a combination of MeSH terms and other key words to develop an effective and efficient PubMed literature search strategy.

Endocrine system	Thyroid gland	Adrenal glands	Premenstrual syndrome
Endocrine glands	Parathyroid glands	Hormones	Puberty
Pineal gland	Thymus gland	Menstruation	Oral contraceptives
Pituitary gland	Pancreas	Menopause	

CHAPTER 53 WORD SEARCH PUZZLE

```
H Y P O K A L E M I A N H A J X Q
I S C G C T Q N E G Y B F E C G E
H I O M R M K S H Y L D L C G A T
P S Y F P N U R C Y V A S W I D E
J H X J L A Z S R N W Q N M Y B N
N R B G P V L F A F O E E D Z Y I
E M G O H A Z J N N V R W W W T R
J N N Q B O W C E H T Y Y E U R H
X E I N J A M B M A O A Z M O E P
M P Y R U X M E N K M R B K O B E
F M X S C S I R O E C Z M B U U N
L V S Q T O E H D S S K V O Z P I
U L K T S P D E R M T G F U N A P
F M E F Y Y X N B T M A B K S E E
O E L H W Y Q H E O R K S W T Q X
E C W M M X V X K Y A G S I M M X
Y N T H Y R O T O X I C Q M S X K
```

Puzzle Clues

1. Catecholamine hormone that causes the "fight-or-flight" response to stress.
2. Pertaining to a substance secreted directly into blood or lymph rather than into a duct.
3. Organ or structure that secretes or excretes substances.
4. Tendency of biologic systems to maintain constant internal stability.
5. Chemical product of an organ or cells within an organ that has a specific regulatory effect upon cells elsewhere in the body.
6. Elevated sodium level in the bloodstream.
7. Lower than normal level of potassium in the bloodstream.
8. Onset of menstruation; may occur from 9 to 17 years of age.
9. Cessation of menstruation in older women.
10. Disease caused by decreased activity of the thyroid gland characterized by dry skin, swellings around the lips and nose.
11. Period during which adolescents reach sexual maturity and become capable of reproduction.
12. Potentially life-threatening crisis during which the thyroid suddenly releases large amounts of thyroid hormone.

The Patient with Diabetes Mellitus

LEARNING OBJECTIVES

Upon successful completion of these exercises, you will be able to:

1. Identify and define the key terms and concepts related to diabetes.
2. Explain the function and effects of insulin.
3. Identify the risk factors for diabetes.
4. Describe etiologic classifications, signs and symptoms, diagnostic procedures, complications, and common

medical treatment for diabetes.

5. React appropriately in a diabetic emergency.
6. Explain the relationship between diabetes and oral health.
7. Plan and document dental hygiene care and oral hygiene instructions for patients with diabetes.

KNOWLEDGE EXERCISES

Write your answers for each question in the space provided.

1. What type of diabetes is related to genetics, obesity, and hormones during pregnancy?

2. Identify the health-related factors besides pregnancy that can result in diabetes.

3. What genetic syndromes are sometimes associated with diabetes?

4. Complete Infomap 54-1 by listing characteristics that will help you learn to differentiate between type 1 and type 2 diabetes.

5. List and describe the types of monogenic diabetes syndromes.

INFOMAP 54-1	COMPARISON OF TYPE 1 AND TYPE 2 DIABETES	
TYPE 1 CHARACTERISTICS		**TYPE 2 CHARACTERISTICS**

6. Match the level of blood glucose to the characteristic.

Level of Blood Glucose	Characteristic
A. Hypoglycemia	_____More common occurrence
B. Hyperglycemia	_____Develops slowly over hours/days
C. Both	_____Fruity smelling breath
	_____Possible convulsions if left untreated
	_____Rapid onset
	_____Anxious, stupor, weakness
	_____Too much insulin
	_____Too much food
	_____Normal to slightly elevated blood pressure
	_____Flushed, dry skin
	_____Fast, irregular pulse

7. Diabetes is characterized by hyperglycemia. In your own words, define the range of measurements for normal glucose blood level and hyperglycemia.

_____

_____

8. Define the following symptoms of hyperglycemia.
- *Polyuria:*

_____

- *Polydipsia:*

_____

- *Polyphagia:*

_____

9. List the common physical complications associated with uncontrolled diabetes.

_____

_____

_____
_____
_____
_____
_____

10. What criteria are used to diagnose diabetes?

_____
_____
_____

11. What does the HbA1c test measure? How is it used?

_____
_____
_____

12. What self-administered tests are used for monitoring blood glucose levels during treatment of diabetes?

_____
_____
_____
_____
_____
_____
_____

13. If your patient tells you that the result of his fasting plasma glucose test this morning was less than_____, you know that his diabetes is well controlled and it is safe to provide dental hygiene treatment today.

14. If your patient tells you that her postprandial glucose level this morning was greater than 200 mg per dL, you know that her diabetes is _____.

15. What is the role of insulin in the human body?

_____
_____
_____

16. Where is insulin produced in the human body?

_____
_____

17. What is exogenous insulin?

_____

18. How is exogenous insulin administered?

_____
_____
_____

19. What factors determine the dose of insulin administered for each patient?

_____
_____
_____

20. Identify the duration of peak action for each of the classes of insulin.

_____
_____
_____
_____
_____

21. What is the relationship of hypoglycemia from an inadequate nutritional intake to the level of insulin in the blood?

_____
_____
_____
_____

22. Describe the consequence when too little insulin is administered to control hyperglycemia.

_____
_____

23. Oral hypoglycemic agents act differently from insulin to control blood glucose levels. What is the mechanism of action of biguanides and thiazolidinediones?

_____
_____

24. If your patient is taking sulfonylureas or meglitinides to control type 2 diabetes, what side effect is important for you to watch for during dental hygiene treatment?

_____

25. Your patient with uncontrolled diabetes is at risk for many long-term health complications. Identify the body systems or organs (other than the mouth) that can be affected.

———————————————————

———————————————————

———————————————————

———————————————————

26. Diabetes can be controlled, but to date, there is no known cure. List five factors important for maintaining the overall good health and well-being of an individual with diabetes or at risk for diabetes.

———————————————————

———————————————————

———————————————————

———————————————————

———————————————————

27. In one sentence, describe the relationship between poorly controlled diabetes and periodontal disease.

———————————————————

———————————————————

———————————————————

———————————————————

28. Uncontrolled glucose levels place your patient at risk for _____, an opportunistic oral infection.

29. What is the role of the dental hygienist in planning care for patients who are at risk for diabetes or who are exhibiting signs and symptoms of diabetes?

———————————————————

———————————————————

———————————————————

30. Why is stress prevention an important component of a dental hygiene care plan for a patient with diabetes?

———————————————————

31. Identify ways that the dental hygienist can reduce stress and prevent an emergency situation during an appointment with the patient with diabetes.

———————————————————

———————————————————

———————————————————

———————————————————

———————————————————

———————————————————

32. Why should you be very careful to avoid undue tissue trauma when providing dental hygiene care for your patient with diabetes?

———————————————————

———————————————————

33. Describe the **Rule of 15**s (fifteens).

———————————————————

———————————————————

———————————————————

———————————————————

———————————————————

✓ COMPETENCY EXERCISES

Apply information from the chapter and use critical thinking skills to complete the competency exercises. Write responses on paper or create electronic documents to submit your answers.

1. In your own words, explain what can happen at the cellular level when glucose needed to supply energy cannot be accessed owing to either decreased supply or action of insulin.

   Read the Section I Patient Assessment Summary to help you answer the following questions.

2. While you are waiting for Mr. Diamandis, your first patient of the day, you look over the health history form he sent to the office a week earlier and note that he has been diagnosed with type 2 diabetes. Mr. Diamandis finally arrives 15 minutes late for the appointment. He is extremely anxious and states he is late because of the traffic. His morning, it seems, has not gone well, and everything is off schedule. As you bring him back to your treatment room, you notice that he is pale and trembling. He is perspiring profusely and seems agitated as he sits in the chair.

   What questions will you ask Mr. Diamandis to add to the information you already know about his medical history?

3. Mr. Diamandis responds irritably to your questions and gives vague answers. He says. "I have been having my teeth cleaned regularly for years and no one has ever asked these kinds of questions." When you take his vital signs, you note that his pulse is rapid

and his blood pressure is a bit elevated. You are really conscious of your appointment time slipping away, so you tilt the dental chair back to do an intraoral examination and begin your oral assessment. After 10 minutes, Mr. Diamandis stops you and says "Please sit me upright." You note that his breath is coming in rapid gasps.

What is most likely to be happening and what will your response be?

4. Using your institution's guidelines for writing in patient records, document Mr. Diamandis's appointment.

5. During a follow-up appointment several weeks later, when Mr. Diamandis's medical situation has been stabilized, you are able to collect the rest of the assessment data. Use the information in Mr. Diamandis's Patient Assessment Summary and a copy of the Patient-Specific Care Plan template in **workbook** Appendix B to develop dental hygiene diagnosis statements and complete a dental hygiene care plan for providing initial therapy dental hygiene interventions for Mr. Diamandis.

6. Discuss options for continuing care if Mr. Diamandis's initial therapy outcomes are not optimal.

CHAPTER 54—PATIENT ASSESSMENT SUMMARY

Patient Name: *Dimitrios Nicholas Diamandis*   Age: *57*   Gender: M   ☑ Initial Therapy
☐ Maintenance

Provider Name: *D.H. Student*   Date: *Today*   ☐ Re-evaluation

Chief Complaint:

Patient presents for new patient examination. "I just want my teeth cleaned."

Assessment Findings

Health History   **At Risk For:**

- Diagnosed several years ago with type 2 diabetes—only monitors blood sugar levels when he isn't feeling well, tries to control the condition through diet and exercise
- No medical visits for 2 years—no current medications
- Blood pressure 145/95 mmHg, pulse 86 beats per minute
- Tobacco use: 1–2 packs per day for 35 years
- Alcohol use: one to two drinks daily (usually beer)
- ASA Classification-III, ADL level-0

Social and Dental History   **At Risk For:**

- 35 years in previous dental practice—dentist was a college roommate of his who recently retired
- No previous periodontal therapy—only received "dental cleanings" every 6 months
- Limited dental knowledge

Dental Examination   **At Risk For:**

- Generalized 6- to 8-mm probing depths
- Generalized recession on mandibular anterior and lingual of maxillary molars—sensitivity in molars
- Generalized slight mobility
- Generalized poor biofilm control
- Calculus lower anteriors
- Generalized bleeding on probing
- Generalized erythematous tissue
- Radiographic findings:
  - Areas of horizontal and vertical bone loss
  - Furcation involvement in mandibular molars
  - Several large amalgam fillings with proximal overhangs
  - Generalized subgingival and interproximal calculus visible on radiographs

EVERYDAY ETHICS

Before completing the learning exercises below, reread and reflect on the Everyday Ethics Scenario and Questions for Consideration in this chapter of the **textbook**. It may also be useful to review the Dental Hygiene Ethics discussion in Chapter 1, the Ethical Applications in the introduction pages for each section in the **textbook**, as well as the Codes of Ethics in **textbook** Appendices I–IV.

Collaborative Learning Activity

Work with another student colleague to role-play the scenario. The goal of this exercise is for you and your colleague to work through the alternative actions in order to come to consensus on a solution or response that is acceptable to both of you.

Discovery Activity

Ask a friend or relative who is not involved in health care to read the scenario and discuss it with you from the perspective of a "patient" who receives services within the healthcare system. Discuss what you learned from the concerns, insights, or difference in perspective that person expressed.

Factors to Teach the Patient

This scenario is related to the following factors listed in this chapter of the **textbook**:

▷ Recognizing early warning signs of diabetes and seeking medical treatment.

▷ Reviewing practice of meticulous oral hygiene to prevent dental and periodontal disease.

Use the information from Chapter 54 in the **textbook** and the principles of motivational interviewing in **workbook** Appendix D as guides to prepare a conversation that you might use to educate Ed (introduced in the **textbook** Everyday Ethics scenario) about the need to consult his physician related to signs and symptoms of diabetes, how diabetes can affect his oral health, and what he can do to prevent further health complications.

Use the conversation you create to role-play this situation with a fellow student. If you are the patient in the role-play, be sure to ask questions. If you are the dental hygienist, try to anticipate questions and answer them in your explanation.

MeSH TERMS

Use a combination of MeSH terms and other key words to develop an effective and efficient PubMed literature search strategy.

Diabetes mellitus, type 1
Hypoglycemia
Diabetes mellitus, type 2
Insulin

Diabetes, gestational
Diabetes complications
Hyperglycemia

The Patient with Cancer

 KNOWLEDGE EXERCISES

Write your answers for each question in the space provided.

1. Match the following terms related to the physical and oral effects of cancer treatment with the correct description.

Term	Description of Effect
___ Mucositis	A. Diminishment or abatement of the symptoms of a disease
___ Dysgeusia	
___ Neurotoxicity	B. Recurrence of a disease after its apparent cessation
___ Alopecia	C. Treatment that provides relief of symptoms but is not intended to cure
___ Palliative	
___ Herpes simplex	D. A loss of hair
	E. Virus that can cause oral infection during or after radiation therapy
___ *Candida albicans*	F. Distortion of the sense of taste
___ Trismus	G. Limited jaw opening because of spasm or fibrosis of muscles or joint; may occur 3–6 months after radiation treatment to the head and neck
___ Immunosuppression	
___ Relapse	H. Fungus that commonly causes oral infection related to treatment for cancer
___ Remission	I. Inhibition of antibody responses resulting from leucopenia related to chemotherapy treatments
	J. Inflammation of the oral mucosa
	K. Can cause a bilateral feeling of toothache related to chemotherapy treatments for cancer

2. What is cancer?

_____

_____

3. How are cancers classified and described?

_____

_____

_____

_____

_____

_____

_____

4. What are the risk factors for developing cancer?

_____

_____

_____

_____

_____

_____

5. Why is it important to plan comprehensive and co-ordinated dental hygiene care for your patient before, during, and after treatment for cancer?

_____

_____

_____

_____

_____

_____

6. Identify the dental hygiene interventions you will most likely provide for your patient before the medical treatment for cancer begins.

_____

_____

_____

_____

_____

_____

7. List oral complications that are commonly the result of any of the various types of treatment for cancer.

_____

_____

_____

_____

_____

8. What are the systemic side effects of chemotherapy cancer treatment?

_____

_____

_____

_____

_____

_____

9. List types of oral infections common during and after treatment for cancer.

_____

_____

_____

10. In your own words, briefly describe a hematopoietic cell transplantation.

_____

_____

_____

_____

_____

11. Describe graft-versus-host disease and list significant oral complications found in affected individuals.

_____

_____

_____

_____

_____

12. _____ is a destructive blood vessel compromise and necrosis of bone that can occur after high-dose radiation treatment in the head and neck area. This condition results in decreased ability to heal and increased susceptibility to infection.

13. What oral changes can influence/restrict nutritional intake and further compromise the health status of a patient who is undergoing cancer therapy?

_____

_____

_____

_____

_____

14. List the symptoms you would expect to observe in all five levels of the World Health Organization scale for oral mucositis.

Level	Clinical Symptoms
0	
1	
2	
3	
4	

15. List personal care recommendations you can make to help the patient who is undergoing treatment for

cancer to reduce the risk for mucositis or to increase ability to maintain daily oral hygiene measures when mucositis is already a problem.

_____

_____

_____

_____

16. Identify measures that could help prevent dental caries in a patient with xerostomia related to cancer treatment.

_____

_____

_____

_____

_____

17. What patient factors can influence your patient's ability to attend to and comply with the counseling and oral hygiene instructions that you provide before, during, and after treatment for cancer?

_____

_____

_____

_____

_____

_____

_____

 COMPETENCY EXERCISES

Apply information from the chapter and use critical thinking skills to complete the competency exercises. Write responses on paper or create electronic documents to submit your answers.

Mrs. Marge Henley is scheduled today in the hospital dental clinic as an emergency patient. After he examines her, Dr. Singh completes the assessment findings component of a patient care plan form and then calls you in to consult with him. Mrs. Henley is currently undergoing chemotherapy for cancer treatment and is experiencing severe oral symptoms related to the treatment. Dr. Singh has already written a prescription to treat the oral candidiasis. He asks you to counsel Mrs. Henley about daily oral care and to write a dental hygiene care plan for her continuing care during the cancer treatment.

When you carefully examine her, you discover that Mrs. Henley's oral tissues are heartbreakingly inflamed, blistered, and dry. She tells you that she has been feeling a bit guilty because her mouth has been so sore that she cannot brush and floss as often or as thoroughly as she used to do. Her sense of humor has remained intact, though, and she tells you with a twinkle in her eye that she eats vanilla pudding for breakfast, lunch, and dinner every day. She asks for any suggestions you have to help her get through this difficult time.

1. What areas of risk are associated with the assessment findings recorded for Mrs. Henley?

2. Write at least two dental hygiene diagnosis statements to include in Mrs. Henley's written care plan.

3. Write a goal for each of the problems identified in the dental hygiene diagnosis statements you wrote for question #2. Include a time frame for meeting each goal. How will you measure whether your patient met the goal?

4. Using your institution's guidelines for writing in patient records, document Mrs. Henley's visit and write a statement regarding her next visit.

 DISCOVERY EXERCISES

1. The National Oral Health Information Clearinghouse (NOHIC) is a resource center for oral health information geared to patients with special needs and the healthcare providers who serve them. Visit their website (www.nohic.nidcr.nih.gov) to discover a wonderful series of education pamphlets about oral cancer and the oral complications of cancer treatment.

2. Investigate the medical and dental literature using a PubMed search to discover which types of cancer may be treated with drugs, such as bisphosphonates, that can have a long-term effect on oral tissues. (Idea: This topic would make an excellent research project.)

 QUESTIONS PATIENTS ASK

What sources of information can you identify that will help you answer your patient's questions in this scenario?

"How can I possibly keep my mouth clean when it is so sore and/or dry that it hurts to use the toothbrush? And why is that so important anyway?" "When is the best time to have my teeth worked on while I am undergoing treatment for my cancer?" "How soon after my radiation treatment can I get my new dentures and/or partial dentures?" "Will the kind of cancer treatment I am receiving now affect my ability to receive dental care, such as having implants placed, later on?"

EVERYDAY ETHICS

Before completing the learning exercises below, reread and reflect on the Everyday Ethics Scenario and Questions for Consideration in this chapter of the **textbook**. It may also be useful to review the Dental Hygiene Ethics discussion in Chapter 1, the Ethical Applications in the introduction pages for each section in the **textbook**, as well as the Codes of Ethics in **textbook** Appendices I–IV.

Discovery Activities

Investigate the practice act in your state to determine the legal issues involved as the dental hygienist in this scenario contemplates what action to take.

Ask a dental hygienist who has been practicing for a year or more to read the scenario. Provide them with a copy of the Code of Ethics as well. Share the responses you have made to answer each question and ask that person to discuss the situation with you. What insights did you have or what did you learn during this discussion?

Factors to Teach the Patient

This scenario is related to the following factors listed in this chapter of the **textbook**:

▷ Why the dental hygienist needs to conduct an oral soft-tissue screening and complete oral examination at regular, frequent intervals.

▷ How and when to use dental biofilm control methods, gel-tray application, use of saliva substitute, and all other details of personal care to reduce oral side effects caused by the disease and/or cancer treatment.

▷ Ideas for remembering to follow the instructions to keep the mouth healthier and more comfortable during cancer treatment.

▷ The reasons why a routine schedule of preventive periodontal scaling, fluoride application, and oral hygiene assessment done by a dental hygienist contributes to the success of cancer treatment.

George Murphy, a 45-year-old construction worker, has recently been diagnosed with parotid gland cancer that has spread into his left neck. He will be having surgery to remove the left parotid gland with a left neck dissection, followed by radiation therapy. He is scheduled today for a pretreatment dental examination. Mr. Murphy has not seen a dentist in more than 10 years and has dental caries lesions, moderately advanced periodontal disease, and very poor oral hygiene. You are asked to prepare a dental hygiene care plan to address Mr. Murphy's oral care needs during and after the radiation treatment.

Mr. Murphy tells you that he hates dentists because they always hurt him and that is why he never comes to see one. The only reason he is here today is because he was told that he could not proceed with his cancer treatment unless he gets his mouth into better shape.

Use the information in the Personal Factors section of Chapter 55 of the **textbook** and the principles of motivational interviewing (see **workbook** Appendix D) as guides to prepare an outline for a conversation you will use to counsel Mr. Murphy regarding his oral condition.

MeSH TERMS

Use a combination of MeSH terms and other key words to develop an effective and efficient PubMed literature search strategy.

Neoplasms	Trismus
Neoplasm staging	Xerostomia
Neoplasm metastasis	Mucositis
Antineoplastic agents	Stomatitis
Osteonecrosis	Candidiasis, oral

CHAPTER 55 CROSSWORD PUZZLE

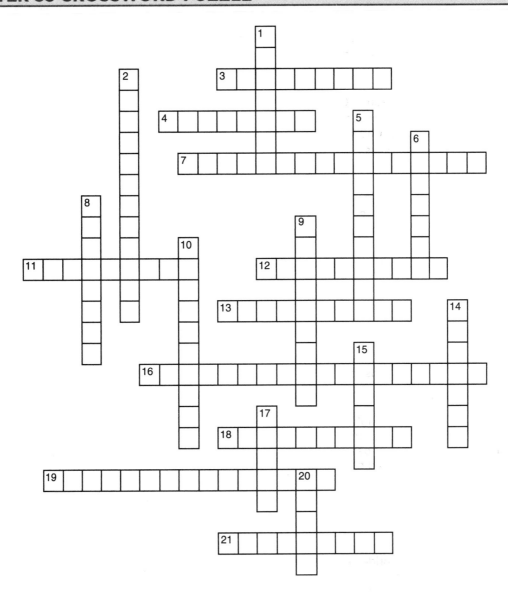

Puzzle Clues

Across

3. Malignant tumor of epithelial origin.

4. The study of tumors.

7. Treatment of disease with ionizing radiation (two words).

11. The irreversible alteration in adult cells toward embryonic cell types, characteristic of tumor cells.

12. The radiation _____ is the member of the cancer care team who is responsible for planning, delivery, and follow-up of radiation therapy.

13. The spread of cancer cells from one body tissue or organ to others through blood and lymph systems.

16. Blood vessel compromise and necrosis of bone exposed to high-dose radiation.

18. A chemical, physical, or biologic agent that may cause cancer.

19. The _____ is a member of the cancer care team with an important role in identifying and managing oral manifestations related to the patient's cancer treatments (two words).

21. Type of tumor that grows at a rapid rate, gains access to blood and lymph channels to metastasize into other areas of the body, and usually causes death unless growth can be controlled.

Down

1. Tumor composed of cells derived from connective tissue.

2. Treatment of an illness by using drugs.

5. Donor for this type of bone marrow transplant is the patient.

6. This condition can limit the patient's ability to open mouth during dental hygiene treatment.

8. Any new and abnormal growth; can be benign or malignant.

9. Inflammation of oral tissues.

10. Intervention to provide relief for symptoms.

14. The _____ oncologist is the member of the cancer care team who manages the patient's chemotherapy treatments.

15. Type of tumor that grows slowly by expansion and does not infiltrate surrounding tissue, does not spread by metastasis, and does not usually cause death unless its location interferes with vital functions.

17. Term for exposed bone in maxilla or mandible that can occur when a patient is taking antiresorptive or antiangenic drugs that are not bisphosphonates (acronym).

20. Clinical classification of a tumor; consists of three components.

The Oral and Maxillofacial Surgery Patient

KNOWLEDGE EXERCISES

Write your answers for each question in the space provided.

1. What is orthognathic surgery?

2. In your own words, define *intermaxillary fixation*.

3. Define *exodontics*.

4. List at least three reasons why it is important to provide dental hygiene care for a patient before oral and maxillofacial surgery, even when all of the patient's teeth will be removed during the surgical procedure.

5. List three personal factors that can affect communication with your patient when you are providing oral hygiene instructions to him or her before oral surgery.

6. List at least three types of printed instructions you would provide as part of your presurgical patient education.

7. Identify specific components to include in instructions which you will provide your patient immediately after a surgical procedure.

_____

_____

_____

_____

_____

_____

_____

_____

8. List postsurgical procedures you may be asked to participate in during follow-up care for your patient.

_____

_____

_____

9. List the important habits patients should avoid after oral surgery.

_____

_____

_____

_____

_____

10. Identify two possible causes of a fractured jaw.

_____

_____

11. List three clinical signs that can aid in recognition of a fractured jaw.

_____

_____

_____

12. Describe a comminuted fracture.

_____

_____

13. Which type of fractured jaw is more likely to occur in a small child?

14. Describe an arch bar and explain how it immobilizes the mandibular jaw.

_____

_____

_____

_____

15. Identify three advantages for using IMF after surgical reduction of a fracture.

_____

_____

_____

16. List three contraindications for using an IMF.

_____

_____

_____

17. List three types of systems/materials used for immobilization after open surgical reduction of a skeletal fracture.

_____

_____

_____

18. List factors that make maxillary fractures more difficult to manage than mandibular fractures.

_____

_____

_____

_____

19. Describe a maxillary alveolar process fracture. (_Hint_: Draw a diagram of what you are trying to describe.) List the components of treatment provided for the patient with this type of fracture.

_____

_____

_____

_____

_____

_____

20. Identify reasons a healthy liquid or soft diet is difficult to plan for a postsurgical patient.

21. List two vitamins that are essential in the diet of a patient who is healing after an oral/maxillofacial surgical procedure.

22. Provide three examples of feeding methods used for patients after a surgical fixation procedure.

23. List at least three foods that can supply needed nutrients as part of a soft diet prepared for a patient with only a single-jaw fixation appliance.

24. When is personal oral care and thorough biofilm removal by the patient resumed after an oral surgical procedure?

25. List three factors that may compromise the patient's own postsurgical biofilm removal or the provision of dental hygiene.

✓ COMPETENCY EXERCISES

Apply information from the chapter and use critical thinking skills to complete the competency exercises. Write responses on paper or create electronic documents to submit your answers.

1. Compare open and closed reduction procedures used for the treatment of a facial fracture.

2. You are asked to provide a presurgical dental hygiene prophylaxis for Mr. Bright, who is scheduled in 2 weeks for oral surgery to remove all of his remaining maxillary teeth and receive an immediate denture. His patient record contains assessment data indicating that teeth 1, 3, 6–9, 13, and 16 are missing; tooth 2 is extremely sensitive owing to a carious lesion; teeth 4 and 5 are mobile; and his gingival tissue is sensitive and bleeds profusely. There is visible calculus and a high level of biofilm on all the remaining teeth. He has not had any regular dental care or oral hygiene instructions for many years. Create an info-map or table that will help you organize the following information.

   • Identify factors from this case scenario that can affect instrumentation techniques when you are providing presurgical scaling for Mr. Bright.

   • Identify why these factors are a problem.

   • Suggest procedures you might use to overcome each problem.

   • Use the format required in your school clinic to write a progress note for an imaginary patient visit that documents the use of one of the potential modifications you have described.

3. Your patient, Alicia Wentworth, is upset today when she comes to the office for her dental hygiene appointment. She tells you that her good friend, David, was recently injured in an automobile accident. She asks you to explain what a simple fracture of the mandible is and what a Le Fort II midfacial fracture is. Draw diagrams you can use to educate Alicia.

4. A week later, Alicia calls and leaves a message on the office voice mail. She says that David is coming home from the hospital and she has agreed to provide meals for him every day. His fracture has been treated using an IMF appliance and he must receive all his nutrition using a straw or a spoon-feeding technique. He is restricted to a full-liquid diet. She asks you to call her back and recommend foods and preparation methods. She wants to know about how he can keep his mouth clean after he eats.

   Make notes that you can refer to when you call her back to give her the information she is asking for.

EVERYDAY ETHICS

Before completing the learning exercises below, reread and reflect on the Everyday Ethics Scenario and Questions for Consideration in this chapter of the **textbook**. It may also be useful to review the Dental Hygiene Ethics discussion in Chapter 1, the Ethical Applications in the introduction pages for each section in the **textbook**, as well as the Codes of Ethics in **textbook** Appendices I–IV.

Individual Learning Activity

Imagine that you have observed what happened in the scenario, but are not one of the main characters involved in the situation. Write a reflective journal entry that:

- Describes how you might have reacted (as an observer—not as a participant),

- Expresses your personal feelings about what happened, or
- Identifies personal values that affect your reaction to the situation.

Discovery Activity

Ask a friend or relative who is not involved in health care to read the scenario and discuss it with you from the perspective of a "patient" who receives services within the healthcare system. Discuss what you learned from the concerns, insights, or difference in perspective that person expressed.

Factors to Teach the Patient

This scenario is related to the following factors listed in this chapter of the **textbook**:

▷ Significance of a clean mouth during general anesthesia.

Mr. Brown is scheduled in about 2 weeks for some very serious surgery that is part of his treatment for pancreatic cancer. His physician has recommended that Mr. Brown visit his dental hygienist for a complete dental assessment before the surgery. As you go over his health history, you discover that he is very confused about why dental hygiene interventions are necessary in his case—after all, his illness has nothing to do with his mouth!

Use the information in Chapter 56 of the **textbook** and the principles of motivational interviewing (see **workbook** Appendix D) as a guide to write a statement explaining to Mr. Brown why this dental hygiene appointment is such an important component of his total health and well-being.

MeSH TERMS

Use a combination of MeSH terms and other key words to develop an effective and efficient PubMed literature search strategy.

Oral surgical procedures
Orthognathic surgical
  procedures
Maxillofacial injuries

Jaw fractures
Mandibular fractures
Maxillary fractures

The Patient with a Seizure Disorder

KNOWLEDGE EXERCISES

Write your answers for each question in the space provided.

1. In your own words, describe a seizure?

2. Although most seizure disorders tend to be stable, some individuals experience a random pattern of seizures that disrupt their lives. List some activities that may be compromised for an individual who experiences recurrent seizures.

3. If your patient has a history of seizure activity, when should you contact/consult with your patient's physician?

4. In what three ways are epileptic syndromes classified?

5. Briefly describe the physical manifestations of a tonic–clonic seizure.

6. In your own words, briefly describe the clinical manifestations of an absence seizure.

_____

_____

_____

_____

_____

_____

7. What is a focal seizure?

_____

_____

8. List some of the medical conditions that can cause seizures.

_____

_____

_____

_____

_____

_____

_____

9. What kinds of stimuli, common in a dental practice, could potentially precipitate a seizure during patient care for a susceptible patient?

_____

_____

10. List other medical conditions you should consider if your patient is manifesting some clinical signs of a seizure, particularly if the patient's medical history does not indicate a seizure disorder. (_Hint:_ Think "differential diagnosis.")

_____

_____

_____

_____

_____

_____

_____

11. If your patient does have a seizure during dental hygiene treatment, what emergency measures will you take to protect your patient from injury?

_____

_____

_____

_____

_____

_____

_____

12. What oral injuries are associated with tonic–clonic seizures?

_____

_____

_____

13. What action should you take in the event that your patient's tonic–clonic seizure continues for longer than 5 minutes?

_____

_____

_____

_____

14. Describe _status epilepticus._

_____

_____

_____

15. List the types of surgical interventions used to medically treat patients with seizure disorders.

_____

_____

_____

16. Your patient with a seizure disorder is likely to be taking an antiepileptic medication. In your own words, briefly describe the mechanism, incidence, appearance, and effects of phenytoin-induced gingival hyperplasia.

_____

_____

_____

_____

_____

_____

_____

_____

_____

_____

_____

_____

17. What medications, in addition to phenytoin, are associated with gingival overgrowth?

_____

_____

_____

18. Identify dental hygiene treatment and education interventions that can prevent or inhibit the growth of gingival tissues in your patient who is taking phenytoin or another medication associated with gingival enlargement.

_____

_____

_____

_____

_____

19. What surgical options are available for treating phenytoin-induced gingival hyperplasia?

_____

_____

_____

_____

_____

✓ COMPETENCY EXERCISES

Apply information from the chapter and use critical thinking skills to complete the competency exercises. Write responses on paper or create electronic documents to submit your answers.

1. You can tell your new patient has a very business-like approach to his health care. Mr. Arakawa is a 45-year-old chief executive officer in a major corporation in town. As you lead him back to your treatment room, he stops briefly at the front desk to make sure of the procedure for submitting today's charges to his dental insurance. He mentions that he is on a tight schedule and wants to be sure about what time his appointment will end.

He fills out the health history form you hand him with short, efficient strokes of his pen and hands it back to you. The only positive answers on the form are for seizure activity and medication, but he does not indicate what drug he is taking. You know that to completely understand Mr. Arakawa's condition, you must ask him more questions. Create a list of questions you will ask Mr. Arakawa as you clarify his health history information.

2. When you begin to ask Mr. Arakawa the questions you formulated, he briskly states that his history of seizures is not relevant to his dental treatment. He states that his previous dental provider never asked such questions, and, besides, he has not had a seizure for a long time. He tells you about the medication he is taking but is clearly not happy about answering the other questions you are asking.

You know he needs to understand why it is important for you to learn about his history of seizures. What information will you include in your discussion with Mr. Arakawa as you convince him to comply with your request for information about his seizures?

3. Your education/counseling approach is successful and you find out Mr. Arakawa has been experiencing seizures for almost 30 years. The severity of the tonic–clonic-type seizures he experiences has decreased since his teenage years, and in fact, the seizures are now fairly well under control.

The medication he is currently taking is an ethosuximide, but his previous prescription was a phenytoin (Dilantin), which he took for almost 20 years. About 10 years ago, he had gingival surgery to control gingival overgrowth he experienced from taking the phenytoin and fears that his gums are growing again.

Mr. Arakawa experienced some fairly serious dental trauma when he lost consciousness and fell during a seizure, and his maxillary anterior teeth have been replaced with a porcelain bridge. He has often bitten his lips and tongue when he is convulsing. One time when he was young, he experienced a seizure during routine dental treatment and that is why he was at first reluctant and embarrassed to share much information about his seizures with you. He describes the aura that he experiences before a seizure, which appears as flashes of light just outside the direct view of his left eye. He also mentions that sometimes changing patterns of light have caused a seizure to happen and asks you to be careful when positioning the dental light during his treatment. His last seizure was about 2 years ago.

Using your institution's guidelines for writing in patient records, document what you have learned about Mr. Arakawa's medical condition.

4. You know that many medications prescribed to control seizures have numerous side effects, other than gingival hyperplasia, that are concerns for dental professionals. Refer to the list of potential side effects in the "Treatment" section of Chapter 57 in the **textbook** and indicate which side effects have implications for patient education or treatment modifications during Mr. Arakawa's dental hygiene appointments.

EVERYDAY ETHICS

Before completing the learning exercises below, reread and reflect on the Everyday Ethics Scenario and Questions for Consideration in this chapter of the **textbook**. It may also be useful to review the Dental Hygiene Ethics discussion in Chapter 1, the Ethical Applications in the introduction pages for each section in the **textbook**, as well as the Codes of Ethics in **textbook** Appendices I–IV.

Collaborative Learning Activity

Answer each of the questions for consideration at the end of the scenario in the **textbook**. Compare what you wrote with answers developed by another classmate and discuss differences/similarities.

Discovery Activity

Ask a dental hygienist who has been practicing for a year or more to read the scenario. Provide a copy of the Code of Ethics as well. Share the responses you have made to answer each question and ask that person to discuss the situation with you. What insights did you have or what did you learn during this discussion?

Factors to Teach the Patient

This scenario is related to the following factors listed in this chapter of the **textbook**:

▷ Relationship of systemic health to oral health.

▷ Importance of careful daily care of mouth.

▷ Antiepileptic medication side effects, including gingival enlargement and how to minimize its growth.

▷ Seek immediate care if any oral change or injury is suspected.

Use the information provided in Chapter 57 in the **textbook** as a guide to prepare a conversation that you could use to provide patient education for Mr. Arakawa (introduced in the Competency Exercises). As you prepare the conversation, remember that you have already observed Mr. Arakawa's businesslike approach to health care. Use the motivational interviewing approach (see **workbook** Appendix D) to be sure your education approach suits his personality and level of readiness for behavior change.

Use the conversation you create to role-play this situation with a fellow student. If you are the patient in the role-play, be sure to ask questions. If you are the dental hygienist, try to anticipate questions and answer them in your explanation.

MeSH TERMS

Use a combination of MeSH terms and other key words to develop an effective and efficient PubMed literature search strategy.

Seizures
Epilepsy, generalized
Epilepsy, absence
Epilepsy, tonic–clonic

Epilepsy, complex partial
Status epilepticus
Anticonvulsants

CHAPTER 57 WORD SEARCH PUZZLE

```
V I M S T A T U S E P I L E P T I C U S V D C H
U N Q A H G P V M G W L G P G M A C R H O M K Y
Y C Y T S Q D V Z D Q B D Z R A I G V F A R U A
C I N O T A V H I E L F C Q Q N G C F P V M L A
A Q H S S Y W L M I B C I T O K K S E U B A U X
M C U J M P Z U G F U R N T M A K A I D U T Q R
Z T R T Y L L M U I O S O R O Q I J I T O I L D
A Z L P O J H I I S A U L V Q B V X O M F C E U
X N P C E P F H I S A V C B D S L N A Q Q T U E
L A T C I T S O P A U I O C R A O T L T T A R P
M S C J U N V A M L M N Y U M M I L R K A L H U
P F A S H P O S G C A K M T I S K T F U E E X Z
K Y K F D M I L I N I M I C M L O D J L N T P Z
T C D E P T N R C U Z T D C A Z S Y A Y F A Y C
C J U C U H M W Z C E T P N K B G U T V R A K A
B L O S J L P E S P I J A D A K S O W O I H Q F
I Q R I Z O A A P L N V G E R I E M D O B C N
A I S N X I P I M I H G O D I N G Y N P C A F E
H L N N L I Z G T U L P O T H B M Q S C V O J Q
V A O I S Y S R V R L E E Y U A I W D P E Z E K
Z D T K I U I X C X A L P Q L F R F I G A U C J
P L G Y M G G R Q T O P Q S R S F D D D S S N E
S Z R G J P W A J A C F F U Y M T U D K M N M Z
A I T S H C X F V L W G G L W X N W D R F E O V
```

Puzzle Clues

1. A life-threatening emergency related to seizure disorders (two words).
2. Refers to a group of functional disorders of the brain characterized by recurrent seizures.
3. Abnormal hairiness.
4. Sudden recurrence or intensification of sharp spasms or convulsions.
5. Seizure that involves only part of the brain.
6. Uncontrolled motor activity, such as repeated swallowing.
7. Period of time after a seizure.
8. A peculiar prodromal sensation experienced by some people immediately preceding a seizure.
9. Former term for a type of tonic–clonic epileptic seizure (two words).
10. Active, acute phase of an epileptic seizure.
11. Shock-like contractions of muscles or groups of muscles.
12. Refers to irregular muscle action.
13. Former term for absence seizure (two words).
14. Class of anticonvulsant drugs highly correlated with gingival hyperplasia.
15. Sudden, involuntary contraction.
16. Drop attacks or drop seizures.
17. Type of seizure in which there is alternate contraction and relaxation of muscles (two words).
18. Term associated with symptoms such as pallor, flushing, sweating, pupillary dilation, cardiac arrhythmia, or incontinence.
19. A type of seizure in which the person experiences a brief impairment of consciousness before a return to awareness with no recollection of the seizure.
20. Nerve that is stimulated by a pacemaker-like device implanted to reduce seizures.
21. Type of contraction that causes the patient to appear stiff.
22. Seizures of unknown onset.

58

The Patient with a Mental Health Disorder

 KNOWLEDGE EXERCISES

Write your answers for each question in the space provided.

1. Why is it more appropriate to refer to your patient as "an individual with bulimia" rather than as "a bulimic"?

2. List the four types of anxiety disorders described in the **textbook**.

3. Briefly describe each of the three types of treatment provided for a patient with anxiety disorder.

4. What oral problems are associated with anxiety disorders?

5. List ways to reduce anxiety and enhance the patient's feeling of being in control while you are providing dental hygiene care.

6. Briefly describe postpartum depression.

7. List the common signs and symptoms that may indicate someone is experiencing an episode of depression.

_____

_____

_____

_____

_____

_____

_____

_____

_____

_____

8. In addition to those discussed for anxiety disorders, what additional treatment modality is sometimes provided for a patient with a depressive disorder?

_____

9. List the types of antidepressant medications you may see on the medical history of a patient being treated for a depressive disorder.

_____

_____

_____

_____

_____

_____

10. What is the most common oral side effect of the antidepressant medications used by patients with depression?

_____

11. Briefly describe why a patient with depression is at higher risk for dental caries.

_____

_____

_____

12. Why might you consider offering tinted protective eyewear for a patient who is taking medications to treat depression?

_____

_____

_____

13. List one specific behavior to avoid in your approach to oral health education for a patient with depression.

_____

14. Define _euphoria_.

_____

_____

15. In what way is bipolar disorder different from a depressive disorder?

_____

_____

16. In your own words, briefly summarize the characteristics common to the manic phase of bipolar disorder.

_____

_____

_____

_____

17. List the categories of drugs used to treat bipolar disorder.

_____

_____

_____

_____

18. What drug used to treat bipolar disorder can impart a metallic taste in your patient's mouth?

_____

19. Define _dysgeusia_.

_____

20. What is _pica_?

_____

_____

21. In your own words, briefly describe and compare the major eating disorders listed below.
  • _Anorexia nervosa:_

_____

_____

- *Bulimia nervosa:*

_____

_____

_____

_____

_____

- *Binge-eating disorder:*

_____

_____

_____

_____

- *Diabulimia:*

_____

_____

_____

_____

_____

- *Orthorexia nervosa:*

_____

_____

_____

_____

_____

22. What medical complication related to the orofacial region can arise from excessive purging behaviors?

_____

_____

23. Discuss the effects of perimolysis as it relates to purging behaviors.

_____

_____

_____

_____

_____

_____

24. Briefly describe factors that increase the risk for negative oral effects when a patient has an eating disorder.

- *Dental caries:*

_____

_____

- *Mucosal lesions:*

_____

_____

- *Periodontal disease:*

_____

_____

- *Hypersensitive teeth:*

_____

_____

- *Trauma:*

_____

_____

_____

25. What changes in saliva contribute to oral problems often identified in patients with an eating disorder?

_____

_____

_____

26. In your own words, define *schizophrenia.*

_____

_____

_____

_____

27. List and briefly describe each of the three categories of symptoms you might observe in a patient with schizophrenia.

_____

_____

_____

_____

_____

_____

_____

28. Identify the concept or term defined by each of the following statements.

- A *false sensory perception in the absence of an actual external stimulus:*

_____

- A *false belief firmly held although contradicted by social reality:*

_____

29. Unfortunately, many people diagnosed with schizophrenia also have high rates of _____.

30. List the major categories of psychotropic medications.

_____

_____

_____

_____

_____

31. List the potential oral effects of antipsychotic medications.

_____

_____

_____

_____

32. List the potential physical side effects of antipsychotic medication that may require modifications during dental hygiene care.

_____

_____

_____

_____

_____

_____

33. In your own words define *dysarthria?*

_____

_____

34. What is tardive dyskinesia?

_____

_____

35. During a scaling and root planing procedure, how can you facilitate safety and comfort of your patient with tardive dyskinesia?

_____

36. In your own words, describe measures you can take to prevent or prepare for a psychiatric emergency.

_____

_____

_____

_____

37. If your patient has a panic attack while you are providing dental hygiene care, what will you do?

_____

_____

_____

_____

_____

_____

COMPETENCY EXERCISES

Apply information from the chapter and use critical thinking skills to complete the competency exercises. Write responses on paper or create electronic documents to submit your answers.

1. Study the list of potential effects of antipsychotic medications in Table 58-1 in the **textbook**. Identify at least three modifications you can make beyond your usual clinical routines to ensure the comfort and safety of your patient who is taking an antipsychotic medication.

2. When you check his health history before calling Jack into your treatment room at the VA hospital, you notice he has been diagnosed with posttraumatic stress disorder. You greet him cheerfully, talk to him brightly all the way down the hall to your room about how beautifully the sun is shining today. You ask him, with a smile, if there have been any changes in his medications since he was last seen in the dental clinic.

But you notice that his only response is to stand beside you trembling and shaking. You immediately suspect that he is displaying symptoms of a panic attack. Describe what additional assessment measures are appropriate to help determine if your suspicion is correct. Describe how you will you react to Jack's obvious distress?

3. After he has calmed down, you and Jack decide together to reschedule his dental hygiene appointment for another day. Use the SOAP note format or your clinic's form for recording a patient visit to develop a progress note to document what happened at today's appointment.

4. Shaun Kennedy, a newspaper reporter, has been your patient for several years. You always enjoy the stories he tells about working for the newspaper. His oral hygiene has never been particularly good, and you have been really working with him each time he comes in to make sure he understands how his risk for oral disease increases when he doesn't thoroughly remove the dental biofilm from his teeth every day. You know that he is receiving treatment for bipolar disorder, but, so far, you have not noticed that he ever displays any symptoms of either the manic phase or the depressive phase of his disease.

Today, Shaun is talking a mile a minute about a new novel he has started writing. As he gets more excited about telling you the plot of the novel, he actually pushes your hands aside, leaps up from the chair, and walks back and forth in your small treatment space! You would really like to convince him to get back in the dental chair so you can complete your oral hygiene instructions in a timely manner. What can happen if you pressure him to comply? Given Shaun's behavior today, how can you sensitively and realistically approach this situation?

5. Isabella Stamos, 13 years old, is a beautiful girl with long curly blond hair, huge green eyes, and an already successful modeling career. You still have not started your intraoral examination, but after talking to her and observing her for several minutes, you suspect that she has an eating disorder. What clinical clues or signs can you look for to help confirm your impressions? What questions will you ask Isabella to help you determine if your suspicions are correct?

6. After you have questioned Isabella and completed an intraoral examination, it becomes clear that she is battling with bulimia nervosa. What ethical factors will you take into consideration when you discuss your assessment findings and Isabella's oral health needs with her mother at the end of the appointment?

Factors to Teach the Patient

This scenario is related to the following factors listed in this chapter of the **textbook**:

▷ The causes and effects of enamel erosion; the high acidity of the vomitus from the stomach.

▷ How to rinse after vomiting but not brush immediately; demineralization begins promptly after the acid from the stomach reaches the teeth, and brushing can cause abrasion of the demineralizing enamel.

▷ The need for multiple fluoride applications through use of home dentifrice, rinse, and brush-on gel, as well as professional application of varnish or gel-tray at regular dental hygiene appointments.

You have talked with Isabella (introduced in the Competency Exercises in this chapter) about some ways she can receive help with her eating disorder, but as a dental hygienist, you know that the most important thing you can do is educate her about the risks to her oral health.

Use the principles of motivational interviewing (see **workbook** Appendix D) as a guide, and taking into account the personal factors that often accompany this disorder, educate Isabella about the negative oral findings common in a patient with bulimia. Discuss strategies for protecting her teeth and gums until she gets her eating behaviors under control.

EVERYDAY ETHICS

Before completing the learning exercises below, reread and reflect on the Everyday Ethics Scenario and Questions for Consideration in this chapter of the **textbook**. It may also be useful to review the Dental Hygiene Ethics discussion in Chapter 1, the Ethical Applications in the introduction pages for each section in the **textbook**, as well as the Codes of Ethics in **textbook** Appendices I–IV.

Individual Learning Activity

Imagine that you are the dental hygienist in this scenario. Answer each of the questions for consideration at the end of the scenario.

Discovery Activity

Ask a dental hygienist who has been practicing for a year or more to read the scenario. Provide them with a copy of the Code of Ethics as well. Share the responses you have made to answer each question and ask that person to discuss the situation with you. What insights did you have or what did you learn during this discussion?

MeSH TERMS

Use a combination of MeSH terms and other key words to develop an effective and efficient PubMed literature search strategy.

Anxiety disorders
Obsessive-compulsive
  disorder
Panic disorder
Stress disorders,
  traumatic
Depression

Depressive disorder
Depression, postpartum
Bipolar disorder
Schizophrenia pica
Anorexia nervosa
Bulimia nervosa
Binge-eating disorder

59

The Patient with a Substance-Related Disorder

 KNOWLEDGE EXERCISES

Write your answers for each question in the space provided.

1. Define the following terms and concepts in your own words to help you differentiate them and understand what they mean.

- *Substance abuse:*

  _____

  _____

- *Dependence:*

  _____

  _____

  _____

- *Addiction:*

  _____

  _____

- *Tolerance:*

  _____

  _____

- *Alcohol use disorder:*

  _____

  _____

- *Detoxification:*

  _____

  _____

2. What is the difference between chemical, physical, and psychological dependence?

_____

_____

_____

_____

_____

_____

3. In your own words, define moderate use of alcohol by women and men.

_____

_____

_____

4. Identify the signs of alcoholism.

_____

_____

_____

_____

_____

5. What is *acne rosacea?*

_____

_____

_____

_____

6. What factors contribute to the etiology of alcoholism?

_____

_____

_____

7. How is the concentration of alcohol in the blood measured?

_____

_____

_____

_____

8. What behavioral characteristics, if you observe them in an otherwise healthy patient, might indicate that your patient is intoxicated?

_____

_____

_____

_____

9. Define *nystagmus.*

_____

_____

10. The liver is the organ most severely affected by chronic alcohol abuse. Briefly describe the adverse effects of excessive or prolonged alcohol use on each of the following body systems.

   • *Immune system:*

   _____

   _____

   • *Digestive system:*

   _____

   _____

   _____

   _____

   • *Cardiovascular system:*

   _____

   _____

   _____

   • *Nervous system:*

   _____

   _____

   _____

   _____

   _____

   • *Reproductive system:*

   _____

   _____

   _____

11. In what ways does excessive alcohol consumption affect nutritional intake?

   _____

   _____

   _____

   _____

12. Describe the two types of complications that can occur if an individual abruptly withdraws from alcohol use.
    - *Alcohol hallucinosis:*

    _____

    _____

    _____

    - *Alcohol withdrawal delirium (DTs):*

    _____

    _____

    _____

    _____

    _____

13. Identify factors that can increase the severity of the symptoms that a person with alcoholism may experience if he or she abruptly ceases drinking.

    _____

    _____

    _____

    _____

14. What is the overall objective of treatment provided to support an individual who is recovering from alcoholism?

    _____

    _____

15. List the four components of an alcohol treatment program.

    _____

    _____

    _____

    _____

16. Your patient who is participating in an alcohol recovery program may be taking an alcohol-sensitizing agent because these drugs act as a deterrent to consuming alcohol. If alcohol is taken, this drug interferes with the conversion of _____ to _____ in the liver and makes the patient very ill.

17. Identify the drug prescribed for the recovering alcoholic to help inhibit or decrease the desire to consume alcohol.

    _____

18. Use of alcohol during pregnancy can seriously threaten the health of the baby because _____.

19. List the other factors that when combined with alcohol use during pregnancy influence the health of the mother and baby.

    _____

    _____

    _____

    _____

    _____

20. Describe the physical features that can be observed in an infant with FASD.

    _____

    _____

    _____

    _____

21. Identify behavioral, cognitive, and psychomotor factors associated with FASD.

    _____

    _____

    _____

    _____

    _____

    _____

22. List the categories of drugs that are most commonly abused.

    _____

    _____

    _____

    _____

23. Describe the characteristics of a drug classified as a U.S. Drug Enforcement Administration Schedule II drug.

    _____

    _____

    _____

    _____

24. Identify oral manifestations associated with the use of each of the following drugs.

- *Methamphetamine:*

_____

_____

_____

_____

_____

- *Speed, ecstasy, and other amphetamine-based drugs:*

_____

_____

_____

_____

_____

_____

- *Cocaine:*

_____

_____

_____

_____

_____

_____

- *Cannabis:*

_____

_____

_____

_____

25. Which body systems can be adversely affected by excessive use of drugs?

_____

_____

_____

_____

_____

_____

26. Identify medications commonly used to assist in lessening withdrawal symptoms during treatment for drug abuse.

_____

_____

_____

27. In your own words, summarize the responsibility of dental team members in managing the risk for prescription drug abuse.

_____

_____

_____

_____

28. List actions that healthcare providers can take to avoid prescription pad theft.

_____

_____

_____

_____

_____

_____

_____

_____

_____

✓ COMPETENCY EXERCISES

Apply information from the chapter and use critical thinking skills to complete the competency exercises. Write responses on paper or create electronic documents to submit your answers.

1. Explain why it is especially important to inspect intraoral tissues each time you assess a patient who has a past or current history of excessive alcohol consumption or drug use.

2. Your afternoon patient is 20 minutes late for her appointment; she is a well-dressed woman in a business suit and is new patient to the office. As you review her medical history, you notice her breath smells of alcohol and she answered "yes" to the question concerning having one or more drinks a day. You explain

the office policy that a "yes" answer to that question requires you to give her an additional questionnaire; you ask if she is willing to answer additional questions and she complies. The patient answers "yes" for all four questions. She immediately engages you in a discussion concerning her answers. The patient admits that she has been trying to stop drinking because she has noticed red areas in her mouth; she states that no matter how much she brushes her gums bleed, they are red and swollen all the time. The patient lives alone and feels very guilty about her habit; lately she needs a drink in the morning before going to work and at night before going to sleep. She has no family.

As you question her further, you determine that her colleagues make annoying comments about her breath and criticize her for drinking. The patient has also answered "yes" to increasing pains in her stomach.

What medical referral would this patient require, and why?

Is this patient at increased risk for drug abuse, and why?

3. Your next patient is Justin Townsley, age 21. He has just returned home from his first year away at college. His mother has made a dental hygiene appointment for him because he has not had his teeth examined in at last 3 years. She also wants him to have his wisdom teeth extracted before he is no longer covered under her dental insurance plan. When you go to greet Justin in the reception area, you overhear the end of a cell phone conversation in which he is planning to meet his buddies later on this evening to go out partying. "And, we'll stay out all night so we can have even more fun *this* time than we did *last* time," he says just before he hangs up the telephone to greet you. He stumbles just a bit as he rises from the chair but recovers quickly to follow you to the treatment room. As he walks past you into the chair, you distinctly catch the odor of alcohol on his breath.

Justin's health history is unremarkable, except for having an arm broken in an automobile accident last year. He states that he does not take any regular medications. When you take his pulse and blood pressure today, both are slightly elevated.

Your intraoral findings include generalized poor oral hygiene, significant calculus deposits, coated tongue, dry oral mucosa, red and swollen gingiva, generalized 4- to 6-mm probing depths, and generalized bleeding on probing. Justin states, "the left side of my jaw has been aching a lot lately, probably from grinding my teeth." A front tooth and the cusp of an upper premolar are both slightly chipped, findings that were not previously noted. As you are working to complete your oral assessment, Justin keeps up a constant conversation about how much fun he has had this year while he was away at college. He sheepishly admits that his daily oral care has suffered, saying, "I stay up all night sometimes—to study for all those mid-term and final exams, you know. Sometimes I just forget to brush."

You decide that you need to ask Justin about his drinking and the possible use of stimulant drugs. Identify the assessment findings that lead you to this decision.

What oral signs and symptoms will you look for as you continue your assessment?

What additional follow-up questions will you ask Justin to help you determine his patterns of alcohol and/or drug use?

4. Your careful and sensitive questioning leads you to believe that Justin's level of alcohol consumption and possible use of street drugs is probably having some detrimental impact on his health status. You are concerned enough that you discuss the matter with him and you give him a brochure about the oral effects of alcohol. You plan to bring your concerns for his health up again at his subsequent appointments. When you write a dental hygiene care plan for Justin, you will plan two additional visits for scaling and root planing his entire mouth. What education/counseling and oral hygiene instructions/home care interventions will you plan to help Justin maximize healing and tissue response during and after oral debridement? (*Hint:* If you write dental hygiene diagnosis statements for Justin, it may help you decide on your planned interventions.)

5. Using your institution's guidelines for writing in patient records, document progress notes for your first appointment with Justin.

EVERYDAY ETHICS

Before completing the learning exercises below, reread and reflect on the Everyday Ethics Scenario and Questions for Consideration in this chapter of the **textbook**. It may also be useful to review the Dental Hygiene Ethics discussion in Chapter 1, the Ethical Applications in the introduction pages for each section in the **textbook**, as well as the Codes of Ethics in **textbook** Appendices I–IV.

Individual Learning Activity

Imagine that you have observed what happened in the scenario, but are not one of the main characters involved in the situation. Write a reflective journal entry that:

- Describes how you might have reacted (as an observer—not as a participant),
- Expresses your personal feelings about what happened, or
- Identifies personal values that affect your reaction to the situation.

Discovery Activity

Summarize this scenario for faculty member at your school and ask them to consider the questions that are included. Is their perspective different than yours or similar? Explain.

Factors to Teach the Patient

This scenario is related to the following factors listed in this chapter of the **textbook**:

▷ Drug abuse is a great risk to overall health.

▷ The risk of oral cancer is increased by the use of alcohol.

▷ Routine oral screening is needed at least twice a year to check for signs of early cancer.

▷ Drinking alcohol and using other drugs (prescription or over the counter) can lead to medical emergencies. Always check each drug and its action before using it in combination with alcohol or in combination with another drug.

Discussing your concerns about potential substance abuse with a patient like Justin Townsley (introduced in Competency Exercises question #3) requires building trust. You will be more successful in educating Justin and changing his health behaviors if you approach him without disapproval or judgment, but instead provide important information that motivates him to make changes in his own behaviors.

Use information in Chapter 59 of the **textbook** and the principles of motivational interviewing (see **workbook** Appendix D) as guides to develop a conversation you will use to discuss the negative effects that alcohol and other drugs can have on Justin's health status.

Use the conversation you create to role-play this situation with a friend or fellow student. If you are the patient in the role-play, be sure to ask questions. If you are the dental hygienist, try to anticipate questions and answer them in your explanation. Modify your conversation based on what you learned.

MeSH TERMS

Use a combination of MeSH terms and other key words to develop an effective and efficient PubMed literature search strategy.

Substance-related disorders
Substance abuse detection
Street drugs
Methamphetamine
Abnormalities, drug-induced
Cocaine-related disorders
Crack cocaine
Marijuana abuse
Amphetamine-related disorders
Alcoholics
Alcoholism
Alcohol drinking
Alcoholic intoxication
Alcohol-induced disorders
Fetal alcohol syndrome

60

The Patient with a Respiratory Disease

KNOWLEDGE EXERCISES

Write your answers for each question in the space provided.

1. Describe four additional infection control practices that can be implemented to help prevent transmission of respiratory infections.

   _____

   _____

   _____

   _____

   _____

2. What vital signs, related to respiratory function, are assessed at each patient visit?

   _____

   _____

   _____

   _____

3. Define *dyspnea*.

   _____

4. What medical test measures various aspects of breathing and lung function?

   _____

5. When performing a pulse oximetry test, what level of blood oxygen saturation signifies poor oxygen exchange?

   _____

6. What should you do if you recognize your patient is experiencing symptoms of respiratory distress during dental hygiene treatment?

   _____

   _____

7. A patient in respiratory distress may experience hypoxia. What patient signs and symptoms characterize hypoxia?

_____

_____

_____

_____

8. _____ is defined as a breathing rate of greater than 20 breaths per minute. A patient who is breathing very rapidly can experience _____, which may lead to dizziness and possible syncope.

9. What body structures are considered to be in the upper respiratory system?

_____

_____

_____

_____

10. What body structures comprise the lower respiratory system?

_____

_____

_____

_____

11. What are the pleura?

_____

12. Identify two functions of the mucus secreted from goblet cells in respiratory mucosa?

_____

_____

13. What happens when an inflammatory disease causes an overproduction of mucus?

_____

_____

14. Identify three upper respiratory diseases more likely to be viral rather than bacterial infections.

_____

_____

_____

15. What medication is used primarily to treat bacterial respiratory infections but is not prescribed for infections caused by a virus or fungus?

_____

16. How are upper respiratory infections transmitted?

_____

_____

17. How can you best prevent transmission of pathogens while you are providing dental hygiene treatment?

_____

_____

18. What type of upper respiratory infection can cause tooth pain?

_____

19. Identify two oral side effects of medications commonly used to treat upper respiratory infections.

_____

_____

20. What oral lesions can accompany the infectious stage of an upper respiratory infection?

_____

_____

_____

_____

21. List the lower respiratory tract diseases described in this chapter.

_____

_____

_____

_____

_____

_____

_____

22. Identify three types of organisms that can cause pneumonia.

_____

_____

_____

23. What medical treatment is provided for each type of pneumonia identified in question 22?

_____

_____

_____

24. What pathogen causes a type of pneumonia most often associated with immune-impaired individuals?

_____

25. Pneumonia infection that occurs from person-to-person transmission (not in a healthcare facility) is called:

_____

26. What is one potential cause for HCAP or NCAP pneumonia?

_____

27. What signs and symptoms are associated with tuberculosis?

_____

_____

_____

_____

_____

_____

28. How is tuberculosis transmitted?

_____

_____

29. How is clinically active tuberculosis diagnosed?

_____

_____

_____

30. What two diagnostic tests are used to determine a latent tuberculosis infection?

_____

_____

31. What medication regimen is used to treat the clinically active stage of tuberculosis?

_____

_____

_____

_____

_____

_____

_____

32. What oral condition is associated with the causative agent of tuberculosis?

_____

33. List five types of asthma based on pathophysiology.

_____

_____

_____

_____

_____

34. List the four National Asthma Education and Prevention Program classifications of asthma.

_____

_____

_____

_____

35. What are the signs and symptoms of an asthma attack?

_____

_____

_____

_____

36. True or False? Corticosteroids and mast call stabilizers are examples of short-term control medications for asthma.

37. List the types of drugs an individual with asthma needs to avoid and briefly describe the reason for each.

_____

_____

_____

_____

_____

_____

38. What ingredient in local anesthetic solutions can be a risk factor for asthma attack?

_____

_____

39. What oral condition(s) may occur in patients being treated for asthma?

_____

_____

_____

_____

_____

40. What is the primary cause of COPD?

_____

_____

_____

41. Patients with COPD who are chronic smokers have an increased risk for which oral conditions?

_____

_____

_____

_____

42. The term blue bloater is related to _____.

43. Describe the cough of an individual with chronic bronchitis?

_____

_____

44. What are the symptoms of emphysema?

_____

_____

_____

_____

_____

_____

45. Cystic fibrosis is an autosomal recessive gene disorder that affects the _____ tract, the _____ tract, and the _____.

46. What oral changes are likely to occur as cystic fibrosis progresses?

_____

47. In your own words, briefly describe sleep apnea and summarize dental hygiene care protocols for the patient who uses a CPAP machine.

_____

_____

_____

_____

_____

_____

_____

48. Complete Infomap 60-1 to compare three types of hypersensitivity reactions.

INFOMAP 60-1		
CONDITION	PATHOGENESIS	SIGNS/SYMPTOMS
Allergic rhinitis (hay fever)		
Atopic asthma		
Anaphylaxis		

COMPETENCY EXERCISES

Apply information from the chapter and use critical thinking skills to complete the competency exercises. Write responses on paper or create electronic documents to submit your answers.

1. Charles Marcin, a handsome blond gentleman who is 67 years old, has been a patient in the practice for many years; however, this is the first time you have met him. His health history confirms your first impression of Mr. Marcin as a patient with COPD, and you are reminded of the term pink puffer. You observe Mr. Marcin carefully as he walks the short distance from the reception room to your treatment room. He rests with his head bent and his hands on the back of the dental chair to catch his breath before he sits down.

   Describe what you observe as you watch Mr. Marcin's breathing pattern and explain how it is different from the breathing pattern of an individual with other respiratory diseases.

2. When he can talk again, Mr. Marcin reminds you to call him Charlie. He says he has recently had a bit of a cold but is feeling somewhat better now. He tells you that his cough has pretty much gone away, and he isn't blowing his nose every 5 minutes any more. He complains that this is already his second cold this year, and once he was treated for a sinus infection. He mentions his teeth are stained because he has been drinking so much hot tea lately, and he is excited about being in your office today so that he can have an especially bright smile for his daughter's wedding this coming weekend. You think back to everything you learned about respiratory diseases as you plan Mr. Marcin's appointment for today. What safety and comfort factors will you need to assess and consider as you provide care during Mr. Marcin's dental hygiene appointment today?

3. Mr. Mitch Angelo is currently taking several medications to treat his asthma. When you are examining his mouth, you notice enamel erosion on the lingual areas of the anterior teeth. Explain what is happening that may be contributing to this oral condition.

4. When you have completed the first quadrant of scaling and root planing, you mention to Mr. Angelo that the gingival tissue in that area might be a bit sensitive later on today. He asks you what he should do if he feels pain. Which analgesics does a patient with asthma need to avoid?

5. When you update his medical history, Mr. Ben Samuelson, a 45-year-old businessman, tells you that he has been taking a new medication called isoniazid. When you question him further, he states that he does not know why he is taking it. What follow-up questions will you ask Mr. Samuelson?

6. What additional steps will you take prior to beginning your assessment of Mr. Samuelson's oral condition?

7. Explain the role of oral bacteria as a potential pathogenic agent in pneumonia, particularly if the patient is debilitated or chronically ill.

Factors to Teach the Patient

This scenario is related to the following factors listed in this chapter of the **textbook**:

▷ The need for frequent handwashing to help prevent transmission of respiratory disease.

▷ The need for thorough daily cleaning of toothbrushes to help prevent spread of infections.

▷ How using a new toothbrush and cleaning dentures/orthodontic appliances after bacterial infections can decrease the possibility of reinfection.

▷ Why elderly patients and those with chronic cardiovascular disease, diabetes, and other immunosuppressed conditions should receive a pneumonia vaccine and annual influenza immunizations.

Because of Mr. Marcin's chronic emphysema (patient introduced in Competency Exercises for this chapter), you are concerned about his recurring upper respiratory infections. Use the information in Chapter 60 in the **textbook** and the principles of motivational interviewing (see **workbook** Appendix D) as guides to write a statement explaining ways that Mr. Marcin can reduce his risk for more serious acute respiratory diseases.

MeSH TERMS

Use a combination of MeSH terms and other key words to develop an effective and efficient PubMed literature search strategy.

Respiratory system	Bronchitis
Asthma	Lung diseases
Respiratory tract diseases	Bronchitis, chronic
Pulmonary emphysema	Pulmonary disease,
Respiratory tract infections	chronic obstructive

EVERYDAY ETHICS

Before completing the learning exercises below, reread and reflect on the Everyday Ethics Scenario and Questions for Consideration in this chapter of the **textbook**. It may also be useful to review the Dental Hygiene Ethics discussion in Chapter 1, the Ethical Applications in the introduction pages for each section in the **textbook**, as well as the Codes of Ethics in **textbook** Appendices I–IV.

Collaborative Learning Activity

Answer each of the questions for consideration at the end of the scenario in the **textbook**. Compare what you wrote with answers developed by another classmate and discuss differences/similarities.

Discovery Activity

Summarize this scenario for faculty member at your school and ask them to consider the questions that are included. Is their perspective different than yours or similar? Explain.

The Patient with Cardiovascular Disease

KNOWLEDGE EXERCISES

Write your answers for each question in the space provided.

1. Explain the two classifications of heart diseases.

_____

_____

_____

_____

2. Identify the various tissues in the heart that can be affected by cardiovascular disease.

_____

_____

_____

_____

3. In your own words, describe the progression and diagnosis of infective endocarditis.

_____

_____

_____

_____

_____

_____

_____

_____

_____

_____

4. List steps you can take to prevent infection during oral assessment and dental hygiene treatment if you suspect your patient is at risk for infective endocarditis.

_____

_____

_____

_____

_____

_____

_____

_____

_____

_____

_____

5. Refer to Figure 61-1 in the **textbook** to help you visualize the veins, arteries, and chambers of a healthy heart. Describe the sequence of the normal flow of blood.

_____

_____

_____

_____

_____

_____

_____

_____

_____

_____

_____

6. Congenital heart disease is the result of anatomic anomalies that occur during the first _____ weeks of fetal development. The exact cause is often unknown but is _____, _____, or a combination of the two.

7. Refer to Figures 61-2 and 61-3 from the **textbook** to help you describe how the normal path of blood flow is compromised in each of the two types of congenital heart disease.

  • _Ventricular septal defect:_

_____

_____

_____

_____

  • _Patent ductus arteriosus:_

_____

_____

_____

_____

8. What symptoms of congenital heart disease may affect the delivery of dental hygiene care?

_____

_____

_____

_____

_____

_____

9. What is the etiology of rheumatic heart disease?

_____

_____

_____

_____

10. Describe how the flow of blood through the heart is altered when there is a mitral valve prolapse.

_____

_____

_____

11. In your own words, explain why screening for hypertension is an essential component of dental hygiene care.

_____

_____

_____

_____

12. Identify the sequelae of long-standing hypertension.

_____

_____

_____

_____

_____

_____

_____

13. From memory (don't look the **textbook**), list the systolic and diastolic values that determine normal adult blood pressure, elevated pressure, and stage 1 and stage 2 hypertension.

_____

_____

_____

_____

14. What systolic and diastolic values indicate a hypertensive crisis?

_____

_____

15. What blood pressure level triggers concern for your child patient? (_Hint:_ You can also see Chapter 12 for specific systolic and diastolic values.)

_____

16. Identify modifiable patient lifestyle risk factors associated with essential hypertension.

_____

_____

_____

_____

_____

17. Ischemic heart disease arises from reduction of _____ to the heart muscle.

18. What is the principle cause of ischemic heart disease?

_____

19. What are the modifiable (lifestyle) risk factors for ischemic heart disease?

_____

_____

_____

_____

_____

20. What are the signs and symptoms of angina pectoris?

_____

_____

_____

_____

_____

_____

21. What is the difference between stable and unstable angina?

_____

_____

_____

_____

_____

22. What is the cause of myocardial infarction?

_____

_____

_____

_____

_____

23. What is the most common artery associated with myocardial infarction?

_____

_____

24. The symptoms of myocardial infarction are similar to the symptoms of angina pectoris. What circumstances indicate that you should summon immediate medical assistance for your patient and be ready to administer basic life support?

_____

_____

_____

_____

25. Explain how the symptoms of myocardial infarction may differ between men and women.

_____

_____

_____

_____

_____

_____

26. Identify the basic steps of patient management during a possible myocardial infarction attack. (*Hint:* Also see Chapter 9.)

_____

_____

_____

_____

27. After a myocardial infarction, your patient's elective dental and dental hygiene treatment is postponed until _____.

28. What is congestive heart failure?

_____

_____

_____

_____

_____

29. Identify the underlying causes and precipitating factors associated with congestive heart failure.

_____

_____

_____

_____

_____

_____

30. If your patient's medical history indicates chronic congestive heart failure, what symptoms can you observe that will indicate whether the right-hand or the left-hand side of the heart is affected?

Left-hand side of heart:

_____

_____

_____

Right-hand side of heart:

_____

_____

_____

_____

31. What are the symptoms of cardiac arrhythmia?

_____

_____

_____

_____

32. What lifestyle changes are commonly recommended for patients with cardiovascular disease?

_____

_____

_____

_____

33. What two categories of surgical intervention can be used to treat heart disease?

_____

_____

34. A coronary stent is put in place to _____ the blocked blood vessel and prevent renarrowing of the lumen.

35. What is the purpose of a cardiac pacemaker or implantable defibrillator?

_____

_____

36. What dental devices are discouraged if the patient has a cardiac pacemaker or implantable defibrillator?

_____

37. Identify clinical procedures that will protect a patient who is receiving anticoagulant therapy during nonsurgical periodontal therapy.

_____

_____

_____

_____

_____

_____

_____

_____

COMPETENCY EXERCISES

Apply information from the chapter and use critical thinking skills to complete the competency exercises. Write responses on paper or create electronic documents to submit your answers.

1. Review your school's dental clinic policy and guidelines for screening and treating patients with hypertension and answer the following questions.

    At what intervals are patients' blood pressure readings recorded in the patient record?

    At what level are patients referred for a physician consult?

    At what level is administration of local anesthetic compromised?

    At what blood pressure classification or level will you suspend planned dental hygiene treatment and reschedule your patient after medical intervention?

2. What is the goal of providing dental hygiene treatment before and after cardiac surgery?

3. When you update her health history at her 3-month dental hygiene visit, Mrs. LaShawn Peal tells you her physician has recently prescribed anticoagulant therapy to treat a cardiac condition. She states that she doesn't really understand what the medication is for, exactly, and that the prothrombin time test you ask her about was not recommended by her physician. She minimizes the issue and tells you if her doctor isn't worried about this kind of thing, then neither is she. She protests vehemently when you mention you need to contact her physician for a consultation before you begin her dental hygiene treatment. Using patient-appropriate language, explain why you will require a physician consult before you begin dental hygiene treatment for Mrs. Peal.

4. When you contact Mrs. Peal's physician, he tells you that he will order the test. Mrs. Peal can stop by any time to have it done. You return to the treatment room to explain the situation to Mrs. Peal. Using your institution's guidelines for writing in patient records, document why Mrs. Peal was dismissed today and her dental hygiene appointment rescheduled.

DISCOVERY EXERCISE

Visit the American Heart Association website at http://www.heart.org and use the website search box to learn more about conditions that put your patient at risk for infective endocarditis and access the latest guidelines for premedication.

MeSH TERMS

Use a combination of MeSH terms and other key words to develop an effective and efficient PubMed literature search strategy.

Cardiovascular diseases	Hypertension
Coronary artery disease	Hypertension, malignant
Myocardial infarction	Prehypertension
Cardiovascular infections	Angina pectoris
Endocarditis, bacterial	Mitral valve prolapse
Atherosclerosis	Pacemaker, artificial
Arteriosclerosis	Rheumatic heart disease

EVERYDAY ETHICS

Before completing the learning exercises below, reread and reflect on the Everyday Ethics Scenario and Questions for Consideration in this chapter of the **textbook**. It may also be useful to review the Dental Hygiene Ethics discussion in Chapter 1, the Ethical Applications in the introduction pages for each section in the **textbook**, as well as the Codes of Ethics in **textbook** Appendices I–IV.

Individual Learning Activity

Imagine that you have observed what happened in the scenario, but are not one of the main characters involved in the situation. Write a reflective journal entry that:

- Describes how you might have reacted (as an observer—not as a participant),
- Expresses your personal feelings about what happened, or
- Identifies personal values that affect your reaction to the situation.

Collaborative Learning Activity

Work with a small group to develop a 2- to 5-minute role-play that introduces the Everyday Ethics scenario described in the chapter (a great idea is to video record your role-play activity). Then develop separate 2-minute role-play scenarios that provide at least two alternative approaches/solutions to resolving the situation. Ask classmates to view the solutions, ask questions, and discuss the ethical approach used in each. Ask for a vote on which solution classmates determine to be the "best."

Factors To Teach the Patient

This scenario is related to the Stress Reduction Procedures listed in the Factors to Teach the Patient section of this chapter in the **textbook**.

When you read the patient record before seating Mr. Pedro Valdez (age 58) for his dental hygiene continuing care appointment, you note that he has a very complex history of cardiovascular disease, including myocardial infarction 6 years ago. When you call his name in the reception area, he looks up at you while coughing into a tissue. He comments that you are not the dental hygienist he usually sees for his appointment. He rises wearily from the chair, complains briefly he has been waiting quite a long time, and walks with you to your treatment room.

As you stroll slowly beside him, you notice he is pale, and the back of his neck is sweating. When he reaches the dental chair, he collapses into it breathing heavily. While you take his blood pressure, you note that his skin feels quite cold, his fingernail beds look bluish, and his wrists and ankles appear quite swollen. You record a blood pressure of 135/95 mmHg on his right arm and a resting pulse of 83 beats per minute. When you begin to lower the dental chair for your intraoral examination, he becomes agitated, leans forward in the chair, and tells you that he has to sit up straight to be comfortable.

Use the information in Chapter 61 in the **textbook** and the motivational interviewing principles in **workbook** Appendix D as guides to prepare an outline for a conversation that you might use to discuss the ways you will help Mr. Valdez to be comfortable and safe during his dental hygiene treatment.

CHAPTER 61 CROSSWORD PUZZLE

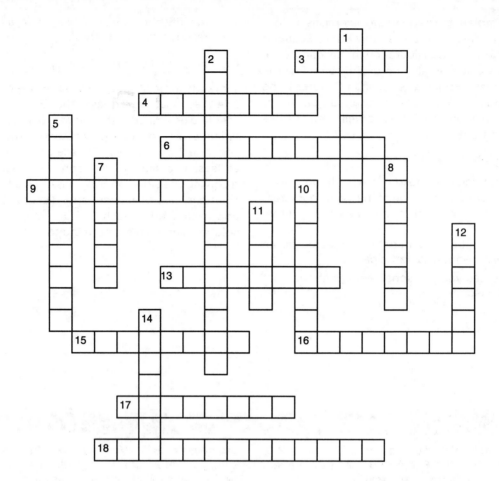

Puzzle Clues

Across

3. Cavity or channel within a tube or tubular organ, such as a blood vessel.

4. Deficiency of blood to supply oxygen resulting from functional constriction or obstruction of a blood vessel.

6. Variation from the normal rhythm, especially with reference to the heart.

9. Induration, hardening.

13. Blood clot attached to the intima of a blood vessel.

15. Narrowing or contraction of a body passage or opening.

16. Lipid (cholesterol) deposit on the intima (lining) of an artery; also called atheromatous plaque.

17. Oxygenated blood carried by an artery away from the heart to nourish the body tissues.

18. Substance that suppresses, delays, or nullifies coagulation of the blood.

Down

1. Sudden blocking of an artery by a detached clot of foreign material carried by the bloodstream.

2. Disease process caused by the deposit of atheromas on the inner lining of arteries.

5. Middle and thickest layer of the heart wall, composed of cardiac muscle.

7. Nonoxygenated blood from the tissues; blood pumped from the heart to the lungs for oxygenation.

8. Labored or difficult breathing.

10. Waking at night one or more times to urinate.

11. Abnormal accumulation of fluid in the intercellular spaces of the body.

12. Acute pain in the chest from decreased blood supply to the heart muscle.

14. Localized area of necrosis produced by occlusion of a blood vessel.

The Patient with a Blood Disorder

LEARNING OBJECTIVES

Upon successful completion of these exercises, you will be able to:

1. Identify and define the key terms and concepts related to hematologic conditions.

2. Recognize blood components and normal reference values.

3. Describe the causes, symptoms, and oral effects of red and white blood cell disorders, bleeding disorders, and clotting deficiencies.

4. Plan and document dental hygiene education and treatment for patients with a blood disorder.

 KNOWLEDGE EXERCISES

Write your answers for each question in the space provided.

1. List seven elements that make up blood.

2. What is the composition of plasma?

3. Identify the function of each of the plasma proteins.

4. Why are red blood cells termed *corpuscles*?

5. What is the purpose of red blood cells?

6. What is a normal hemoglobin value?

7. When the diagnosis is anemia, what has happened to the hemoglobin value?

_____

_____

8. Identify five basic causes of anemia.

_____

_____

_____

_____

9. Iron-deficiency anemia is more often seen in younger people than in older people; more often in _____ than in _____.

10. What can cause iron-deficiency anemia?

_____

_____

11. Identify two main types of anemia disorders in which red blood cells are destroyed.

_____

_____

12. Identify two causes of diminished production of red blood cells.

_____

_____

13. What genetic disorders are characterized by absent or decreased production of normal hemoglobin?

_____

_____

_____

_____

14. Which megaloblastic anemia is caused by a vitamin B₁₂ deficiency?

_____

15. What oral findings are related to anemia?

_____

_____

_____

16. Which foods can you suggest to your patients as good sources of vitamin B_{12}?

_____

_____

17. Dietary factors are important in the treatment of folate-deficiency anemia, but this type of megaloblastic anemia may be more frequently related to _____ than to inadequate intake.

18. What severe condition affecting newborns is also a result of folic acid deficiency?

_____

19. Sickle cell disease is a form of _____ anemia.

20. Individuals from which ethnic populations are most at risk for sickle cell disease?

_____

_____

21. In your own words, briefly describe the clinical course of the chronic and acute phases of sickle cell disease.
    - *Chronic anemia:*

    _____

    _____

    _____

    _____

    _____

    - *Acute vaso-occlusion or crisis:*

    _____

    _____

    _____

    _____

22. Briefly describe preventive and disease state treatments for sickle cell disease.
    - *Preventive:*

    _____

    _____

    _____

    _____

- *During a crisis:*

_____

_____

_____

_____

23. List oral manifestations associated with sickle cell disease that can be identified by the dental hygienist.

_____

_____

_____

_____

_____

_____

24. A red blood cell count _____ normal levels is characteristic of polycythemia.

25. List symptoms of polycythemia that may be noted by the dental hygienist during an oral examination.

_____

_____

_____

26. Identify two main types of white blood cells.

_____

_____

27. What is the main function of leukocytes?

_____

_____

_____

Erythrocytes   Neutrophil   Eosinophil   Basophil   Monocyte   Lymphocyte   Plasma cell

28. Match the name of the correct cell in the drawing above to the description of each white blood cell in the list below.

Functions to increase vascular permeability so that phagocytic cells can pass into inflamed areas.

_____

Stains bright pink under the microscope; increases markedly during allergic conditions.

_____

Multiplies when needed and moves back and forth between vessels and extravascular tissue.

_____

Actively phagocytic; changes into macrophage in connective tissue.

_____

Also called PMN; first in line to phagocytosis when the body is invaded by bacteria.

_____

29. What is the normal reference value of leukocytes in the blood?

_____

30. White blood cell counts can be used to detect and monitor disease because each cell type either _____ or _____ in association with certain conditions.

31. Identify the specific type of white blood cell associated with these approximate percentages of the total WBC count.

- 60%–70%:

_____

- 20%–35%:

_____

- 2%–6%:

_____

- *1%–3%:*

  _____

- *1%:*

  _____

32. Match each descriptive statement with the correct white blood cell disorder.

Disorder	Descriptive Statement
A. Neutropenia	___Caused by defects in myeloid cells
B. Lymphocyto-penia	___Abnormally low number of lymphocytes
C. Leukocytosis	___Increase in circulating white blood cells
	___Oral stomatitis and lymph mode enlargement are symptoms
	___Symptoms include petechiae and mouth ulcers
	___Can happen for many reasons including infection and excess exertion
	___Symptoms include bruising and gingival bleeding
	___Can be caused by protein-energy malnutrition or infection
	___Decrease in numbers of neutrophils
	___Can be associated with malignant neoplasms of immature white blood cells
	___Can be caused by chemotherapy or radiation therapy

33. List and briefly describe three platelet disorders.

_____

_____

_____

_____

34. List and briefly describe the cause of two types of coagulation disorders.

_____

_____

_____

_____

35. In your own words, describe the effects of hemophilia.

_____

_____

36. List at least five common herbs associated with increased bleeding if taken as a nutritional supplement.

_____

_____

_____

_____

_____

_____

_____

_____

37. What common pain medications affect coagulation?

_____

38. Cancer treatments with chemotherapeutic agents put your patient at risk for which two blood disorders?

_____

_____

39. Consultation with the patient's primary care provider or _____ may be a necessary component of a complete pretreatment assessment if the patient has a blood disorder.

40. What common dental hygiene interventions or actions can inadvertently cause increased risk for bleeding when the patient has a blood disorder?

_____

_____

_____

_____

✓ COMPETENCY EXERCISES

Apply information from the chapter and use critical thinking skills to complete the competency exercises. Write responses on paper or create electronic documents to submit your answers.

1. When you update his health history, Jeremiah Bell tells you that his gums, which have always been healthy, have been bleeding profusely when he flosses. Once he woke up in the morning with blood in his mouth and on his pillow. What questions will you ask him?

2. Mr. Bell replies that he has seen his physician to be tested for a blood disorder and hands you a sheet of paper reporting the results of four tests. Which tests

would you expect to see included in the report that evaluate bleeding time? (*Hint*: Table 62-1 in the **textbook** will help you to answer this question.)

3. If the report handed to you by Mr. Bell indicates a diagnosis of leukemia, what results would you expect to see for the blood tests?

4. You and the attending dentist decide together to postpone clinical dental hygiene treatment for Mr. Bell until you can arrange a telephone consultation with his physician. You provide oral hygiene instruction for Mr. Bell with an emphasis on what he can do on a daily basis to minimize oral effects of his blood disorder. Using your institution's guidelines for writing in patient records, document this appointment.

5. Mr. Weber presents for his continuing care appointment. He states that since his myocardial infarction 8 months ago, he is taking Warfarin daily. He is not sure of the amount nor his last anticoagulation test. What laboratory test(s) would you need to know before proceeding? What levels would be recommended for you to proceed today with treatment? What questions will you ask when you consult with his physician?

DISCOVERY EXERCISE

Explore the American Dental Association website or do a PubMed literature search to find information about the latest guidelines for management of dental patients who are taking anticoagulant or antiplatelet medications.

EVERYDAY ETHICS

Before completing the learning exercises below, reread and reflect on the Everyday Ethics Scenario and Questions for Consideration in this chapter of the **textbook.** It may also be useful to review the Dental Hygiene Ethics discussion in Chapter 1, the Ethical Applications in the introduction pages for each section in the **textbook**, as well as the Codes of Ethics in **textbook** Appendices I–IV.

Individual Learning Activity

Imagine that you are the dental hygienist in this scenario. Answer each of the questions for consideration at the end of the scenario.

Collaborative Learning Activity

Work with another student colleague to role-play the scenario. The goal of this exercise is for you and your colleague to work through the alternative actions in order to come to consensus on a solution or response that is acceptable to both of you.

Factors to Teach the Patient

This scenario is related to the following factors listed in this chapter of the **textbook**:

▷ Meticulous hygiene techniques to practice daily: toothbrushing, flossing, and other interdental cleaning devices.

▷ How to self-evaluate the oral cavity for deviations from normal; any changes should be reported to the dentist and dental hygienist.

When Mr. Bell (introduced in Competency Exercises in this chapter) returns in a few weeks for his follow-up appointment, he tells you that he has just started treatment for leukemia. He has been advised that it is very difficult to control all of the symptoms of his condition. He is very concerned about his oral health.

Use the information in Chapter 62 in the **textbook** and the motivational interviewing principles in **workbook** Appendix D to outline your education plan for Mr. Bell.

Use the outline you created to role-play this situation with a fellow student. If you are the patient in the role-play, be sure to ask questions. If you are the dental hygienist, try to anticipate questions and answer them in your explanation.

CHAPTER 62 WORD SCRAMBLE PUZZLE

1. RAEFTDFLIIEN _____
2. GLSOTISIS _____
3. SDNSLGOOAIY _____
4. MORAHEHSISTR _____
5. RAEOTHTIMC _____
6. NGOBOLEIMH _____
7. LOMSSYEIH _____
8. CLOHIEMYT _____
9. IYAHXPO _____
10. YOESSTKLICOU _____
11. KPOINELAUE _____
12. PUEENIRNOAT _____
13. CPTEAHEI _____
14. SGIOSPYTCAOH _____
15. PUPURRA _____
16. CAOLUSOOISCN-V _____
17. VGEIROT _____

Puzzle Clues

1. Cell count of white blood cells, including determination of the percentage of each type of cell.
2. Inflammation of the tongue.
3. Pain in the tongue.
4. Blood in a joint cavity.
5. Volume percentage of erythrocytes (red blood cells) in whole blood.
6. Protein in the erythrocyte that transports molecular oxygen to body cells.
7. Rupture of erythrocytes with the release of hemoglobin into the plasma.
8. Destruction of blood cells, resulting in liberation of hemoglobin.
9. Diminished availability of oxygen to body tissues.
10. Increase in the total number of leukocytes.
11. Reduction in total number of leukocytes in the blood; count under 500 per mL.
12. Diminished number of neutrophils (polymorphonuclear leukocytes or PMNs).
13. Minute, pinpoint, round, nonraised, purplish-red spot in the skin or mucous membrane, caused by hemorrhage.
14. Engulfing of microorganisms and foreign particles by phagocytes, such as macrophages.
15. Hemorrhage into the tissues, under the skin, and through the mucous membranes; produces petechiae and ecchymoses.
16. Blood vessel blockage resulting in organ damage.
17. Dizziness.

 MeSH TERMS

Use a combination of MeSH terms and other key words to develop an effective and efficient PubMed literature search strategy.

Blood cells	Hemocytes	Neutropenia	Anemia
Blood platelets	Leukocytes	Thrombocytopenia	Hemorrhagic disorders
Erythrocytes	Hematologic diseases	Thrombocytosis	Blood platelet disorders
Neutrophils	Leukocyte disorders	Hemoglobins	

63

The Patient with an Autoimmune Disease

LEARNING OBJECTIVES

Upon successful completion of these exercises, you will be able to:

1. Identify and define the key terms and concepts related to the patient with an autoimmune disease.

2. Identify clinical considerations and oral health factors related to autoimmune diseases.

3. Plan and document dental hygiene care for a patient with autoimmune disease.

KNOWLEDGE EXERCISES

Write your answers for each question in the space provided.

1. What characteristic of the immune system is unique to an autoimmune disease?

2. What is the difference between the innate immune system and the acquired immune system?

3. What are lymphocytes and where in the body are they produced?

4. Differentiate between the two types of autoimmune diseases.

5. List two predispositions to autoimmune diseases.

6. Glucocorticosteroids and NSAIDs are two treatment options for systemic autoimmune diseases. List four additional treatment options.

7. List three connective tissue autoimmune diseases.

8. Match the shapes of oral lichen planus (OLP) to their associated characteristic.

Type of OLP	Characteristic
_____Atropic	A. Central ulceration in lesion
_____Bullous	B. Slightly raised lacey white threads
_____Papular	C. May look like oral leukoplakia
_____Plaque-like	D. Separation of oral epithelium from underlying connective tissue
_____Reticular	E. Typically bilateral and symmetric
_____Ulcerative	F. Round, raised elevation of skin

9. What is *oral lichen planus*?

_____

_____

_____

_____

10. List two ingredients found in some oral healthcare products that may be contraindicated in a patient with OLP.

_____

_____

11. List two pharmacologic approaches to symptom for OLP.

_____

_____

12. What recommendations might you include in dietary counseling for a patient with OLP?

_____

_____

_____

_____

13. In your own words, describe the symptoms of rheumatoid arthritis.

_____

_____

_____

_____

_____

_____

14. What is juvenile rheumatoid arthritis?

_____

_____

15. What orofacial structure can be affected by rheumatoid arthritis?

_____

_____

16. What is the relationship between rheumatoid arthritis and periodontal disease?

_____

17. What is the meaning of the acronym DMARDs?

_____

_____

18. In what ways might rheumatoid arthritis affect the patient's personal oral care and/or dental hygiene treatment?

_____

_____

_____

_____

19. What is the most significant environmental factor associated with rheumatoid arthritis?

_____

20. What body tissues are affected by systemic sclerosis?

_____

_____

21. Match the type of systemic scleroderma with the characteristic. Some characteristics apply to more than one type.

Type of Systemic Scleroderma	Characteristic
_____Systemic	A. Thick skin on fingers or face
_____Diffuse cutaneous systemic	B. Loss of blood supply to the fingers
	C. Affects internal organs but not the skin
_____Limited cutaneous	D. Targets women more than men
	E. Progresses more quickly
	F. Milder form
	G. Large areas of body are thick and tight

22. Orofacial manifestations of systemic sclerosis may create challenges for oral care by both the patient and the dental hygienist. Without looking at the **textbook**, list as many of these oral manifestations as you can.

_____

_____

_____

_____

_____

_____

_____

_____

_____

23. CREST syndrome is another term for limited cutaneous scleroderma. In your own words, define each letter of the acronym CREST.

_____

_____

_____

_____

_____

_____

_____

24. What is the primary cause of a gastrointestinal autoimmune disease?

_____

_____

25. Fill in the table below to compare these gastrointestinal autoimmune diseases.

Disease	Tissues Affected	Causes/Triggers
Celiac disease		
Crohn's disease		
Ulcerative colitis		

26. What is the only effective treatment for celiac disease?

_____

_____

27. Describe the long-term consequence of inflammation and destruction of the intestinal villi in celiac disease.

_____

_____

_____

28. Describe the orofacial manifestations of Crohn's disease.

_____

_____

_____

_____

29. Pyostomatitis vegetans is a symptom related to ulcerative colitis. Describe the appearance of pyostomatitis vegetans in the oral cavity.

_____

_____

30. List the tissues impacted by neurologic autoimmune diseases.

_____

_____

31. Describe multiple sclerosis?

_____

_____

32. Briefly describe the four categories/types of multiple sclerosis.

_____

_____

_____

_____

_____

_____

_____

_____

33. List the oral manifestations of multiple sclerosis.

_____

_____

_____

_____

_____

_____

34. Why is a medical consultation necessary for a patient with multiple sclerosis?

_____

_____

_____

_____

_____

35. What are the expected outcomes of drug therapies for multiple sclerosis?

_____

_____

_____

_____

36. What are the characteristics of myasthenia gravis?

_____

_____

_____

_____

_____

37. Describe what happens during a myasthenic crisis.

_____

_____

_____

_____

_____

38. Why are anxiety management strategies important during a dental hygiene appointment with a patient with myasthenia gravis?

_____

_____

39. In Sjogren's syndrome, autoantibodies attach to _____ in _____, followed by _____.

40. List three symptoms of Sjogren's syndrome.

_____

_____

_____

_____

_____

_____

41. List three potential oral manifestations of Sjogren's syndrome.

_____

_____

_____

42. Describe systemic lupus erythematosus.

_____

_____

_____

_____

43. What oral lesions may be associated with systemic lupus?

_____

_____

_____

44. Describe the appearance of a malar rash.

COMPETENCY EXERCISES

Apply information from the chapter and use critical thinking skills to complete the competency exercises. Write responses on paper or create electronic documents to submit your answers.

1. Design an infomap with just enough information to help you identify and differentiate among the autoimmune diseases discussed in the **textbook**. To get you started, consider the following design for your infomap. List the autoimmune disease in the first column. Next, add additional column headers such as Cause/Occurrence, Organ/System Targeted, Basic Characteristics, and Considerations for Dental Hygiene Care. This project could also be divided into four individual infomaps, one for each of the four categories of autoimmune diseases discussed in the **textbook**. Creating an infomap is an excellent method of organizing and integrating your knowledge.

Read the Chapter 63 patient assessment summary to help you answer questions #2 through #4.

2. Mandy Justerman presents for an initial visit dental hygiene appointment. Theodora, Mandy's caregiver, introduces herself as she assists Mandy into the chair. While you are helping to transfer Mandy to the dental chair, you notice bilateral parotid area swelling, very dry facial skin, tight skin about her lips, angular chelitis on the left side, and labored breathing. Her hands appear deformed, without strength, and Mandy requires assistance to lift her legs onto the dental chair. Describe steps you will take to determine modifications in your usual patient care procedures that will help to keep Mandy safe and comfortable during dental hygiene treatment.

3. When she is trying to communicate, it takes Mandy a long time to say anything and you cannot understand her very well. What communication strategies will help you successfully complete your patient assessment?

4. As you complete the assessment data, you determine that Mandy has enjoyed regular professional and personal dental care throughout her life. But for the last several years, her caregiver Theodora has always provided daily oral biofilm removal. Theodora admits to having very little dental knowledge, but she very much wants to learn how to keep Mandy's mouth as healthy as possible. Use the assessment summary data for Mandy and a copy of the Dental Hygiene Care Plan template (**workbook** Appendix B) or the care plan form used by your school clinic to complete a dental hygiene care plan for Mandy that includes appropriate education for Theodora.

EVERYDAY ETHICS

Before completing the learning exercises below, reread and reflect on the Everyday Ethics Scenario and Questions for Consideration in this chapter of the **textbook**. It may also be useful to review the Dental Hygiene Ethics discussion in Chapter 1, the Ethical Applications in the introduction pages for each section in the **textbook**, as well as the Codes of Ethics in **textbook** Appendices I-IV.

Cooperative Learning Activity

Answer each of the questions for consideration at the end of the scenario in the **textbook**. Compare what you wrote with answers developed by another classmate and discuss differences/similarities.

Discovery Activity

Ask a dental hygienist who has been practicing for a year or more to read the scenario. Provide a copy of the Code of Ethics as well. Share the responses you have made to answer each question and ask that person to discuss the situation with you. What insights did you have or what did you learn during this discussion?

Factors to Teach the Patient

This scenario is related to the following factors listed in this chapter of the **textbook**:

▷ Maintain recommended recare intervals to keep biofilm at a low level.

▷ What are the autoimmune disease-specific oral manifestations?

▷ What can be done at home to reduce symptoms?

▷ The dental office is a safe place to share concerns and ask questions.

Use the information in the Factors section of Chapter 63 of the **textbook** and the principles of motivational interviewing (see **workbook** Appendix D) to develop a conversation explaining to Theodora (introduced in question #2 of the Competency Exercises) how to perform daily oral care for Mandy and the reasons for maintaining the recommended recare interval.

Use the conversation you create to role-play this situation with a fellow student. If you are the patient in the role-play, be sure to ask questions. If you are the dental hygienist, try to anticipate questions and provide evidence-based answers for them in your explanation.

CHAPTER 63—PATIENT ASSESSMENT SUMMARY

Patient Name: *Mrs. Mandy Justerman*   Age: *40*   Gender: F   ☑ Initial Therapy

☐ Maintenance

Provider Name: *D.H. Student*   Date: *Today*   ☐ Re-evaluation

Chief Complaint:

Patient has recently moved into the area. She presents for routine 3-month maintenance and new patient examination.

Assessment Findings

Health History   **At Risk For:**

- Medical diagnosis of Sjogren's syndrome
- Limited mouth opening, bilateral parotid enlargement, dry skin, joint damaged hands
- No intellectual or cognitive disability.
- Takes methotrexate and a long-term corticoidsteroid, but caregiver who accompanies her to the appointment is not sure what it is nor the dosages for both medications.
- ASA Classification-III
- ADL level 3

Social and Dental History   **At Risk For:**

- Previous history of excellent professional dental care
- Personal dental literacy is high
- New caregiver with low dental knowledge

Dental Examination   **At Risk For:**

- Difficulty opening and fatigue with staying open for long periods
- Generalized visible biofilm and debris in all areas of the mouth
- Generalized erythematic and bleeding gingival tissue
- Generalized 3- to 4-mm probing depths; generalized bleeding
- Xerostomia
- Increased gag reflex
- Current posterior restorations in good repair; no anterior restorations
- History of orthodontia

CHAPTER 63 CROSSWORD PUZZLE

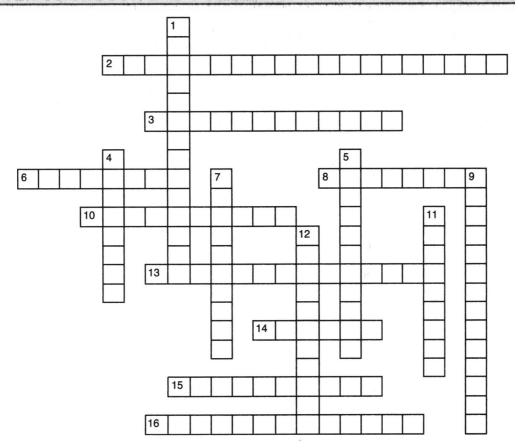

Puzzle Clues

Across

2. Adrenal gland substance (or medication) involved in anti-inflammatory activity through catabolism of proteins, carbohydrates, and fat.

3. Any disease affecting blood vessels.

6. Inflammation of a peripheral nerve.

8. Seeing double.

10. Joint pain.

13. Small red or purple cluster that may have a "spidery" appearance.

14. Droopy eyelid.

15. Difficult or unclear speech caused by muscle weakness.

16. Thickening and tightening on the skin of extremities.

Down

1. An appearance found in OLP (two words).

4. Thickening and scarring of connective tissue.

5. Small mouth opening.

7. Care to reduce pain without worrying about the cause.

9. Substance produced by the immune system against the individual's own body proteins/tissues.

11. Refers to a drug or therapy that is the first choice for treatment (two words).

12. Elimination of large quantities of fat with the feces as a result of malabsorption.

 MeSH TERMS

Use a combination of MeSH terms and other key words to develop an effective and efficient PubMed literature search strategy.

Immune system	Autoimmune diseases,	Celiac disease	Multiple sclerosis
Diseases of immune system	nervous system	Crohn's disease	Myasthenia gravis
Lichen planus, oral	Scleroderma, systemic	Inflammatory bowel	Sjogren's syndrome
Arthritis rheumatoid	Scleroderma, localized	disease	Lupus erythematosus,
	Scleroderma, limited	Colitis, ulcerative	systemic

IX Summary Exercises

Patients with Special Needs

Chapters 46–63

 COMPETENCY EXERCISES

Apply information from the chapters in this section of the **textbook** and use critical thinking skills to complete the competency exercises. Write responses on paper or create electronic documents to submit your answers.

1. The best way to become competent in planning and providing dental hygiene care for patients with special needs is, of course, to practice planning and providing care. The learning that comes from practicing your skills is always enhanced by taking time to record the process in some sort of written format so that you can later reflect on what you have done, how you did it, and why things did or did not work out as you had planned.

   Select one or more patients for whom you provide care in your school clinic who have one (or more) of the special needs identified in the **textbook**. To complete this exercise, gather the assessment data from each patient's record, a copy of the patient-specific dental hygiene care-plan template in Appendix B (or from your clinic), the information from the appropriate chapters in the **textbook**, and any other source of information you think might be important (such as a drug reference book).

   Use the patient-specific care-plan template to develop a comprehensive written dental hygiene care plan for each patient you select.

 DISCOVERY EXERCISES

1. Gather as much information as you can about a specific special-need condition that interests you. Use PubMed (and the appropriate MeSH terms from the chapters in the **textbook**) to help you search the professional literature and/or look for online sources of information about the condition. The information in the scientific literature will probably be the most valid

and reliable about the condition you select. Online sources can be variable, and it is important to determine that the host of the website is a reliable source of data and provides information about the condition that is supported by scientific principles.

2. You and your student colleagues can share information and learn from each other if you each present a different type of case and discuss the cases in a sort of case-presentation seminar. Each patient case you present should contain the following information:

   - *Patient background and demographics*
   - *A general description of your patient, including name, age, race, sex, height, weight, blood pressure, pulse, and respiration*
   - *Other information about your patient that is important for understanding the special condition*
   - *A statement describing the significance of these data for planning and providing dental hygiene care*
   - *Medical history*
   - *A definition of each medical problem with an explanation of its significance to the delivery of dental care*
   - *A description of your patient's ASA level*
   - *A statement of the physical and oral manifestations of your patient's conditions*
   - *A note about the anticipated complications associated with patient management during dental hygiene care*
   - *A statement of the anticipated complications or potential emergency situations that are related to your patient's medical history*
   - *A description of the actions needed to prevent complications and emergencies during dental hygiene care*
   - *Pharmacological and therapeutic considerations*
   - *Refer to a Physicians Desk Reference (PDR) or other accepted drug information reference as a guide.*
   - *Identification of specific medications your patient is taking currently and how they relate to the medical history*

- *A list containing the commercial and generic name of each drug, class or mechanism of action, usual dosage, indications for use, and anticipated adverse side effects for dentistry*
- *An evaluation of your patient's local anesthesia considerations*
- *Dental hygiene care delivery considerations*
- *A description of the general physical and oral manifestations of your patient's condition that affect dental hygiene care*
- *A description of your patient's ADL and IADL levels*
- *A description of your patient's OSCAR considerations*
- *Identification of and rationale for modifications to standard dental hygiene treatment procedures needed to meet your patient's special needs during dental hygiene care*
- *Identification of and rationale for modifications in providing oral hygiene instructions*
- *Identification of and rationale for modifications of oral hygiene aids*
- *A description of behavioral and psychosocial considerations for planning and providing care for your patient*
- *Identification of communication issues and needed actions to ensure that your patient is fully informed before he or she consents to the planned dental hygiene treatment.*

FOR YOUR PORTFOLIO

1. Include your written responses to the Everyday Ethics questions from any of the chapters in this section.

2. It is likely that while you are a student, you will develop many dental hygiene care plans for a variety of patients with a wide range of special needs. Include all of these written care plans in your portfolio. Also include the care plans you developed using the patient-assessment data summaries when completing the competency exercises in this workbook; be sure to indicate which care plans were developed for practice patient cases and which were developed for individuals for whom you provided dental hygiene care in your school clinic.

3. An effective way to document your growing knowledge about planning patient care is to include a written reflection that describes, in detail, how the care plans you developed later in your student career are different from the care plans you developed when you were first providing patient care.

   Cite specific examples from your earlier and later care plans to document your increased competency in planning individualized, patient-specific dental hygiene care. The examples should show how your later plans are more complete, more comprehensive, and more professional than your earlier plans.

4. If you develop and present a case presentation, include your presentation outline, along with any PowerPoint presentation or handouts you created to accompany the presentation. Or include a photograph that shows you and your coauthor colleagues presenting your information to your classmates or other learners. A brief written reflection of what you learned from the experience of preparing and presenting the case study will add depth to your documentation.

SPECIAL PATIENT CARE KEY WORDS BINGO

Learning the meaning of all of the key terms associated with each chapter in this section of the **textbook** can be overwhelming. Active learning activities that encourage you to practice and recall definitions can help enhance your ability to learn these terms. The BINGO game can be played a couple of different ways, but the instructions here can help you get started.

The first step is to study the word lists provided here for each category by consulting the **textbook** glossary and making a separate slip of paper containing each of the terms and a relevant short definition. These slips of paper can be folded in half and then put into a large container from which one slip will be randomly drawn at a time.

Individual players, each of whom selects one of the BINGO cards in a category, can compete against each other. Teams of several players can also work together to compete against other teams. A "moderator" selects and reads out loud the definition of various terms in the category selected. An individual player, who recognizes which term is being referred to, can mark it, if it appears on the BINGO card. Team members can discuss and come to consensus about which word on their card the moderator has defined. (*Note: Every card in each category contain a different selection of words, and not all the words in the list will appear on any given card.*)

When a player or team marks all five squares in a horizontal, vertical, or diagonal line, a "winner" is announced by calling out BINGO! At that point, all of the words marked on the card can be checked to be sure the moderator called them out. The game may continue being played, with "winners" periodically calling out BINGO! until one of the cards is completely marked. That person or team can be declared the "grand winner" of that round of the game.

Get creative! You might decide to play the game by having the "moderator" call out terms, and a participant can mark it on the card if the player or team can say the correct definition for the term loudly. You can easily develop a whole new set of BINGO cards for these categories or combine all three categories into one game. Another idea is to find the key words in every chapter and look up their definitions in the glossary to make up a BINGO game for other sections of the **textbook**. Can anybody figure out a way to use this kind of game to practice SPELLING the terms??

Have fun! Knowing the key words throughout all the chapters in the **textbook** is definitely a plus in your quest to become a professional dental hygienist.

BINGO GAME – WORD LISTS

Through the Ages	Systemic Conditions		Disabilities
Aging	Alopecia	Palliative	ADA (or AwDA)
Anticipatory guidance	Alveolitis	Pallidotomy	Adaptive behavior
Adolescent	Anaphylaxis	Pancytopenia	Akinesia
Biological age	Anaplasia	Pathognomonic	Ankylosis
Chronological age	Apoptosis	Pathophysiology	Aphasia
Dementia	Arrhythmia	Pervasive	Applied behavioral analysis
Dental home	Arthralgia	Petechia	Ataxia
Developmental disability	Atrophy	Polydipsia	Barrier free
ECC	Carcinoma	Polyphagia	Blind
Fetus	Comorbid	Polyuria	Bradykinesia
Functional age	Cyanosis	Postprandial	Braille
Gerontology	Detoxification	Prodrome	Cataract
Gestation	Diplopia	Ptosis	Clonic
Infant	Dysgeusia	Purpura	Cochlear implants
Lifestyle	Dysphagia	Retinopathy	Decompensate
Low birth weight	Dyspnea	Sclerosis	Disability
Menarche	Edema	Sialorrhea	Dysarthria
Menopause	Endocrine	Stenosis	Dysmorphic
Nonnutritive sucking	Endometrium	Tachycardia	Dystonia
Osteoporosis	Epinephrine	Tachypnea	Epicanthic fold
Polypharmacy	Exacerbation	Tardive dyskinesia	Hearing impairment
POSA	Fibrosis	Thrombus	Hemiparesis
Presbycusis	Gastroparesis	Thyroiditis	Hemiplegia
Presbyopia	Glossitis	Thyrotoxic crisis	Hirsutism
Preschooler	Glossodynia	Trismus	Ictal (or Ictus)
Puberty	Glycemia		Impairment
Retinopathy of prematurity	Hematopoiesis		Intellectual functioning
School-age	Homeostasis		Kyphosis
SECC	Hormone		Macroglossia
Sippy cup	Hyperinsulinemia		Medical disability
Toddler	Hyperkalemia		Microcephalus
	Hypernatremia		Musculoskeletal disability
	Hyperpnea		Neurodevelopmental disability
	Hypogeusia		Neurologic disabilities
	Hypoxia		Paralysis
	Infarct		Paresthesia
	Ischemia		Paroxysm
	Ketones		Spasm
	Leukopenia		Status epilepticus
	Metastasis		Stereotypic movement disorder
	Myalgia		Tic
	Myxedema		Tinnitus
	Neoplasm		Tonic
	Neuritis		Tonic–clonic
	Neutropenia		Visual impairment
	Norepinephrine		
	Nosocomial		
	Nystagmus		
	Oral mucositis		
	Osteoradionecrosis		
	Osteosynthesis		

Through the Ages

Retinopathy of prematurity	Menarche	SECC	Puberty	Preschooler
Osteoperosis	Functional Age	Dementia	Low Birth Weight	Developmental disability
Presbycusis	Presbyopia	**FREE**	Toddler	Menopause
Fetus	POSA	Nonnutritive Sucking	Polypharmacy	School-age
Lifestyle	Aging	Chronological Age	Dental Home	Gestation

Through the Ages

Low Birth Weight	Puberty	Osteoperosis	Menarche	Gerontology
Developmental disability	ECC	School-age	SECC	Biological Age
Presbyopia	Infant	**FREE**	Menopause	Polypharmacy
Dementia	Fetus	Preschooler	POSA	Retinopathy of prematurity
Lifestyle	Aging	Functional Age	Chronological Age	Gestation

Through the Ages

Lifestyle	Nonnutritive Sucking	Presbycusis	Dental Home	Functional Age
ECC	School-age	Menarche	Toddler	Aging
Chronological Age	Puberty	**FREE**	Gestation	Retinopathy of prematurity
Polypharmacy	Gerontology	Presbyopia	Fetus	Dementia
Low Birth Weight	Biological Age	Infant	Sippy Cup	Osteoperosis

Through the Ages

Menarche	Presbyopia	Chronological Age	Polypharmacy	Functional Age
Preschooler	Gestation	Menopause	Dental Home	Osteoperosis
Sippy Cup	School-age	**FREE**	Biological Age	Developmental disability
Toddler	Aging	POSA	Fetus	Retinopathy of prematurity
SECC	Presbycusis	Lifestyle	Nonnutritive Sucking	Gerontology

Systemic Conditions

Purpura	Palliative	Ischemia	Sialorrhea	Prodrome
Comorbid	Carcinoma	Hormone	Tachypnea	Ketones
Alopecia	Homeostasis	**FREE**	Hematopoiesis	Glossodynia
Anaplasia	Exacerbation	Hyperinsulinemia	Arrhythmia	Thyroiditis
Postprandial	Detoxification	Retinopathy	Glossitis	Norepinephrine

Systemic Conditions

Hypoxia	Comorbid	Palliative	Tardive dyskinesia	Anaplasia
Carcinoma	Nystagmus	Glossodynia	Cyanosis	Ketones
Pathognomonic	Glycemia	**FREE**	Homeostasis	Fibrosis
Endometrium	Hematopoiesis	Dyspnea	Ptosis	Norepinephrine
Nosocomial	Sialorrhea	Alveolitis	Polydipsia	Hypernatremia

Systemic Conditions

Nystagmus	Postprandial	Edema	Neutropenia	Polydipsia
Trismus	Dysphagia	Comorbid	Arrhythmia	Alveolitis
Pathognomonic	Pervasive	**FREE**	Homeostasis	Purpura
Thyroiditis	Pathophysiology	Osteosynthesis	Cyanosis	Polyuria
Hypoxia	Thrombus	Glossitis	Leukopenia	Endometrium

Systemic Conditions

Exacerbation	Hyperpnea	Postprandial	Trismus	Anaphylaxis
Hypernatremia	Leukopenia	Dysgeusia	Dyspnea	Neutropenia
Carcinoma	Thyroiditis	**FREE**	Sialorrhea	Sclerosis
Ketones	Oral mucositis	Neoplasm	Arthralgia	Homeostasis
Pancytopenia	Comorbid	Pallidotomy	Hematopoiesis	Cyanosis

Systemic Conditions

Anaphylaxis	Osteosynthesis	Edema	Leukopenia	Myxedema
Dyspnea	Trismus	Retinopathy	Gastroparesis	Oral mucositis
Hypogeusia	Comorbid	**FREE**	Dysgeusia	Metastasis
Sclerosis	Alveolitis	Glossodynia	Sialorrhea	Polydipsia
Epinephrine	Endocrine	Pervasive	Arrhythmia	Thrombus

Systemic Conditions

Sialorrhea	Sclerosis	Myalgia	Polyuria	Cyanosis
Tardive dyskinesia	Metastasis	Exacerbation	Neuritis	Tachycardia
Petechia	Pathophysiology	**FREE**	Hypogeusia	Postprandial
Trismus	Hyperkalemia	Purpura	Dysgeusia	Thyroiditis
Homeostasis	Glossitis	Comorbid	Hematopoiesis	Retinopathy

Systemic Conditions

Nosocomial	Pervasive	Ptosis	Dysphagia	Oral mucositis
Trismus	Pathophysiology	Endocrine	Neoplasm	Hypoxia
Diplopia	Hormone	**FREE**	Gastroparesis	Dyspnea
Apoptosis	Neutropenia	Anaphylaxis	Exacerbation	Polydipsia
Glossodynia	Pancytopenia	Tardive dyskinesia	Myalgia	Anaplasia

Systemic Conditions

Palliative	Prodrome	Dyspnea	Pathognomonic	Diplopia
Carcinoma	Comorbid	Fibrosis	Polyphagia	Polyuria
Myalgia	Oral mucositis	**FREE**	Cyanosis	Hypernatremia
Anaplasia	Stenosis	Pallidotomy	Infarct	Ketones
Retinopathy	Nystagmus	Epinephrine	Hormone	Neoplasm

Disabilities

Applied Behavioral Analysis	Barrier free	Macroglossia	Ankylosis	Stereotypic movement disorder
Cochlear implants	Tic	Intellectual functioning	ADA (or AwDA)	Impairment
Paralysis	Cataract	**FREE**	Hemiparesis	Visual impairment
Clonic	Dysarthria	Epicanthic fold	Dystonia	Musculoskeletal disability
Neurologic Disabilities	Disability	Braille	Tonic	Tonic–Clonic

Disabilities

Aphasia	Paresthesia	Paralysis	Neurologic Disabilities	Stereotypic movement disorder
Hemiplegia	Decompensate	Tic	Musculoskeletal disability	Hirsutism
Blind	Tinnitus	**FREE**	Applied Behavioral Analysis	Braille
Adaptive behavior	Visual impairment	Ankylosis	Medical Disability	Status epilepticus
Tonic–Clonic	Kyphosis	Tonic	Barrier free	Intellectual functioning

Disabilities

Hemiplegia	Decompensate	Epicanthic fold	Bradykinesia	Aphasia
Blind	Barrier free	Musculoskeletal disability	Status epilepticus	Clonic
Paralysis	Kyphosis	**FREE**	Hemiparesis	Impairment
Dysarthria	Braille	Adaptive behavior	Ataxia	Intellectual functioning
Hirsutism	Akinesia	Cataract	Neurodevelopmental disability	Dysmorphic

Disabilities

Ankylosis	ADA (or AwDA)	Decompensate	Ictal (or Ictus)	Paralysis
Neurodevelopmental disability	Adaptive behavior	Tonic	Macroglossia	Bradykinesia
Dysmorphic	Disability	**FREE**	Braille	Dysarthria
Tonic–Clonic	Visual impairment	Blind	Neurologic Disabilities	Tinnitus
Status epilepticus	Cataract	Intellectual functioning	Hemiparesis	Stereotypic movement disorder

ADEA Competencies for Entry into the Profession of Dental Hygiene

CORE COMPETENCIES (C)

C.1 Apply a professional code of ethics in all endeavors.

C.2 Adhere to state and federal laws, recommendations, and regulations in the provision of dental hygiene care.

C.3 Use critical thinking skills and comprehensive problem-solving to identify oral healthcare strategies that promote patient health and wellness.

C.4 Use evidence-based decision making to evaluate emerging technology and treatment modalities to integrate into patient dental hygiene care plans to achieve high-quality, cost-effective care.

C.5 Assume responsibility for professional actions and care based on accepted scientific theories, research, and the accepted standard of care.

C.6 Continuously perform self-assessment for lifelong learning and professional growth.

C.7 Integrate accepted scientific theories and research into educational, preventive, and therapeutic oral health services.

C.8 Promote the values of the dental hygiene profession through service-based activities, positive community affiliations, and active involvement in local organizations.

C.9 Apply quality-assurance mechanisms to insure continuous commitment to accepted standards of care.

C.10 Communicate effectively with diverse individuals and groups, serving all persons without discrimination by acknowledging and appreciating diversity.

C.11 Record accurate, consistent, and complete documentation of oral health services provided.

C.12 Initiate a collaborative approach with all patients when developing individualized care plans that are specialized, comprehensive, culturally sensitive, and acceptable to all parties involved in care planning.

C.13 Initiate consultations and collaborations with all relevant healthcare providers to facilitate optimal treatments.

C.14 Manage medical emergencies by using professional judgment, providing life support, and utilizing required CPR and any specialized training or knowledge.

HEALTH PROMOTION AND DISEASE PREVENTION (HP)

HP.1 Promote positive values of overall health and wellness to the public and organizations within and outside the profession.

HP.2 Respect the goals, values, beliefs, and preferences of all patients.

HP.3 Refer patients who may have a physiological, psychological, and/or social problem for comprehensive evaluation.

Reprinted with permission from American Dental Education Association (ADEA). Competencies for entry into the allied dental professions (as approved by the 2010 House of Delegates). *J Dent Educ.* 2017;81(7):853–860.

HP.4 Identify individual and population risk factors and develop strategies that promote health-related quality of life.

HP.5 Evaluate factors that can be used to promote patient adherence to disease-prevention or health maintenance strategies.

HP.6 Utilize methods that ensure the health and safety of the patient and the oral health professional in the delivery of care.

COMMUNITY INVOLVEMENT (CM)

CM.1 Assess the oral health needs and services of the community to determine action plans and availability of resources to meet healthcare needs.

CM.2 Provide screening, referral, and educational services that allow patients to access the resources of the healthcare system.

CM.3 Provide community oral health services in a variety of settings.

CM.4 Facilitate patient access to oral health services by influencing individuals or organizations for the provision of oral health care.

CM.5 Evaluate reimbursement mechanisms and their impact on the patient's access to oral health care.

CM.6 Evaluate the outcomes of community-based programs, and plan for future activities.

CM.7 Advocate for effective oral health care for underserved populations.

PATIENT/CLIENT CARE (PC)

Assessment

PC.1 Systematically collect, analyze, and record diagnostic data on the general, oral, and psychosocial health status of a variety of patients using methods consistent with medicolegal principles.

PC.2 Recognize predisposing and etiologic risk factors that require intervention to prevent disease.

PC.3 Recognize the relationships among systemic disease, medications, and oral health that impact overall patient care and treatment outcomes.

PC.4 Identify patients at risk for a medical emergency, and manage the patient care in a manner that prevents an emergency.

Dental Hygiene Diagnosis

PC.5 Use patient assessment data, diagnostic technologies, and critical decision-making skills to determine a dental hygiene diagnosis, a component of the dental diagnosis, to reach conclusions about the patient's dental hygiene care needs.

Planning

PC.6 Use reflective judgment in developing a comprehensive patient dental hygiene care plan.

PC.7 Collaborate with the patient and other health professionals as indicated to formulate a comprehensive dental hygiene care plan that is patient-centered and based on the best scientific evidence and professional judgment.

PC.8 Make referrals to professional colleagues and other healthcare professionals as indicated in the patient care plan.

PC.9 Obtain the patient's informed consent based on a thorough case presentation.

Implementation

PC.10 Provide specialized treatment that includes educational, preventive, and therapeutic services designed to achieve and maintain oral health. Partner with the patient in achieving oral health goals.

Evaluation

PC.11 Evaluate the effectiveness of the provided services and modify care plans as needed.

PC.12 Determine the outcomes of dental hygiene interventions using indices, instruments, examination techniques, and patient self-reports as specified in patient goals.

PC.13 Compare actual outcomes to expected outcomes, reevaluating goals, diagnoses, and services when expected outcomes are not achieved.

PROFESSIONAL GROWTH AND DEVELOPMENT (PGD)

PGD.1 Pursue career opportunities within health care, industry, education, research, and other roles as they evolve for the dental hygienist.

PGD.2 Develop practice management and marketing strategies to be used in the delivery of oral health care.

PGD.3 Access professional and social networks to pursue professional goals.

Patient-Specific Dental Hygiene Care Plan Template

PATIENT SPECIFIC DENTAL HYGIENE CARE PLAN

Patient Name: Age: Gender: Record #:   Date:

Initial Therapy   Maintenance   Re-evaluation

Health/Social History Findings Impacting Treatment:

ASA Classification:

Systemic Disease:

Medications:

Health Behaviors/Cultural Factors:

Modifiable Risk Factors:

Related to Dental Hygiene Diagnosis:

Related to Periodontal Diagnosis:

Dental Hygiene Diagnosis (Related to Risk Factors and Etiology):

Periodontal Diagnosis and Status (Active or Stable, Classification, Extent, Severity):

Caries Management Risk Assessment (CAMBRA) Level: ☐ Low   ☐ Moderate   ☐ High   ☐ Extreme

Medical and Dental Referrals Required:

Radiographic Exposures Completed/Interpreted: (identify film or digital)

☐ PAN   ☐ FMX   ☐ 2 BWX   ☐ 4/6 BWX

Initial Biofilm Score:

Planned Interventions (to arrest or control disease and regenerate, restore, or maintain health)		
Clinical **Address DH Diagnosis and** **Periodontal Diagnosis**	**Education/Counseling**	**Oral Hygiene Instruction/** **Oral Self-Care (evidence-based &** **patient-centered rationale)**

Recommended Oral Self-Care Aids:

<u>**Recommended Preventive Agents and Chemotherapeutics (include type and percentage) (home use)**</u>

☐ Dentifrices: ☐ Mouthrinses: ☐ Fluoride:

Expected Outcomes		
Patient-Centered	**Evaluation Methods**	**Time Frame**

<u>**Previous Treatment Goals Met/Not Met:**</u>

<u>**Recommended Dental Hygiene Treatment:**</u>

☐ Prophylaxis ☐ Selective Polish Agent:

☐ Periodontal Maintenance ☐ Topical Fluoride: Agent:

☐ Non-Surgical Periodontal Therapy: ☐ Sealants: Tooth #(s)

  Quadrant(s): _____ ☐ Custom Tray: Type

☐ Non-Surgical Periodontal Therapy 1–3 Teeth ☐ Education

  _____ ☐ Nutritional Analysis

☐ Scaling in the Presence of Inflammation ☐ Other:

☐ Anesthesia:

☐ Power Scaling

Estimated Number of Treatment Appointments:

Recommended Re-care Interval with Rationale:

Appointment Plan (sequence of planned interventions)	
Appt#	**Plan for Treatment, Services** **Plan for Education, Counseling, and Oral Hygiene Instruction**
1)	
2)	
3)	

Example Dental Hygiene Care Plan

PATIENT SPECIFIC DENTAL HYGIENE CARE PLAN

Patient Name: *Mrs. Lorna Patel* Age: *49*   Gender: *F*   Record #: *XXX01*   Date: *Today*

(**Initial Therapy**)   Maintenance   Re-evaluation

Health/Social History findings impacting treatment:

ASA Classification: *II*

Systemic disease: ***PENICILLIN ALLERGY** Hypertension, increased cholesterol*

Medications: *Lisinopril 20mg, Amlodipine Besylate 5mg, Statin (Zocor) 20 mg, chewable (gummy bear) daily vitamin*

Health behaviors/Cultural factors: *1.5 years since last dental visit, brushes daily and flosses occasionally, uses candy/mints daily for dry mouth, uses bottled water with no fluoride.*

Modifiable Risk Factors:

Related to Dental Hygiene Diagnosis: *Use of candy/mints for xerostomia, use of sticky daily vitamin*

Related to Periodontal Diagnosis: *Poor daily oral biofilm control*

Dental Hygiene Diagnosis (Related to Risk Factors and Etiology): *Need for oral health education based on increased risk for dental caries and periodontal disease due to behavioral habits*

Periodontal Diagnosis and Status (Active or Stable, Classification, Extent, Severity): *Generalized biofilm-induced gingivitis*

Caries Management Risk Assessment (CAMBRA) Level: ☐ Low ☐ Moderate ☐ High ☑ Extreme

Medical and Dental Referrals Required: *Restorative dental care for assessment and management of faulty restorations.*

Radiographic Exposures Completed/Interpreted: (identify film or (digital))

☐ PAN   ☐ FMX   ☐ 2 BWX   ☑ 4/6 BWX

Initial Biofilm Score: *65%*

Planned Interventions
(to arrest or control disease and regenerate, restore, or maintain health)

Clinical Address DH Diagnosis and Periodontal Diagnosis	Education/Counseling	Oral Self-Care (evidence-based & patient-centered rationale)
Scaling and root planning with selective polishing *Fluoride application*	*Importance of oral biofilm control* *Importance of fluoride in caries control* *Importance of daily fluoride rinse* *Use of fluoridated water* *Use of Xylitol gum/candies instead of sugar-based sweets.* *Use of alternative (non-sticky) daily vitamins* *Need for dental intervention to manage faulty restorations*	*Reinforce sulcular brushing technique* *Review flossing technique* *Review daily fluoride rinse.*

Recommended Oral Self-Care Aids: *Soft toothbrush and waxed dental floss*

Recommended Preventive Agents and Chemotherapeutics (include type and percentage) (home use)

☐ Dentifrices: *Tartar-control fluoridated toothpaste* ☐ Mouthrinses: *Daily over-the-counter fluoride rinse* ☐ Fluoride: *In-office fluoride application*

Expected Outcomes		
Patient-Centered Goals	**Evaluation Methods**	**Time Frame**
1. Eliminate gingivitis/control periodontitis	Reduction of oral biofilm, gingival redness, gingival bleeding, and periodontal probing depths	4-week re-evaluation
2. Increase use of sugarless mints/gum and replacement of sticky daily vitamin with non-cariogenic type	Patient discussion	4-week re-evaluation
3. Increase fluoride exposure; use of daily fluoride rinse and fluoridated water	Patient discussion	4-week re-evaluation
4. Eliminate faulty restorations	Refer for restorative dental care	4-week re-evaluation and reassessment at 3-month re-care appointment
5. Maintain patient comfort and safety throughout treatment	Patient Discussion	On-going at all appointments

Previous Treatment Goals Met/Not Met: *N/A*

Recommended Dental Hygiene Treatment:

☐ Prophylaxis

☐ Periodontal Maintenance

☐ Non-Surgical Periodontal Therapy:

   Quadrant(s): _____

☐ Non-Surgical Periodontal Therapy 1–3 teeth

_____

☑ Scaling in the presence of inflammation

☑ Anesthesia: *Topical or local as needed for patient comfort*

☑ Power Scaling

☑ Selective Polish Agent: *Superfine pumice*

☑ Topical Fluoride: Agent: *5% NaF Varnish*

☐ Sealants: Tooth #(s)

☐ Custom Tray: Type

☑ Education

☐ Nutritional Analysis

☐ Other:

Estimated Number of Treatment Appointments: *2 treatment appointments plus re-evaluation appointment*

Recommended Re-care Interval with Rationale: *3 month re-care appointment to re-assess and control gingival infection*

Appointment Plan (sequence of planned interventions)	
Appt#	**Plan for Treatment, Services** **Plan for Education, Counseling, and Oral Hygiene Instruction**
1)	Assessment, Education: managing xerostomia, importance of biofilm removal, systemic impact of periodontal disease. Self care: demonstrate oral biofilm removal –tooth brushing
2)	Scaling, all 4 quadrants, polish. Education: importance of fluoride and managing xerostomia to control dental caries, importance of follow-up for management of faulty restorations, Self care: review biofilm removal techniques—brushing, demonstrate flossing
3)	Re-evaluation—in 4 weeks. Education: answer patient questions and reinforce patient previous education and self care instructions based on re-evaluation assessment findings.

Understanding the Motivational Interviewing (MI) Approach to Patient Counseling

The purpose of all patient education and counseling is to help your patient adopt healthy behaviors that ensure positive health outcomes.

Motivational interviewing (MI) is a patient-centered, goal-directed approach to communicating that:

- Engages the patient
- Provides continuous support and feedback

- Encourages an exchange of information
- Stimulates the patient's own motivation for change
- Leads to development of a commitment to healthy behavior change

Brief motivational interviewing (BMI) uses the MI tools during short conversations (5–10 minutes) during patient care.

The Spirit of MI	Guiding Principles
P Partnership	**R** Resist righting reflex
A Acceptance	**U** Understand
C Compassion	**L** Listen
E Evocation	**E** Empower

Four processes of the MI approach

- **Engaging** the patient's attention and interest
- **Focusing** the discussion
- **Evoking** the patient's own responses about health goals, reasons for, and ambivalence toward change
- **Planning** behavior change for health

To implement the MI approach, use the following MI tools:		The MI approach offers continuous support and feedback to help your patient:		

Core skills that lead to good information exchange:
 	
O Open-ended questions
 	
A Affirmations
 	
R Reflective listening
  • Simple
  • Complex
 	
S Summary
	Components that facilitate **information exchange:**
	
	• **Ask permission**
	• **Elicit, provide, elicit**
	• **Agenda setting**
	• **Use of MI core skills**
		Explore ambivalence: sustain talk vs. change talk
		
		(Readiness ruler)
		
		Decisional balance
		
		(pro/con matrix)
			Initiate change talk: preparatory change talk
			
			Patient expresses the *desire, ability, reasons, or need* for change (DARN)
			
			Mobilizing change talk
			
			Patient expresses *commitment, actions, or steps taken* toward change (CAT)
				Express commitment through development of a plan:
				
				• Clear plan
				• Several clear options
				• Brainstorming

APPENDIX E

Evaluation Rubric for Competency Exercises

Competence is the ability to apply knowledge and skills in a relevant way to solve problems, answer questions, or make decisions.

Objectively evaluating a learner's ability to recall factual information is relatively easy. Evaluation of student responses to exercises/learning activities that are intended to assess competence is often significantly more difficult. Competence is a complex interaction of skills that begins with an understanding of basic facts (*knowledge*) and incorporates the *analysis* of all relevant factors in a specific situation and *synthesis* of information in order to answer questions or solve problems. Competence also includes being able to *support* or clearly explain the rationale for decisions and effectively *communicate* the plan for action.

An academic grading rubric provides objective criteria useful for evaluating student work that has been submitted to demonstrate competence. The assignment of points for each of the criteria stated in the rubric will aid the faculty member in providing an objective grade or score. When the evaluation rubric is provided along with instructions for the assignment, students receive a guide to faculty expectations. When the finished assignment is graded, focused feedback will help the students understand errors or omissions that result in a lower score or grade for the assignment.

The example evaluation rubric on the next page can be used as a template for evaluating student responses to all of the competency exercises, including those related to Factors to Teach the Patient and Everyday Ethics, in each chapter of the Student Workbook.

Evaluation Rubric for Competency Exercises

CATEGORIES	EXCELLENT 3 POINTS	ACCEPTABLE 2 POINTS	UNSATISFACTORY 0–1 POINTS
Knowledge Familiarity with and understanding of concepts and information. Points _____	Student includes relevant and accurate information from the main chapter. And Student includes relevant information from related chapters in the **textbook**.	Student includes relevant and accurate information from the main chapter.	Significant relevant information from the main chapter is missing. Or Misunderstanding of one or more basic concepts is evident.
Analysis Breaking down a complex topic into its component parts. Points _____	All components of the question, case scenario, or patient assessment data are considered in the student's answer.	Only minor details or components of the question, case scenario, or patient assessment data have not been addressed in the student's answer.	At least one major component has not been addressed.
Synthesis Combining ideas to form a complex, cohesive whole using logical reasoning and deduction. Points _____	Connections or comparisons made between factors, concepts, and facts/knowledge from the **textbook** chapter are very clear.	Connections or comparisons between factors, concepts, and facts/knowledge from the chapter **textbook** are apparent, but not completely explained.	Important or obvious connections are missing from the student's answer.
Support Providing rationale for statements. Points _____	Student provides clear explanations that support conclusions, statements, or connections made. Examples: • Linking basic information and intended actions or conclusions drawn • Explaining personal perspective • Defining controversy that requires further investigation.	Explanations are provided that support conclusions, statements, or connections, but could be more completely or clearly explained.	Little evidence is provided to support conclusions, statements, or connections.
Communication Conveying information. Points _____	Meets professional writing standards for: • Grammar • Spelling • Appropriate use of either a formal or "patient-friendly" writing style (based on the focus of the exercise).	Minor errors in professional writing standards for: • Grammar • Spelling • Appropriate use of either a formal or "patient-friendly" writing style (based on the focus of the exercise).	Errors in spelling or grammar. Or Writing style is too casual/conversational for professional writing. Or Inappropriate professional jargon is used for a patient discussion.

Total points _____/15 possible points

Faculty Feedback:

Functional Movement Exercises

A. Sitting in neutral position, close eyes, do full diaphragm breathing. Allow abdomen to be full as lungs become full. Exhale with lips slightly parted.

B. Standing or sitting in neutral position, stretch both arms up, interlace fingers, turn interlaced fingers so that palms are up. Look at hands and follow with eyes as you pull hands backward (spinal extension). Return to neutral.

C. Standing or sitting in neutral position, interlace fingers and place on back of head; push elbows backward while slowly looking upward then slowly return to neutral. Chin moves up toward ceiling. Inhale as you look up and exhale as you return to neutral (thoracic extension).

D. Standing in neutral position, slowly bend forward, rounding the back, gently bring the chin in the direction of the chest, letting the arms and hands hang down freely (spinal flexion).

E. Standing in neutral position, raise left arm, palm facing toward midline; right arm hangs by side, palm facing hip. Bend trunk to the right and return to neutral. Right ribs flex and come closer together. Left ribs extend and move away from each other.
Repeat on opposite side.

F. As chest moves forward and upward allow the head to move back (thoracic extension); chin moves in an upward direction. Inhale fully, count to five; exhale as you slowly return to neutral. Jaw remains relaxed.

G. Sitting in neutral position, palms resting on thighs. Very gently look over right shoulder and allow right shoulder to move back as left shoulder moves forward (spinal rotation). Right palm will move along thigh back toward hip. Left palm will move forward along thigh toward knee.
Repeat on opposite side.

H. Shoulders relaxed in neutral position. Move right shoulder up toward right ear, backward and down. Do this movement in a clockwise direction 10 times and in a counter-clockwise direction 10 times. This movement should be done slowly and with awareness of movement of shoulder in all directions.
Repeat on opposite side.

I. Standing, roll onto balls of feet, roll back onto heels of feet. Stand near wall for support.

J. Tendon gliding exercise for fingers, hand, and wrist. This is a fluid movement involving movement of wrist as you perform the sequence, left to right.